Thomas Szasz

International Perspectives in Philosophy and Psychiatry

Series editors: Bill (K.W.M.) Fulford, Lisa Bortolotti, Matthew Broome, Katherine Morris, John Z. Sadler, and Giovanni Stanghellini

Thomas Szasz
An appraisal of his legacy

Edited by
C.V. Haldipur, James L. Knoll IV,
and Eric v.d. Luft

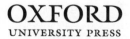
OXFORD
UNIVERSITY PRESS

OXFORD

UNIVERSITY PRESS

Great Clarendon Street, Oxford, OX2 6DP,
United Kingdom

Oxford University Press is a department of the University of Oxford.
It furthers the University's objective of excellence in research, scholarship,
and education by publishing worldwide. Oxford is a registered trade mark of
Oxford University Press in the UK and in certain other countries

© Oxford University Press 2019

The moral rights of the authors have been asserted

First Edition published in 2019

Impression: 2

Published in the United States of America by Oxford University Press
198 Madison Avenue, New York, NY 10016, United States of America

British Library Cataloguing in Publication Data
Data available

Library of Congress Control Number: 2018949660

ISBN 978-0-19-881349-1

Printed and bound by
CPI Group (UK) Ltd, Croydon, CR0 4YY

Advanced Praise

Thomas Szasz was one of the most influential critics of psychiatry in the late twentieth century. He offered not merely a libertarian political critique of mainstream mental health care but conceptually based arguments against the very idea of mental illness, coercive care, and the insanity defence in law, amongst other things. These wide-ranging and stimulating chapters, by both philosophers and psychiatrists, responds to Szasz's legacy by taking his arguments seriously—through their critical reassessment, development of some of their consequences, and re-examination of mental health care more broadly in response to Szaszian concerns. As one of the authors in this collection argues, whether or not Szasz's answers to them were the most plausible, he asked the right questions of psychiatry. This book is both a contribution to academic psychiatry and the philosophy of psychiatry, but of broader interest to anyone with a stake in understanding the fundamental and vital issues raised by mental health care.

Tim Thornton, Professor of Philosophy and Mental Health, Faculty of Health and Wellbeing, University of Central Lancashire, U.K.

A comprehensive, scholarly examination of one of the most influential social scientists of the late twentieth century, *Thomas Szasz: An Appraisal of His Legacy* should be on the bookshelf of anyone interested in the social history, philosophy, or practice of psychiatry. While most discussions of Szasz either lionize, renounce, or trivialize him, the authors in this important collection present reasoned assessments of the importance and limitations of his work.

Barry Glassner, Professor of Sociology, Lewis & Clark College, U.S.A. and author of *The Culture of Fear* (Basic, 2010)

As the climate of psychiatry changes, this carefully crafted book—that delves into Thomas Szasz's prescient ideas—is needed now, perhaps more so than ever. Drawing on the illuminating words of a stellar cast of authors to light up the imagination and neuronal pathways, Haldipur, Knoll, and Luft have to be applauded for guiding us expertly through the labyrinthine thought processes of their mentor and colleague. The result, a marvellous 'appraisal of his legacy', is an erudite and stimulating amalgamation of philosophy and psychiatry. This beautifully composed symphony of thought is essential 'listening' for anyone intending to navigate the mind and fathom the human condition.

Gin S. Malhi, Distinguished Professor of Psychiatry, University of Sydney, Australia

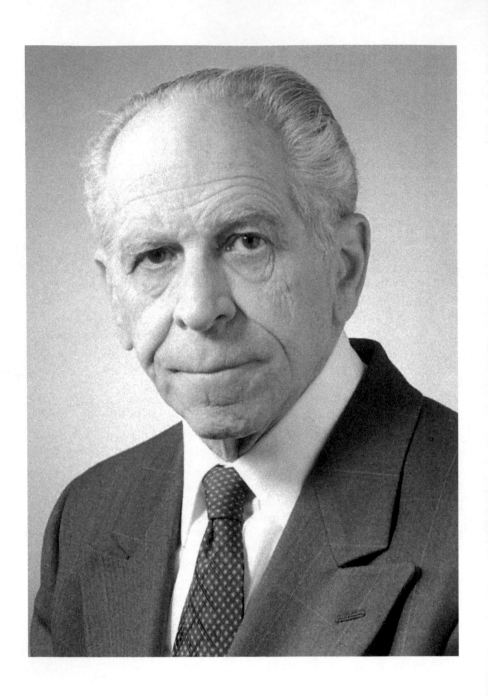

Contents

List of Editors

C.V. Haldipur is Emeritus Professor in the Department of Psychiatry, SUNY Upstate Medical University. He met Thomas Szasz, then already at Upstate, when he was a trainee in England in the 1960s, maintained correspondence with Szasz, and eventually joined the same faculty after completing his psychiatric training in Cambridge and Edinburgh. Haldipur has held various academic and administrative positions at Upstate, including Director of Medical Student Education in the Department of Psychiatry and Co-Director of the required Practice of Medicine (POM) course for all first- and second-year medical students. He is a Member of the Royal College of Psychiatrists and a Distinguished Fellow of the American Psychiatric Association.

James L. Knoll IV is Director of Forensic Psychiatry and Professor of Psychiatry at SUNY Upstate Medical University. He has worked as a forensic evaluator for state and federal courts, corrections, and the private sector. He is Editor-in-Chief Emeritus of *Psychiatric Times* and a contributing editor for the *Correctional Mental Health Report*. He has authored over 150 journal articles and book chapters. His afterword to David Kaczynski's memoir, *Every Last Tie: The Story of the Unabomber and His Family*, was published by Duke University Press in 2016. He has authored chapters in two well-received books from Oxford University Press: *Stalking: Psychiatric Perspectives and Practical Approaches*, edited by Debra A. Pinals (2007), and the *Oxford Textbook of Correctional Psychiatry*, edited by Robert L. Trestman et al. (2015). Knoll developed an academic friendship with Szasz in Upstate's Department of Psychiatry.

Eric v.d. Luft earned his B.A. *magna cum laude* in philosophy and religion at Bowdoin College in 1974, his Ph.D. in philosophy at Bryn Mawr College in 1985, and his M.L.S. at Syracuse University in 1993. From 1987 to 2006 he was Curator of Historical Collections at SUNY Upstate Medical University. He has taught at Villanova University, Syracuse University, Upstate, and the College of Saint Rose. He is the author, editor, or translator of over 640 publications in philosophy, religion, librarianship, history, history of medicine, and nineteenth-century studies, including *Hegel, Hinrichs, and Schleiermacher on Feeling and Reason in Religion: The Texts of Their 1821–22 Debate* (1987), *God, Evil, and Ethics: A Primer in the Philosophy of Religion* (2004), *A Socialist Manifesto* (2007), *Die at the Right Time: A Subjective Cultural History of the American Sixties* (2009), *Ruminations: Selected Philosophical, Historical, and Ideological Papers* (volume 1, 2010; volume 2, 2013), and *The Value of Suicide* (2012). He owns Gegensatz Press and is listed in *Who's Who in America*.

All three editors knew Tom Szasz personally as a friendly, charming, outgoing exponent of his own thought. CVH shared an office for over a decade with him, offering a unique opportunity for ongoing dialogues and discussions about various topics. JLK enjoyed collegial friendship with Szasz for many years, including private teaching sessions with students. EvdL (a trained philosopher in the speculative tradition) had frequent philosophical conversations with Szasz, but scarcely agreed with him about anything—except suicide.

List of Contributors

George J. Annas is the Warren Distinguished Professor at Boston University and Director of the Center for Health Law, Ethics, and Human Rights at Boston University School of Public Health. He is the author or editor of twenty books on health law and bioethics, including *The Rights of Patients: The Basic ACLU Guide to Patient Rights* (1989), *American Bioethics: Crossing Human Rights and Health Law Boundaries* (2004), and *Worst Case Bioethics: Death, Disaster, and Public Health* (2010). He has written regularly for the *New England Journal of Medicine* since 1991; served on boards of concern for the dying in the 1980s and 1990s; and wrote amicus briefs for a series of "right to die" cases, including Spring v. Geriatric Authority of Holyoke, Brophy v. New England Sinai Hospital, Bartling v. Glendale Adventist Medical Center, Bouvia v. County of Riverside, Cruzan v. Harmon et al., and two assisted suicide cases— Compassion in Dying v. State of Washington and Vacco v. Quill.

Jennifer Church is Professor of Philosophy at Vassar College. She obtained her B.A. from Macalester College and her Ph.D. from the University of Michigan, Ann Arbor. She was a graduate student at Somerville College at Oxford and a postdoctoral fellow at the University of Chicago. Her many publications address topics in the philosophy of mind, including consciousness, the emotions, irrationality, and the imagination. She is also interested in Kant, Freud, feminist theory, and the philosophy of music.

Marisola Xhelili Ciaccio is a Ph.D. candidate and lecturer in the Philosophy Department at Marquette University. Prior to graduate school, she received her B.A. in government and philosophy from Skidmore College, where she studied political theory and social identity as it pertains to the Balkan region of Europe. Her current academic research focuses on topics ranging from social identity to moral psychology. She is also co-founder and co-director of Engendering Dignity in Philosophy (EDIP), a classroom-based program that brings together faculty, graduate students, incarcerated women, and undergraduate students to develop collaborative solutions to shared issues in social justice. She was recently declared an Arthur J. Schmitt Leadership Fellow in recognition of her innovative approaches to diversifying academic philosophy.

Robert W. Daly is Professor Emeritus of Psychiatry and of Bioethics and Humanities at SUNY Upstate Medical University. He was the original Chair of the Upstate University Hospital's Ethics Committee and Consultation Service; founded the Consortium for Culture and Medicine; co-edited *The Cultures of Medicine* (1989); and was an editorial consultant for the *Journal of the American Medical Association* (*JAMA*) and *Philosophy, Psychiatry, and Psychology* (*PPP*). His work has appeared in such journals as *Psychiatry, The Psychoanalytic Review*, and *The Journal of the American Psychiatric Association*. He was a Senior Fellow of the National Endowment for the Humanities; practiced clinical psychiatry for forty years; held academic appointments at Cornell, Syracuse, and Cambridge (Kings College) Universities; and lectured extensively in Europe, China, and the United States. LeMoyne College made him a Doctor of Humane Letters (*honoris causa*) in 2007.

Mantosh J. Dewan is SUNY Distinguished Service Professor and former Chair of the Department of Psychiatry at Upstate Medical University, where he also served as Director of Undergraduate Education and of Residency Training. His published work ranges from brain imaging and the economics of mental health care to psychotherapy. He co-edited two books: *The Difficult-to-Treat Psychiatric Patient* (2008) and *The Art and Science of Brief Psychotherapies: A Practitioner's Guide* (2004). He is a Distinguished Life Fellow of the American Psychiatric Association; received the Scientific Achievement Award from the Indo-American Psychiatrists Association, the Exemplary Psychiatrist Award from the National Alliance on Mental Illness, and the 2010 George Tarajan Award from the American Psychiatric Association; was designated Exemplary Chair by SUNY in 2011; and served on the editorial boards of *Annals of Clinical Psychiatry* and *Surgical Neurology*.

Allen Frances is Professor Emeritus and former Chair of the Department of Psychiatry at Duke University, did his medical and subsequent psychiatric training at Columbia University. He founded two journals, *Journal of Personality Disorders* and *Journal of Psychiatric Practice*; has published extensively in refereed journals; and has authored several books. He chaired the task force that produced the fourth edition of the *Diagnostic and Statistical Manual of Mental Disorders* (DSM-IV), but has been a vocal critic of DSM-V (i.e., the fifth edition), and has warned against expanding the boundaries of psychiatry, which he sees as causing diagnostic inflation and as distracting the attention of clinicians from treating more serious mental disorders. Among his books is *Essentials of Psychiatric Diagnosis: Responding to the Challenge of DSM-V* (2013).

K.W.M. ("Bill") Fulford is a fellow of St. Catherine's College and member of the philosophy faculty of the University of Oxford; Emeritus Professor of Philosophy and Mental Health, University of Warwick Medical School; and Director of the Collaborating Centre for Value Based Practice, St. Catherine's College, Oxford. He has published widely in the philosophy of psychiatry, including *Moral Theory and Medical Practice* (1989), co-authored the *Oxford Textbook of Philosophy and Psychiatry* (2006), and served as lead editor of *The Oxford Handbook of Philosophy and Psychiatry* (2015). He is lead editor for the Oxford University Press book series International Perspectives in Philosophy and Psychiatry, and founding editor and chair of the advisory board of the international journal, *Philosophy, Psychiatry and Psychology* (PPP). His co-authored *Essential Value-Based Practice* (2012) is the launch volume for a new series from Cambridge University Press on value-based medicine. The recently endowed Oxford tutorial post in philosophy of mind with special relevance to psychiatry and cognitive neuroscience has been named the Fulford Clarendon Lectureship and Fellowship in recognition of his contributions to the field.

Mona Gupta is a consultation-liaison psychiatrist at the Centre Hospitalier de l'Université de Montréal (CHUM) and a researcher at the Centre de Recherche du CHUM (CRCHUM) in Montreal. She is also Associate Professor in the Department of Psychiatry at the University of Montreal. She received her medical degree from McGill University and completed her residency and fellowship training in psychiatry at the University of Toronto, where she also did a Ph.D. in bioethics. Her academic interests are bioethics and the philosophy of psychiatry. She is the author of several articles and book chapters, particularly on ethics and evidence-based medicine in psychiatry. Her research monograph on this topic was published in the "International Perspectives in Philosophy and Psychiatry" series by Oxford University Press in 2014 and nominated for a BMA Medical Book of the Year award in 2015.

Eugene A. Kaplan is a member of the SUNY Upstate Medical University class of 1957, joined Upstate's Department of Psychiatry in 1961 and served as its Chair from 1986 to 1999. Thus, insofar as Szasz had arrived at Upstate in 1956, Kaplan enjoys the unique distinction of having been first Szasz's student, then his colleague and close personal friend. Kaplan is mainly known as a teacher with a national reputation for having trained and supervised hundreds of psychiatrists. Among his many pedagogical awards is, in 2015 at Upstate, the President's Award for Teaching. As he inculcated in students and residents an ethical and noncoercive approach to psychotherapy, he based many of his innovations in psychiatric education on the theories, habits, and methods of Szasz.

Neil Pickering is Associate Professor in the Bioethics Center at the University of Otago, Dunedin, New Zealand. He is the author of *The Metaphor of Mental Illness*, published in the "International Perspectives in Philosophy and Psychiatry" series of Oxford University Press in 2006, and of a number of articles on the concept of mental illness. He is a regular contributor to the International Network for Philosophy and Psychiatry conferences and convened the organizing committee for the 2012 conference in Dunedin on culture and mental health.

Ronald W. Pies is Professor of Psychiatry and Lecturer in Bioethics and Humanities at SUNY Upstate Medical University, Clinical Professor of Psychiatry at the Tufts University School of Medicine, and Editor-in-Chief Emeritus of *Psychiatric Times*. His undergraduate degree is from Cornell University and he earned his M.D. and did his psychiatric residency both at Upstate. His most recent book is *Psychiatry on the Edge* (2014). Among his others are *The Judaic Foundations of Cognitive-Behavioral Therapy: Rabbinical and Talmudic Underpinnings of CBT and REBT* (2010) and *The Three-Petalled Rose: How the Synthesis of Judaism, Buddhism, and Stoicism can Create a Healthy, Fulfilled, and Flourishing Life* (2013).

Jan Pols obtained his medical and Ph.D. degrees from Leiden University and completed his psychiatric training at the University of Groningen. He has published books on the history of psychiatry in the Netherlands, training supervision, and "coercion in psychiatry," as well as articles in Dutch scholarly journals, and is widely credited in the Netherlands for bringing ethical issues to the attention of practitioners. He is now retired from clinical practice, but continues to espouse less coercive treatment of psychiatric patients. His revised 1984 doctoral thesis, "Mythe en Macht: Over de Kritische Psychiatrie van Thomas S. Szasz," has been translated into English by Mira de Vries as *The Politics of Mental Illness: Myth and Power in the Work of Thomas Szasz* (2006).

Nancy Nyquist Potter is Professor of Philosophy and Associate with the Department of Psychiatry and Behavioral Sciences at the University of Louisville. She has published extensively in the interdisciplinary field of philosophy and psychiatry in anthologies as well as journals such as *Philosophy, Psychiatry, and Psychology* (PPP), *Journal of Personality Disorders*, and *Current Opinion in Psychiatry*. She wrote *How Can I Be Trusted? A Virtue Theory of Trustworthiness* (2002), *Mapping the Edges and the In-Between: A Critical Analysis of Borderline Personality Disorder* (2009), and *The Virtue of Defiance and Psychiatric Engagement* (2016). She also co-edited *Trauma, Truth, and Reconciliation: Healing Damaged Relationships* (2006). She is a senior editor of *PPP*. Her current research is on connections between theories of knowledge and ethics, with special attention to nosological and diagnostic issues, and on the relationship among voice, silence, and uptake, in particular for patients living with mental illness.

Jennifer Radden is Professor of Philosophy Emerita at the University of Massachusetts, Boston. She received her graduate training at Oxford University, and has published extensively on mental health concepts, the history of medicine, and ethical and policy aspects of psychiatric theory and practice. Her books include *Madness and Reason* (1986), *Divided Minds and Successive Selves: Ethical Issues in Disorders of Identity and Personality* (1996), *Moody Minds Distempered: Essays on Melancholy and Depression* (2009), *The Virtuous Psychiatrist: Character Ethics in Psychiatric Practice*, co-authored with John Sadler (2010), and *On Delusion* (2011), as well as two collections of which she was editor—*The Nature of Melancholy* (2000) and *Oxford Companion to the Philosophy of Psychiatry* (2004). Her most recent work is *Melancholic Habits: Burton's Anatomy and the Mind Sciences* (2017). Her positions have included President of the Association for the Advancement of Philosophy and Psychiatry, and Ethics Consultant at MacLean Hospital in Belmont, Massachusetts.

John Z. Sadler is the Daniel W. Foster Professor of Medical Ethics, Psychiatry, and Clinical Sciences at the University of Texas Southwestern Medical Center; Editor-in-Chief of *Philosophy, Psychiatry, and Psychology (PPP)*; an editor for Oxford University Press's "International Perspectives in Philosophy and Psychiatry" book series; and a Distinguished Life Fellow of the American Psychiatric Association. He is the author of *Values and Psychiatric Diagnosis* (2005) and co-author (with Jennifer Radden) of *The Virtuous Psychiatrist: Character Ethics in Psychiatric Practice* (2009). The Texas Society of Psychiatric Physicians awarded him its Psychiatric Excellence Award in 2001.

Thomas Schramme is Chair in Philosophy at the University of Liverpool. His main research interests are in moral philosophy, political philosophy, and the philosophy of medicine. He has published widely on numerous topics in the philosophy of medicine and psychiatry, mainly regarding the concepts of health and disease, and notably the *Handbook of the Philosophy of Medicine*, co-edited with Steven Edwards, which was released in February 2017. He has edited several collections of essays, for instance, *Philosophy and Psychiatry* (with Johannes Thome) in 2004.

E. Fuller Torrey is an eminent psychiatrist and schizophrenia researcher who earned his bachelor's degree from Princeton University and his medical degree from McGill University, and trained in psychiatry at the Stanford University School of Medicine. He is Executive Director of the Stanley Medical Research Institute, and also heads the Treatment Advocacy Center, whose main activity is promoting the passage and implementation of outpatient and civil commitment laws and standards. He has conducted numerous studies, including one on possible infectious causes of schizophrenia. Among his many books are *Surviving Schizophrenia* (1983; 5th edition, 2006), *The Insanity Offense* (2008), and *The Roots of Treason: Ezra Pound and the Secret of St. Elizabeths* (1984). Despite their differences in ideology, Torrey maintained a cordial friendship with Szasz. They met frequently and corresponded with each other regularly.

Stephen Wilson is a psychiatrist, psychoanalyst, and writer. He qualified in medicine in 1968 and spent most of his professional life in Oxford, England. He has held consultant posts at the Littlemore and Warneford hospitals and honorary appointments at the University of Oxford and Oxford Brookes University. He is the author of numerous articles and academic papers, as well as ten books, including *The Cradle of Violence: Essays on Psychiatry, Psychoanalysis, and Literature* (1995), *The Bloomsbury Book of the Mind* (2003), and *Introducing the Freud Wars* (2002). He has also translated the works of Irene Nemirovsky.

Introduction

C.V. Haldipur, James L. Knoll IV,
and Eric v.d. Luft

Thomas Szasz (1920–2012) was born in Budapest, Hungary, immigrated to the United States in 1938, earned his M.D. in 1944 at the University of Cincinnati, and completed his psychoanalytic training at the University of Chicago and the Chicago Institute for Psychoanalysis. He joined the psychiatry faculty of Upstate Medical University in 1956, retired in 1990, but remained at Upstate until his death. He was a Distinguished Life Fellow of the American Psychiatric Association.

In 1961 he published his magnum opus, *The Myth of Mental Illness*, which catapulted him to fame. This book was translated into many languages and spawned an eponymous ideology which challenges the notion of mental illness, the insanity defense, and involuntary psychiatric treatment. His other, mostly subsequent, writings comprise over thirty books and several hundred articles in scientific as well as popular periodicals.

His works are peppered with acerbic wit and trenchant criticism of psychiatry and much else. Insofar as he was an uncompromising libertarian, his books and articles are best read as written by an ideologue rather than by a practicing psychiatrist. Hence, in taking a critical look at his legacy, it made sense to invite not only psychiatrists, but also philosophers, sociologists, and ethicists to contribute to this volume.

There is much to admire about Szasz, but also much to disagree with. Many of the contributors to this volume knew him, respected him, and counted him as a major intellectual influence on them. A few may have been merely tempted to add something here as a paean to an iconoclast. We three editors were all his colleagues at Upstate and found him quite charming and friendly, which is not to say either agreeable or conciliatory. Indeed, our combative encounters with Szasz remain among our fondest memories of him. We strive in this book to be critical in examining his legacy and to portray him "warts and all," just as he would have wanted us to do.

He never shied away from a good debate either in print or in person. Most of the issues raised in this volume were familiar to him. Readers can easily imagine how he would have responded to the arguments in these chapters.

Szasz may be credited, at least partially, obliquely, or negatively, with influencing some of the recent changes in society's attitude toward the mentally ill. He railed against medicalizing the individual's problems of living in society. In trying to stop the inexorable move toward considering such human follies as diseases, he has been compared to King Canute trying to stop the sea. Psychotherapy continues to thrive as a popular treatment modality. His theories were somewhat successful in reducing the frequency of involuntary treatment and forced commitment, but we are now seeing a gradual backlash against deinstitutionalization. The debate about the insanity defense is unresolved in jurisprudence.

Szasz's singular, and most lastingly important, contribution may well be that he provoked the psychiatric profession to take a good look at itself and to question its role in society. He certainly believed that each of his readers should have conceded *rem acu tetigisti*. Surely some did just that, and the controversy continues. We hope that this volume will encourage that controversy, raise further questions, and keep the debate productive.

Part I

Intellectual roots of Szasz's thought

Chapter 1

Study on the Szaszophone: Theme and variations

Stephen Wilson

1.1 Introduction

What has been plain to the rest of the world since antiquity is not obvious to Thomas Szasz, and what Szasz deems self-evident is not so for most other people. I am talking about the attribution of free will to madmen and its corollary, criminal responsibility. More than 2,300 years ago, Plato put the following words into the mouth of an "Athenian Stranger" in a discussion concerning offenses such as robbery (of the Gods), treachery, and corrupt practices aimed at civil subversion: "Now a man might conceivably commit an act of one of these kinds from insanity, or when so disordered by disease, so extremely aged, or of such tender years, as to be virtually insane. If one of these pleas can be established to the satisfaction of the court . . . he shall in any case pay full compensation to any party endamaged by his act, but the rest of the sentence shall be remitted, unless, indeed, he have taken a life and incurred the pollution of homicide" (Plato, 1973, p. 1425; *Laws* 864d–e). In all such cases, the Athenian suggested that the law should recognize an exemption from normal punishment. Similarly, echoing a letter from Emperor Marcus Aurelius and his son Commodus (ca. 177–180), Modestinus Herennius (fl. ca. 250) wrote: "Truly, if anyone kills a parent in a fit of madness, he shall not be punished . . . for it was enough for him to be punished by the madness itself, and he must be guarded the more carefully, or even confined with chains" (Watson, 1998, p. 336).

Illness is indeed generally accepted as a factor that can mitigate personal responsibility. We make allowances for an ill person. Although modern law takes a commonsense view of free will, embracing the normative assumption that adults are responsible for their behavior, illness can vitiate or diminish that responsibility. A strong case can be made against all human free will, which appears to hold irrespective of determinism or indeterminism. It is based on the notion that the choices we make are a product of whatever we are—and what we are is essentially given: "Nothing can be *causa sui*—the cause of itself" (Strawson, 1994, p. 5). Szasz would find nothing to disagree with the commonsense view of illness and free will. Indeed he seems to accept *physical* illness as an uncomplicated value-free entity. But the theme that runs through his voluminous writings hinges on the assertion that madness is mistakenly described as *mental* illness. For Szasz, madness exists, mad behavior certainly occurs, but it is not subsumed under the rubric of illness. To place it there is to fall into a category error. It is to confuse a linguistic trope, a metaphor, a socially constructed label, with a substantive entity.

1.2 **Madness and responsibility**

If a madman is not ill, if he is simply pursuing his own unusual, mendacious, misguided, or antisocial agenda, then he must be responsible for everything he does. Thus a person who asserts he is God or claims to have fifteen different personalities is interpreted on the Szaszophone as being simply—"a liar" (Szasz, 2004, p. 33). But a liar is someone who knowingly deceives, not someone who states a falsehood believing it to be true. By denying this distinction Szasz manages to "normalize" delusion and prevent it from mitigating personal responsibility. Szasz's view diverges from that of the ancients, but he shares it in common with those fundamentalists who think that human free will is a universal God-given absolute. There is always method in Szasz's madness. "Like sane persons," Szasz says, "madmen and mad women have reasons for their actions. They can and do control their behavior. If they could not do so, they would not engage in the criminal conduct in which they sometimes engage. Nor could they then be so easily controlled in insane asylums" (Szasz, 2004, p. 4).

But wait a minute. If the question at issue is whether a madman has full responsibility for his criminal conduct, it is not good enough to simply cite the conduct itself in evidence that it was freely chosen and clearly intended. *Mens rea* does not automatically follow from *actus reus*. Szasz's circular rhetoric begs the question. Moreover, if it be true that some madmen are easily controlled in insane asylums, might this not be due to an abnormality of volition characteristic of their mental condition, suggesting a lack of control over behavior, a constraint on their ability to choose?

1.3 **Definition of illness**

Diseases which can give rise to psychological disturbance (and there are many), such as diabetic hypoglycemia or hypothyroidism, malarial fever, influenza, or dementia, are real for Szasz, not because they produce signs and symptoms, discomfort and malfunction, but because an underlying pathology can be found. When the same symptoms and signs occur in the absence of detectable organic pathology—for example, irritability or agitation or psychomotor retardation in depression; hallucinations and delusions in schizophrenia; or confusion in an anxiety state—the illness is, for Szasz, "mythological," which is to say not an illness at all but some other kind of entity, a deviant mode of expression for problems in living, or just an unusual language equivalent perhaps to the text of James Joyce's *Finnegans Wake* (Joyce, 2012).

Szasz is clearly right when he states: "My claim that mental illnesses are fictitious . . . rests on the . . . materialist-scientific definition of illness as the structural or functional alteration of cells, tissues, and organs. If we accept this definition of disease, then it follows that mental illness is a metaphor—asserting that view is stating an analytic truth, not subject to empirical falsification" (Szasz, 2011, pp. 179–80). However, it is blindingly obvious that if the term "illness" is limited, by definition, to the structural pathology of the body, then the mind, which has no corporeal structure or local habitation, cannot be ill. I am not taking an idealist position here; I am simply recognizing that the term "mind" is abstract, denoting the quality and organization of experiences, thoughts, intentions, subjective awareness, etc., whereas the term "body" denotes material substance. Whatever the relation between the one and the other, the two are not coterminous. But the mind can be disordered! If a wider definition of illness is embraced, one based on subjective dis-ease combined with functional impairment, then the mind too can be said to be ill, leaving open the question as to how the illness is generated; and this is the sense in which psychiatrists, lawyers, and most other people use the word. As Ronald Pies tells us in Chapter 12 of this volume, to use the vocabulary of "mental illness" is not to point to the existence of some metaphysical or actual entity called "mind" which is held to be ill, but rather to use "ordinary language" (Wittgenstein, 1958) in order to describe a particular kind of psychological suffering (Pies, 2015).

By defining illness solely according to its biopathological cause rather than its clinical manifestation, Szasz dismisses, in a stroke, all possibility of social or psychological etiology. Take the case of a woman who murders her husband in an unfounded fit of jealousy. If her delusional jealousy was caused by "organic degeneration," as was commonly believed to be the case during the nineteenth century, it would be an illness according to Szasz, and as such might mitigate personal responsibility (Pick, 1989). But if it resulted from a purely psychological process, say the unconscious attribution of the wife's own adulterous wishes to her husband, then it would cease to be so (Freud, 1917).

Conditions once thought of as illnesses by the psychiatric profession and no longer included in the diagnostic lexicon—homosexuality, hysteria, or the possession of black skin which Benjamin Rush, signatory to the American Declaration of Independence and "father of American psychiatry," believed to be a mild form of leprosy (Stanton, 1960, pp. 6–13; Szasz, 1970b, pp. 153–9)—are cited by Szasz in order to demonstrate the arbitrary status of mental illness in contrast to the supposedly unshakable biomedical bedrock of physical illness. However, the social construction of illness entities is no news to medical historians, sociologists, or bioethicists. Illness, both physical and mental, and the perceived need for treatment, can be shown to be value-dependent (Agich, 1983; Fulford, 1989). But Christopher Boorse (1975) argues that while the *application* of medicine is value-laden, its underlying scientific and technical aspects are value-free. Moreover, definitions of health (not just mental health) vary both geographically and cross-culturally, as do a range of "normal" physiological parameters such as blood pressure, hemoglobin level, or the body mass index (Wood et al., 2012; Bindon et al., 2007). The fact is that the existence of illness is a gradually evolving process which starts with an undesirable state of affairs demanding amelioration and leads to a search for causes and cures. Bill Fulford argues that, although physical and psychological medicine are both value-dependent, there is a greater consensus over the "badness" of bodily pain and "the risk of death" than there is over the "badness" of the emotions, desires, affects, and beliefs with which psychiatry concerns itself (Fulford, 2004). Uncertainty over the credibility of a diagnostic entity often persists for a long time while the relation between experienced illness, causal factors, and underlying pathology is being elaborated. It is not just a matter for scientists and physicians; the reality of a diagnosis is often promoted or rejected through political processes, pressure groups, and patient associations. One only has to think of chronic fatigue syndrome (CFS), myalgic encephalomyelitis (ME), fibromyalgia, irritable bowel syndrome, etc.

To take a more nuanced view of how medicine actually works, consider an example drawn from a specialty far from psychiatry: specific antibody deficiency, a putative immunodeficiency disease whose existence continues to be debated by physicians. Here, total antibody levels are normal, yet patients suffer an increased susceptibility to infection. It is thought that they have a specific inability to produce antibodies in response to encapsulated bacteria such as pneumococcus. This can be demonstrated by immunizing the patient with a vaccine. However, in the U.K., the "normal" response to immunization is usually taken to be 0.35 ug/L, whereas in the U.S., the threshold is generally set at 1.3 ug/L. In other words, patients in the U.K. who are deemed to be "well" are "diseased" in the U.S. (Perez, 2013). Not only are there differences in diagnostic criteria among and between American and European immunologists, but there are also marked divergences in treatment practice and the perceived risk to patients' health of policies adopted by health-care funders (Hernandez-Trujillo et al., 2012). The point is that the higher threshold in the U.S., where health care is rationed by insurance companies, enables physicians to claim expensive immunoglobulin treatment for more patients, whereas in the U.K., where health care is rationed by the state, the lower threshold results in the treatment of fewer patients and a smaller burden on the health-care budget. So, socioeconomic factors may well be determining the definition of biomedical disease.

1.4 **Personal and political consequences**

Part of the problem is the general terms in which Szasz's argument is habitually conducted. All the variations, all the critiques of institutional psychiatry, all the polemical attacks on mental health legislation, drug legislation, the social sciences, economics, collectivist politics, etc., stem from the coupling of one untenable idea—the idea of universal unimpeachable individual responsibility—with a strict libertarian political and economic philosophy. Because political freedom in Szaszophone music is indissolubly linked to the attribution of personal responsibility in every individual, there can be no exception, no question of degree without unacceptable diminution of liberty. Liberty is a *bonum in se,* a good in itself, which ranks above mental health and individual well-being. According to Szasz, people should have "a right to be mentally ill" (Szasz, 2004, p. 20) or even to subject themselves to financial ruin or physical danger while in an unbalanced state of mind. But they should not have a right to be treated for that illness when their own judgment is clouded.

Szasz, Peter Sedgwick says in *Psychopolitics*, "attains his role as proxy spokesperson for the rights of the mental patient by ignoring, simply, what it is to be a mental patient" (Sedgwick, 1982, p. 158). What it is to be a mental patient is sometimes to experience oneself as—and to be experienced by others as—out of control. The traditional bracketing together of children and the mentally ill, both of whom enjoy exemption from responsibility and as a result suffer a reduction in liberty, recognizes the need for protective coercion. John Stuart Mill saw that the self-determination which he valued so highly could not be universally applied. Indeed, political thinkers from ancient to modern times have subscribed to the view that children and madmen cannot be free. However, Szasz thinks otherwise: "Mill's argument is valid only if his premise is valid, that is, only if insane adults resemble children so significantly that it is legitimate to subject them to 'benevolent' rather than 'punitive' coercion. This premise is patently invalid" (Szasz, 2004, p. 90). But is it?

Here Szasz suggests that Mill's attitude to children and the insane is as unfounded as his (now outdated) colonial paternalism. Mill thought that human beings in so-called "backward" states of society might need to be coerced *for their own good*. Szasz reminds us that slavery was similarly justified by its adherents. The point is well taken. But one can acknowledge the kernel of truth in Maxim CLX of French moralist Luc de Clapiers, Marquis de Vauvenargues: "Le prétexte ordinaire de ceux qui font le malheur des autres est qu'ils veulent leur bien [The usual pretext of those who do harm to others is that they wish them well]" without dismissing all cases of benign intervention (Vauvenargues, 1747, p. 290).

Clearly there are differences between children and mentally disturbed adults, but there are also similarities. Just as a child might fail to appreciate the danger posed by stepping into road traffic without looking, so might an adult in an omnipotent state of hypomanic excitement. Just as an unsupervised child in play might injure him or herself or others, so might the impulsive or deluded behavior of a psychotic adult result in injury. The premise that links children's vulnerability to that of certain mentally-ill adults is far from invalid, and in both cases, but not all cases, can justify protective intervention.

Few thinkers come higher in the pantheon of Szasz's political philosophers than Edmund Burke. His classic caveat on freedom, contained in *Letter to a Member of the National Assembly*, written two years into the French Revolution, reads as follows: "Society cannot exist unless a controlling power upon will and appetite be placed somewhere, and the less there is within, the more there must be without. *It is ordained in the eternal constitution of things, that men of intemperate minds cannot be free. Their passions forge their fetters*" (Burke, 1791, p. 69; italics added).

Szasz thinks this statement so important that he suggests it should be called the "First Law of Political Philosophy" (Szasz, 2004, p. 59). Yet does it speak in favor of freedom for the mentally ill? What minds can be more intemperate than those designated ill? If only men of temperate minds can be free, it follows that the mentally ill cannot be. Still the question remains whether any special legislation is required "from without," over and above that which applies to the general population. This is a question to which Szasz would answer a resounding "No!" (Szasz, 1970a, pp. 113–37). As he emphasizes, there is no objective evidence that the average severely mentally-ill patient is dangerous (Szasz, 1970a, p. 33). In fact, as a group, the mentally ill are more likely to fall victim to other people's violence (Hiroeh et al., 2001). However, they are more likely to commit violence against themselves, and a significant subgroup can be shown to be more violent than the general population (Torrey, 1994). Noncompliance with medication and comorbid substance abuse are important factors here. According to Szasz, there can be no justification for what amounts to preventive detention before a crime has been committed.

1.5 **Conclusion**

Szaszophone music is a kind of strident, freedom-loving, anti-authoritarian, punk. If its profound political individualism denies the real nature of psychiatric illness, rides roughshod over the suffering of patients and their families, stigmatizes the physicians who care for them, promotes the dissolution of mental health services, and mistakenly embraces "the contract" as a legalistic paradigm for all human freedom (Sedgwick, 1982, p. 156), then it has also acted as a lesson for legislators against the arbitrary incarceration of people designated mentally ill, directed attention to the political abuse of psychiatry at home as well as abroad, punctured the scientific pretensions of mental health-care professionals, and sounded a warning bell over the ever-growing "identification" of new mental disorders without adequate justification (Kendell, 2004). To conclude as I began, I think that Szasz would have been pleased to be compared to the gadfly which Plato's Socrates suggested that Athenian society needed in order to sting the "thoroughbred horse" of state into a proper acknowledgment of its duties and responsibilities (Plato, 1973, pp. 16–17, *Apology* 30e).

Acknowledgments

The author wishes to thank his daughter, Dr. Anna Shrimpton, for sharing immunologic expertise and Professor Tony Hope for pointing to the Socrates "gadfly" analogy.

References

Agich, George J. 1983. "Disease and Value: A Rejection of the Value-Neutrality Thesis." *Theoretical Medicine* **4** (1) (February): 27–41.

Bindon, Jim, et al. 2007. "A Cross-Cultural Perspective on Obesity and Health in Three Groups of Women: The Mississippi Choctaw, American Samoans, and African Americans." *Collegium Antropologicum* **31** (1) (March): 47–54.

Boorse, Christopher. 1975. "On the Distinction Between Disease and Illness." *Philosophy and Public Affairs* **5** (1) (Autumn): 49–68.

Burke, Edmund. 1791. *A Letter from Mr. Burke, to a Member of the National Assembly in Answer to Some Objections to His Book on French Affairs*, 2nd edn. Paris, London: J. Dodsley.

Freud, Sigmund. 1917. "Psycho-Analysis and Psychiatry." In *The Standard Edition of the Complete Psychological Works of Sigmund Freud, Volume 16 (1916–1917): Introductory Lectures on Psycho-Analysis, Part III*, pp. 243–56. London: Hogarth, 1963.

Fulford, K.W.M. 1989. *Moral Theory and Medical Practice*. Cambridge: Cambridge University Press.

Fulford, K.W.M. 2004. "Values-Based Medicine: Thomas Szasz's Legacy to Twenty-First Century Psychiatry." In *Szasz Under Fire: The Psychiatric Abolitionist Faces His Critics*, edited by Jeffrey Schaler, pp. 57–92. Chicago: Open Court Publishing.

Hernandez-Trujillo, Hillary Sunamoto, et al. 2012. "Comparison of American and European Practices in the Management of Patients with Primary Immunodeficiencies." *Clinical and Experimental Immunology* **169** (1) (July): 57–69.

Hiroeh, Urara, et al. 2001. "Death by Homicide, Suicide, and Other Unnatural Causes in People with Mental Illness: A Population-Based Study." *Lancet* **358** (9299) (December 22–29): 2110–12.

Joyce, James. 2012. *Finnegans Wake*. Oxford: Oxford University Press.

Kendell, Robert Evan. 2004. "The Myth of Mental Illness." In *Szasz Under Fire: The Psychiatric Abolitionist Faces His Critics*, edited by Jeffrey Schaler, pp. 29–48. Chicago: Open Court Publishing.

Perez, Elena Elizabeth. 2013. "Use and Interpretation of Pneumococcal Vaccination and Specific Antibody Deficiency." Paper presented at the "Current Challenges in Primary Antibody Deficiencies" symposium, Royal College of Pathologists, London, U.K. (September 5).

Pick, Daniel. 1989. *Faces of Degeneration: A European Disorder, c. 1848 – c. 1918*. Cambridge: Cambridge University Press.

Pies, Ronald. 2015. "Mind-Language in the Age of the Brain: Is 'Mental Illness' a Useful Term?" *Journal of Psychiatric Practice* 21 (1) (January): 79–83.

Plato. 1973. *The Collected Dialogues, Including the Letters*, edited by Edith Hamilton and Huntington Cairns. Princeton: Princeton University Press.

Sedgwick, Peter. 1982. *Psychopolitics*. New York: Harper & Row.

Stanton, William Ragan. 1960. *The Leopard's Spots: Scientific Attitudes Toward Race in America, 1815–59*. Chicago: University of Chicago Press.

Strawson, Galen. 1994. "The Impossibility of Moral Responsibility." *Philosophical Studies* 75 (1–2) (August): 5–24.

Szasz, Thomas S. 1970a. *Ideology and Insanity: Essays on the Psychiatric Dehumanization of Man*. Garden City, New York: Doubleday Anchor.

Szasz, Thomas S. 1970b. *The Manufacture of Madness: A Comparative Study of the Inquisition and the Mental Health Movement*. New York: Harper & Row.

Szasz, Thomas S. 2004. *Faith in Freedom: Libertarian Principles and Psychiatric Practices*. New Brunswick, New Jersey: Transaction.

Szasz, Thomas S. 2011. "The Myth of Mental Illness: 50 Years Later." *The Psychiatrist* 35: 179–82.

Torrey, E. Fuller. 1994. "Violent Behavior by Individuals with Serious Mental Illness." *Hospital and Community Psychiatry* 45 (7) (July): 653–62.

Vauvenargues, Luc de Clapiers, Marquis de. 1747. *Introduction à la Connoissance de l'Esprit Humain, suivie de Réflexions et de Maximes*. Paris: Chez Antoine-Claude Briasson.

Watson, Alan (ed.). 1998. *The Digest of Justinian, Volume 4*. Philadelphia: University of Pennsylvania Press.

Wittgenstein, Ludwig. 1958. *The Blue and Brown Books: Preliminary Studies for the Philosophical Investigations*. New York: Harper & Row.

Wood, Sally, et al. 2012. "Blood Pressure in Different Ethnic Groups (BP-Eth): A Mixed Methods Study." *BMJ Open* 2 (6). Accessed April 11, 2018. <bmjopen.bmj.com/content/bmjopen/2/6/e001598.full.pdf>

Chapter 2

Leading up to *The Myth of Mental Illness*

Jan Pols

2.1 Szasz's publications before 1961

Szasz's later critical attitude toward psychiatry is hardly discernible in his publications between 1950 and 1956, while he was at the Chicago Institute for Psychoanalysis. In accordance with that institution's research program, he wrote almost exclusively on psychosomatic illness from a psychoanalytical viewpoint. Psychosomatic illness was then perceived as a physical illness caused largely or entirely by psychical determinants. Szasz, in reporting his psychoanalytical research on patients who underwent vagotomy for stomach ulcers, attempted to find explanations of their results that fit Franz Alexander's theories (Szasz, 1948a, 1948b, 1949a, 1949b). He also studied patients with hypersalivation (Szasz, 1949c, 1950), diarrhea, and constipation (Szasz, 1951). This research led to a conclusion about psychoanalysis and the autonomic nervous system (Szasz, 1952) and a chapter co-authored with Alexander (Alexander and Szasz, 1952).

Thereafter, he wrote articles about pain, culminating in his first book, *Pain and Pleasure: A Study of Bodily Feelings* (1957a), which was also a psychoanalytic study. Little in this book hinted at the turn Szasz would later take. He did, however, make this interesting comment in a footnote: "It seems to me that from the point of view of scientific clarity it would help to restrict the scope of 'medicine' to those sciences and techniques that are based on and that use the physico-chemical frame of reference. Other sciences, which study human experiences in different frames of reference (such as those of history, sociology, linguistics) would be subsumed under the label 'socio-psychology' and would complement 'medicine' in the study and change of man" (Szasz, 1957a, p. 242).

Because he believed that science requires reductionism, Szasz's proposal to distinguish between exact and social sciences seems not particularly revolutionary. Perhaps that is why he relegated it to a footnote. But he went further. His studies of psychosomatic issues confronted him with a scientific domain in which the spheres of psyche, soma, and society were considered—at the time—to be intimately related within all their dualistic confusion. His attempt to reduce this confusion by demarcating these scientific domains led him to describe pain as a psychological phenomenon. Therefore, he rejected the distinction between "organic" and "psychogenic" pain. For Szasz, the decisive criterion of such a distinction would be each researcher's judgment about the cause of each pain. This he considered senseless and, from the patient's point of view, discriminatory, because it suggests that "organic" pain is credible, clear, and justified, while "psychogenic" pain is incredible, suspect, and unjustifiable. Thus motivated, he sided with the patient, who would not wish to be discriminated against, but found a role for "scientific clarity" in the background. How the patient would take this distinction, however, is questionable, considering that it would be in the patient's interest to identify the source of pain correctly. Szasz regarded pain as a psychological phenomenon, of interest to the somatic physician only insofar as it indicates a bodily lesion. In 1959, he concluded that the physical concept of pain should be abandoned and that pain should be understood as solely psychological (Szasz, 1959a).

A problem with Szasz's position is that it pressures one to choose between two approaches. Purely physical science requires reductionism, whereas medical practice requires the integration of social and psychological factors with bodily lesions indicated by the phenomenon of pain. It becomes a choice between the perspective of the scientist and the perspective of the practitioner. For the latter, the concept of physical pain is, after all, vital. Also, an individual's personality and response to bodily pain often have pivotal roles. It is essential for the practicing physician and the patient to keep the physically indicative side of pain foremost in mind. The duality between these two concepts of pain, as Szasz interpreted it, exposes the contrast between medicine as a science and medicine as a helping profession. He showed awareness of this contrast in 1958, when he rejected the traditional definition of psychiatry as a branch of medicine that involves studying and treating psychological illness. He described this definition as "generally comforting and often useful, in a practical sense. It is inadequate, however, from the viewpoint of scientific accuracy" (Szasz, 1958, p. 229). Szasz chose two points of departure in his effort to resolve this dilemma: (1) the scientific or theoretical perspective (i.e., the methods and frame of reference which psychiatry employs); and (2) the practical perspective (i.e., what clinical psychiatrists actually do).

From the scientific theoretical perspective, he described psychiatry as "the science and practical application of those disciplines which use the psychological method and language (in a medical setting). Their object is man as a social being, his development, social identity, self-concept, and his relationships with his fellow men" (Szasz, 1959a, p. 985). This description is unsurprising given the time, when (certainly for Szasz himself) psychoanalysis dominated psychiatry, and given that he made his career practicing psychoanalysis: "Modern psychiatry is said to consist of a body of knowledge upon which there is more or less general agreement. This knowledge consists of, or is derived from, the theory and practice of psychoanalysis" (Szasz, 1956, p. 301). His description conspicuously omits the role that the body can have in the cause and course of psychiatric disorders. Later, he would defend this position by claiming that, when the body is involved, the case should be categorized as somatic, not psychiatric.

From the practical perspective, Szasz (1958) posited two kinds of psychiatrists. One group, whom he called physicians, not psychiatrists, used physicochemical treatment methods (e.g., electroshock, medication, psychosurgery). The other group used sociopsychological treatment methods, and they were the real psychiatrists. His ideal, as expressed in *Pain and Pleasure*, became for him the actual state: "Now, it is clear that medicine is concerned with the workings of the human (and animal) body as a physicochemical machine" (Szasz, 1958, p. 230). He considered this choice inescapable: "We cannot have both, or a combination of the two, either by simply wishing or by coining a word like psychosomatic" (Szasz, 1957b, p. 405).

It is difficult to repudiate some inversions of reality, including this one, without setting up straw-man arguments. Szasz began by denying the status quo, then characterizing it as wishful thinking. The line he drew, based on scientific theory, has since then been running smack through the entire field of medicine and psychiatry. To defend his position and to ground it in the beginning of scientific medicine in the nineteenth century, he cited Rudolf Virchow's principle that illness is just damage to the body's cells or functions. Virchow's biomedical concept of illness has become the dominant model in somatic medical specialties. Nevertheless, this concept is inadequate, especially for family practice and clinical psychiatry, and to some extent dangerous, since it leads to unilateral focus on bodily lesions while losing sight of the person who is ill.

Disability, temporary or not, has existed since time immemorial. Efforts to provide a single definition covering all these situations have led to a variety of ideas, each based on particular arguments. Some fall out of favor, others retain their value (for some length of time), but in the end none of them prove comprehensive or even satisfactory (Pols, 1984, 2005). There is no doubt that the biomedical concept, by promoting the empirical scientific study of illness, fostered revolutionary development of medical science, therapy, and prevention. Psychiatry and family practice are thus each in an exceptional position because, for them, the biomedical concept of illness does not suffice. Practitioners of medical specialties regularly hear and express dissatisfaction with the biomedical view, which has too much focus on the body and too little on the patient as a human being.

Szasz encountered this deficiency in trying to bring order out of this conceptual confusion. His solution was perhaps cogent, given his own training and the psychoanalytic domination of psychiatric thought in his day. But in retrospect, it reveals a psychiatric unilateralism that limits itself to psychoanalysis. Against Szasz, I believe that a multifaceted approach is essential to psychiatry, not only because intrapsychic, social, and cultural factors can be involved, but also because physical factors may play a role, as I have argued elsewhere (Pols, 2015). Psychiatry's mission is to employ all these heterogeneous aspects to achieve optimal therapy. However, a seemingly endless series of one-dimensional explanatory models has been in vogue. Insofar as science's biomedical concept of disease has accomplished enormous and beneficial successes in strictly somatic medicine, the trend (at least at the time of this writing) is to expect further advances in psychiatry only from neurobiology and other neurosciences. Szasz represents one extreme, while neuroscience represents the other extreme. Yet there is ample evidence that practice, not science, is the best guide for finding therapeutic solutions. In practice, *people* become ill, not just their bodies (or their psyches).

One of Szasz's typical methods of argumentation was to dissociate complex issues, such as the difference between the physicochemical and sociopsychological sides of psychiatry. But he did not leave it at that; rather, he presented divergent aspects as contrasting opposites, each a separate reality. He lamented losing the family physician of yore, who "combined the social roles of physicochemical scientist vis-à-vis the body and psychotherapist vis-à-vis the person" (Szasz, 1959b, p. 358). To distinguish between these two faces of the family physician is reasonable; but to split the complex mission of this practitioner into two separate roles, divorced from each other, is another matter entirely. Unlike Szasz, most medical practitioners would find these roles not only compatible, but also well-nigh inseparable. Occasionally, from either a scientist's or a practitioner's point of view, it may be desirable to emphasize one while temporarily keeping the other low-key, but we must keep in mind that this is an artificial construct. To equate such reductionism with reality would encourage a purely physical medicine, concerned little with the actual fate of ill people, but restricted to studying and affecting their bodily lesions. Also in Szasz's later writings, this divorce between distinguishable yet inseparable aspects occurs as rhetorical direction which sometimes clarifies but sometimes confuses.

To return now from this digression to 1956–1961 (i.e., the period leading up to *The Myth of Mental Illness*), Szasz first differentiated the sphere of physicochemistry from that of sociopsychology, assigning medicine to the former and psychiatry to the latter. Then he severed these two spheres from each other with regard to the roles of professionals. It was just a small yet spectacular step to section off the concept of illness as belonging to physicochemistry, thus letting sociopsychology fall outside the domain of medicine. This step left psychiatric disorders as only metaphorical disorders. The consequence for Szasz is that the psychiatric concept of illness falls by the wayside. This is the subject of *The Myth of Mental Illness*.

2.2 **Sociopolitical background**

Szasz was a staunch libertarian and did not conceal his political views. Many of his later ideas were based on libertarian values. Such works as Friedrich August von Hayek's *The Counter-Revolution of Science* (1952) and *The Road to Serfdom* (1944) influenced him. Szasz favored a very small government, limited to protecting and defending citizens' imperiled freedom through armed forces and to establishing a system of justice to punish criminals. Anything else that government undertakes is undesirable. He maintained that socially disadvantaged people are better assisted by empowerment than by being pampered with welfare benefits and protective measures: "Legislative prescriptions, no matter how enlightened, will not create a good society. Our best chance for success still lies in a political system that is consistently noncoercive, limiting its power to the prevention and punishment of crime, and deploying its resources to providing relatively equal opportunities for various kinds of personal self-development" (Szasz, 1963, p. 222).

He developed this idea further in later writing (Szasz, 1977, pp. 145–62). Above all, in this regard, he favored a complete separation of medicine and state. People offering healing services should have equal rights to compete in a free market. Adults should be free to choose whichever health-care services they wish, provided they pay for them themselves. Children should be educated in health care as part of their basic schooling. Unfortunately, Szasz did not go into detail about who should provide such education or how the relationship between conventional and alternative medicine should be shaped.

This extreme free-market principle converts the relationship between health-care supplier and health-care demander into a contract which each is free to begin and end.

This contractual relationship makes compulsory psychiatric care inconceivable. When such coercion occurs, it is an unjustified deprivation of liberty.

Szasz revealed to me in a personal communication, June 1982, that, during his training, he avoided interning in a mental hospital because he did not want to be compelled to administer electroshock treatments to involuntary patients. It is significant that he already objected on principle to compulsory treatment in the early 1950s. Despite his department's close association with Hutchings Psychiatric Center, a mental hospital in Syracuse, he did not work in a mental hospital at any time in his career as a psychiatrist, nor was he involved in any way with compulsory commitment, except to oppose it.

Humans, according to Szasz, have a duty to develop themselves. Their own efforts determine what station in life they will achieve. I find that idea difficult to accept. Some people's talents and learning abilities are limited by, for instance, low intelligence, physical disability, illness, psychiatric disorder, environmental factors, or plain bad luck, so that they cannot achieve their station—no matter how much effort they put in. I believe that we are obligated to extend assistance to such people when they experience problems in living. Otherwise, society would be inhumane and callous.

Szasz *did* recognize that people can experience problems in living—and that psychiatry can help with such problems on a private, individual, contractual, and confidential basis. But he considered the social function of psychiatry to be a misleading dodge, a fraud, because it polishes away these problems by renaming them mental illness.

2.3 **Sociological background**

The period in which it appeared was another factor that contributed to reverberations following the publication of *The Myth of Mental Illness*. The early sixties were a time of social change, perhaps even more so in Europe than in the United States. In Europe, societal reconstruction in the wake of World War II, aided in part by the Marshall Plan, and the accompanying nostalgia for the prewar era, were drawing to a close. Unprecedented social change was dawning, which involved, among other things, heightened individualism, altered views about sexuality influenced by new contraceptive inventions, rebellion against hierarchy and authority, the generation gap, the ascendancy of racial and ethnic minorities, and widespread drug use.

1961 was a significant year in the history of psychiatry because it spawned a proliferation of critical books by psychiatrists, sociologists, and philosophers in both the United States and Europe—launching psychiatry into crisis. Several factors lay at the heart of this wave of criticism. Customary biomedical treatments in psychiatry, with the exception of some psychopharmaceuticals serendipitously discovered during this period, were producing disappointing outcomes. Shock treatment, insulin coma, and prefrontal lobotomy not only produced poor results but also were increasingly condemned as inhumane. Conditions in mental hospitals were exposed as hideously disgraceful, in the United States more than in Europe (Ridenour, 1961). Sociologist Erving Goffman's book (1961, 2007), which dealt with psychiatric facilities as "total institutions," was received with enthusiasm and approval. Such works helped to give birth to a tempestuous critical movement, echoed in a broad spectrum of social echelons outside psychiatry. Issues arose: Are psychiatry and/or mental hospitals injurious and/or inhumane? Do psychiatric disorders actually exist, or is schizophrenia, for instance, a consequence of long-term psychiatric hospitalization? What justification exists for compulsory commitment? Why do fellow humans in mental hospitals receive no or hardly any treatment?

As the concepts, foundations, and practices of psychiatry were attacked in various ways, the almost revolutionary zeitgeist that ensued was given a name, in 1967, when David Cooper correlated these maverick critical theories as "antipsychiatry" (Cooper, 1967). Observers ascribed similarities to antipsychiatry theoreticians who in fact were quite dissimilar. In this atmosphere of unmasking and protest, Szasz, as a rebel, was mentioned in the same breath with popular figures such as Cooper and R.D. Laing in the United Kingdom, Michel Foucault in France, Franco Basaglia and the movement for democratic psychiatry that he spurred in Italy, various leftist initiatives in Germany, Timothy Leary in the United States, and Jan Foudraine in the Netherlands. Persons of utterly disparate plumage were identified as antipsychiatrists. Many of their books became bestsellers and were consumed avidly. Cooper's honorary title, antipsychiatry, proved to be a gimmicky term that would soon become a means to discredit those who presented themselves as belonging to that group, or were assigned to it by others.

Shortly after *The Myth of Mental Illness* appeared, Szasz was absorbed into this surge of rebellion and was welcomed as an antipsychiatrist. Leary, for example, hailed it (in a personal letter to Szasz, July 17, 1961) as "the most important book in the history of psychiatry" (Luft, 2009, p. 15). Szasz rode on this tide of publicity for this and his later critical books. Many people identified his themes—the metaphorical character of the concept of mental illness, the criticism of psychiatric hospitals, the categorical rejection of compulsory commitment and treatment—as "antipsychiatric" topics. But in many reviews of his writing, his libertarian motives remained conspicuously unmentioned. He was the only major critical psychiatrist on the political right wing.

In his 1976 book, *Schizophrenia*, Szasz rejected the term "antipsychiatry." He called it "imprecise, misleading, and cheaply self-aggrandizing" (Szasz, 1976, p. 48) and considered the application of this concept to himself thoroughly misplaced. Other famous "antipsychiatrists" also later opposed this label, feeling ostracized by it. Szasz's protest against being called an "antipsychiatrist" was mainly because it included him in movements in which he had no part and in the company of those with whom he wished no association. For instance, in *Schizophrenia* he favorably cited David Martin's interpretation of Laing as "an angry prophet, an intolerant religious fanatic" (Szasz, 1976, p. 55).

The tumult raised by *The Myth of Mental Illness* cannot be properly understood without first understanding this historical context.

2.4 Summary

In his early years as a psychiatrist, Szasz was a dedicated psychoanalyst. His scientific research on psychosomatic disorders confronted him with the problem of the body versus the mind. He then, from a scientific-theoretical perspective, advocated separating biomedicine from sociopsychology (i.e., psychoanalysis) and separating physicians from psychiatrists. *The Myth of Mental Illness* further supported this proposed separation by disqualifying the concept of illness in psychiatry. In this light, his rebellion within psychiatry can be seen as a consequence of his earlier opinions and persuasions about the nature of illness.

More or less independently, his libertarian political views led him to condemn coercion categorically—except as retribution for criminal behavior. This condemnation had not yet come to fruition in his publications before *The Myth of Mental Illness*. His classifying of psychiatric disorders outside psychiatry gave him the opportunity to expose the whole psychiatric industry as deception.

His belief that "psychiatric disorder" was a deceptive medical concept included him in the wave of critics who debunked psychiatric theories and practices in the early 1960s. He thus rapidly became well known as an advocate of non-medical psychiatry, which partly explains why, on the one hand, the general public enthusiastically endorsed his views, while, on the other hand, the psychiatric establishment initially ignored and then vehemently dismissed them.

Nonetheless, Szasz's ideas, though springing from an unconventional political position, rendered many fruitful and inspiring ideas, which constitute a warning against unilateral approaches within a profession characterized by complexity. This warning can also be applied to the current unilateral neurobiological direction, which renders many scientific but few pragmatic results.

References

Alexander, Franz, and Thomas S. Szasz. 1952. "The Psychosomatic Approach in Medicine." In *Dynamic Psychiatry*, edited by Franz Alexander and Helen Ross, pp. 369–400. Chicago: University of Chicago Press.

Cooper, David G. 1967. *Psychiatry and Anti-Psychiatry*. London: Tavistock.

Goffman, Erving. 1961. *Asylums: Essays on the Social Situation of Mental Patients and Other Inmates*. New York: Doubleday.

Goffman, Erving. 2007. *Asylums: Essays on the Social Situation of Mental Patients and Other Inmates*. New Brunswick, New Jersey: Aldine Transaction.

Hayek, Friedrich August von. 1944. *The Road to Serfdom*. Chicago: Economic Institute for Research and Education.

Hayek, Friedrich August von. 1952. *The Counter-Revolution of Science: Studies on the Abuse of Reason*. Glencoe, Illinois: Free Press.

Luft, Eric v.d. 2009. *Die at the Right Time: A Subjective Cultural History of the American Sixties*. North Syracuse, New York: Gegensatz Press.

Pols, Jan. 1984. *Mythe en Macht: Over de Kritischepsychiatrie van Thomas S. Szasz*. Nijmegen: SUN.

Pols, Jan. 2005. *The Politics of Mental Illness: Myth and Power in the Work of Thomas S. Szasz*, translated by Mira de Vries. Accessed April 6, 2018. <www.janpols.net>

Pols, Jan. 2015. *Veertig jaar Psychiatrie: Een Dynamisch Doolhof*. Utrecht: De Tijdstroom.

Ridenour, Nina. 1961. *Mental Health in the United States: A Fifty Year History*. Cambridge, Mass.: Harvard University Press.

Szasz, Thomas S. 1948a. "Psychiatric Aspects of Vagotomy: A Preliminary Report." *Annals of Internal Medicine* **28** (2) (February): 279–88.

Szasz, Thomas S. 1948b. "Psychiatric Aspects of Vagotomy, II: A Psychiatric Study of Vagotomized Ulcer Patients with Comments on Prognosis." *Psychosomatic Medicine* **11** (4) (July–August): 187–99.

Szasz, Thomas S. 1949a. "Factors in the Pathogenesis of Peptic Ulcer: Some Critical Comments on a Recent Article by George F. Mahl." *Psychosomatic Medicine* **11** (5) (September–October): 300–4.

Szasz, Thomas S. 1949b. "Psychiatric Aspects of Vagotomy, IV: Phantom Ulcer Pain." *Archives of Neurology and Psychiatry* **62** (6) (December): 728–33.

Szasz, Thomas S. 1949c. "Psychosomatic Aspects of Salivary Activity, I: Hypersalivation in Patients with Peptic Ulcer." *Research Publications of the Association for Research in Nervous and Mental Disease* **29** (December): 647–55.

Szasz, Thomas S. 1950. "Psychosomatic Aspects of Salivary Activity, II: Psychoanalytic Observations Concerning Hypersalivation." *Psychosomatic Medicine* **12** (5) (September–October): 320–31.

Szasz, Thomas S. 1951. "Physiological and Psychodynamic Mechanisms in Constipation and Diarrhea." *Psychosomatic Medicine* **13** (2) (March–April): 112–6.

Szasz, Thomas S. 1952. "On the Psychoanalytic Theory of Instincts." *Psychoanalytic Quarterly* **21** (1) (January): 25–48.

Szasz, Thomas S. 1956. "Some Observations on the Relationship Between Psychiatry and the Law." *AMA Archives of Neurology and Psychiatry* **75** (3) (March): 297–315.

Szasz, Thomas S. 1957a. *Pain and Pleasure: A Study of Bodily Feelings*. New York: Basic Books.

Szasz, Thomas S. 1957b. "The Problem of Psychiatric Nosology: A Contribution to a Situational Analysis of Psychiatric Operations." *American Journal of Psychiatry* **114** (5) (November): 405–13.

Szasz, Thomas S. 1958. "Scientific Method and Social Role in Medicine and Psychiatry." *AMA Archives of Internal Medicine* **101** (2) (February): 228–38.

Szasz, Thomas S. 1959a. "Language and Pain." In *American Handbook of Psychiatry: Volume One*, edited by Silvano Arieti, pp. 982–99. New York: Basic Books.

Szasz, Thomas S. 1959b. "Psychoanalysis and Medicine." In *Readings in Psychoanalytic Psychology*, edited by Morton Levitt, pp. 355–74. New York: Appleton-Century-Crofts.

Szasz, Thomas S. 1963. *Law, Liberty, and Psychiatry: An Inquiry into the Social Uses of Mental Health Practices*. New York: Macmillan.

Szasz, Thomas S. 1976. *Schizophrenia: The Sacred Symbol of Psychiatry*. New York: Basic Books.

Szasz, Thomas S. 1977. *The Theology of Medicine: The Political-Philosophical Foundations of Medical Ethics*. New York: Harper & Row.

Chapter 3

Philosophical influences on Thomas Szasz

Eric v.d. Luft

3.1 Introduction

Insofar as Thomas Szasz describes himself as a libertarian (Luft, 2001), a conservative, and a Republican, one would naturally expect to find among his philosophical influences: defenders of individual freedom such as Jean-Jacques Rousseau, conservative theorists such as Edmund Burke, libertarian theorists such as Friedrich A. Hayek (Vatz and Weinberg, 1983, pp. 139–43), laissez-faire economists such as Ludwig von Mises (Vatz and Weinberg, 1983, pp. 117, 137–9), champions of civil disobedience such as Henry David Thoreau, inveterate questioners such as Socrates (Vatz and Weinberg, 1983, p. 110), absurdists such as Albert Camus, existentialists such as Jean-Paul Sartre, liberal utilitarians such as John Stuart Mill (Vatz and Weinberg, 1983, pp. 117–24), conservative commentators such as H.L. Mencken, unswerving Stoics such as Seneca, radical individualists and neo-Stoics such as Friedrich Nietzsche, and perhaps even anarchist individualists such as Max Stirner. But this is generally not the case. Szasz does not explicitly deny any of these, but his influences are much broader. Although he is somewhat of a philosophical rogue, and certainly no one's disciple or apologist, still there is occasional evidence that he incorporates—or perhaps we should say scatters—contributions of many other thinkers into his philosophy, though none in depth. His philosophical influences are subterranean, selective, and so eclectic that we could almost accuse him of cherry-picking.

Szasz cannot use many philosophers to his advantage since almost all of them— whatever they may deem to be the entity status of "illness" or "disease" in general— accept the reality of mental illness, while Szasz, of course, as a central ideological point, does not. Hence, throughout his corpus, he makes only minimal use of explicit philosophical citations. Moreover, most such references are out of context. For example, in *The Therapeutic State* (1984, p. 120), in support of his analysis of the Patty Hearst case, Szasz quotes Nietzsche twice without citing the exact sources. The former is § 109 of *Beyond Good and Evil*, which suggests that the crime is often greater than the criminal who commits it. The latter is the next aphorism, § 110, which says that lawyers must be artists to defend criminals properly. To be fair to Szasz, this section of *Beyond Good and Evil* is just a series of disconnected epigrams under the collective title, "Judgments (*Sprüche*) and Intermezzos (*Zwischenspiele*)." To illustrate this disconnection, § 108 presents G.E. Moore's naturalistic fallacy seventeen years before *Principia Ethica* and § 111 is a witty twist on the notions of pride and vanity.

Nevertheless, before publishing *The Therapeutic State*, Szasz should have examined Nietzsche's other passages about criminals and criminality. For example, in his discussion of law and punishment in the "Wanderer and His Shadow" section of the second volume of *Human, All Too Human*, Nietzsche asserts (§24 and § 28) that punishment is meted out, not to have any effect on the convicted criminal, but to please and pacify society; then (§ 186) he decries this practice as counterproductive for everyone involved. In *Daybreak*, § 202, interrelating the ideas of health, disease, guilt, revenge, sin, punishment, and crime, Nietzsche concludes that, rather than declare sick criminals guilty and punish them, we should declare guilty criminals sick and treat them or, in extreme cases, facilitate their suicide. Pursuing similar lines in § 366 of the same book, Nietzsche advocates getting rid of the concept of shame, just as, in § 202, he had advocated getting rid of the concept of sin. Finally, in the famous discourse on "The Pale Criminal" in *Thus Spake Zarathustra*, I, § 6, Nietzsche's persona, the prophet Zarathustra, states unequivocally that all originative deeds, including crimes, arise from madness (*Wahnsinn*). Nietzsche's association of madness with crime is clear throughout, as is his condemnation of self-righteous judges for not recognizing their own madness. For him, madness is not undesirable, but is, in most instances, the source of true individuality and high cultural creativity, which are paramount Nietzschean virtues. The criminal, after committing his crime, "hereafter always saw himself as the Doer of That One Deed. I call this madness. The exception has turned into his essence . . . He did not want to be ashamed of his madness . . . What is this man? A pile of diseases which spill over into the world through his spirit . . . Whoever now becomes sick is called evil by those who are evil. He wants to harm those who have harmed him . . . Formerly the sick were seen as heretics and witches. As heretics and witches they suffered and wanted to make others suffer" (Nietzsche, 1980, pp. 46–7, my translation). Nietzsche (1980, p. 45) would like to do away with the whole "good/evil" dichotomy and replace it with "strong/weak," "healthy/sick," "austere/decadent," etc. Society is insane to tell the mentally ill that they are evil and to call criminals "vicious, evil sinners" instead of "sick, foolish enemies."

Szasz's larger purpose here, for which he enlists Nietzsche, is to debunk the concept of brainwashing. But Nietzsche is not his ally in this quest. In fact, Nietzsche's main points are actually the opposite of what Szasz intends, insofar as Nietzsche grounds his theory of criminality in a worldview which includes the reality of mental illness, hence mind control (i.e., the control of weak minds and wills by stronger ones, hence brainwashing).

Yet Szasz is equally capable of making judicious use of another thinker's words. For example, while arguing that oppressed classes of people (e.g., witches) are not real classes in themselves, but rather the creations of those who wish to persecute, control, and sometimes kill them, Szasz cites favorably and accurately Sartre's analysis of the persecution of Jews: "Sartre views anti-Semitism as I view the persecution of witches and madmen . . . [His] existentialist interpretation of anti-Semitism closely resembles the sociologic interpretation of deviance: in both, the deviant—scapegoat or victim—is regarded as partly the creation of his persecutors . . . In saying that the anti-Semite 'makes' the Jew, he means the Jew *qua* social object upon whom the anti-Semite proposes to act in his own self-interest. This point cannot be emphasized too strongly about mental illness" (Szasz, 1970, pp. 269, 273). Szasz, by birth himself Jewish, would have felt this topic keenly and would have been naturally sensitive to anyone who might be a kindred spirit in this experience, especially in view of the oncoming Nazism which led him to leave his native Hungary and settle in the United States. Accordingly he writes: "All scapegoat theories postulate that if only the offending person, race, illness, or what-not could be dominated, subjugated, mastered, or eliminated, all manner of problems would be solved" (Szasz, 1972, p. 193).

In 2001, when I was writing a biographical cover story about Szasz for the Upstate Medical University *Alumni Journal*, he told me that he considered that his life's mission was to wrest artificial control of people's lives away from bureaucracies, government, religion, the medical profession, the legal profession, the insurance business, etc., which had usurped it, and give it back to individuals so that they could again enjoy their natural freedom as individuals. Also at that time, he told me that, of the twenty-five books he had already published, only three were essential to understand his thought: *The Myth of Mental Illness: Foundations of a Theory of Personal Conduct* (1961), *Insanity: The Idea and its Consequences* (1987), and *Fatal Freedom: The Ethics and Politics of Suicide* (1999). I doubt that he would subsequently have added any titles to these three. Hence I will focus on them.

3.2 *The Myth of Mental Illness*

The first of these three major works is a vigorous and notorious polemic against the reality or pathology of what is typically called "mental illness." This thesis seems original with Szasz, but powerful figures nevertheless lurk behind it. Karl Popper's rejection of historicism and social determinism is among Szasz's most fundamental premises. Historicism is the belief that there is a connective logic to history and that trajectories into the future can be described and predicted by studying the past. Historicism is not necessarily deterministic. It admits of degrees—depending upon, among other things, whether our topic is the near or the far future and whether the power of the past over the future amounts to inexorable force or only to probable or even just possible influence. Szasz (1972, p. 21) gives the impression that Popper coined the term and originated the concept, but this is not true. The term (*Historismus*) and concept were both current in German philosophy throughout the nineteenth century, particularly in the work of Friedrich Schlegel (1772–1829), who coined the term in 1797, Leopold von Ranke (1795–1886), and Ernst Troeltsch (1865–1923). Even the year that Popper published *The Poverty of Historicism*, Friedrich Engel-Jánosi's *The Growth of German Historicism* (1944) also appeared. But in *The Poverty of Historicism* (1944) and *The Open Society and its Enemies* (1945), Popper presents only an extreme version of historicism as if it comprised all historicism. Szasz, closely following Popper, writes that historicism is the "application of the principle of physical determinism to human affairs . . . a doctrine according to which historical prediction is essentially no different from physical prediction. Historical events are viewed as fully determined by their antecedents, just as physical events are by theirs" (Szasz, 1972, p. 21). This is not classical German historicism, but rather the extreme kind that Marx and Engels espoused and called "historical materialism." Popper's critique of what he calls "historicism" is more applicable to orthodox Marxism-Leninism. Despite what both Popper and Szasz (1972, pp. 21–2) suggest, it is not applicable to either Nietzsche or Plato, the latter of whom did not even have a philosophy of history. Scholars generally agree that the first genuine philosophy of history was Augustine's *City of God*, which, insofar as it sees history in terms of Christian soteriology, might be vulnerable to Popperian charges of historicism.

The Popper/Szasz definition of historicism is so extreme that it sets up a straw-man argument. No serious thinkers except Marxists and other strict determinists believe that historical causality either resembles physical causality or is predictable to the same high level of certainty as physical causality. Historical events, processes, and "forces" are not billiard balls. Szasz admits that "historical constancy and predictability are of the utmost importance for all of psychiatry" and suggests that a more reasonable view of "the effects and significance of past experiences . . . must be conceptualized and understood not in terms of antecedent 'causes' and subsequent 'effects,' but rather in terms of modifications in the entire organization and functioning of the subject acted upon" (Szasz, 1972, pp. 21–2). But such conceptualizing and understanding in terms of organization, function, and logical structure is precisely what Hegel advocates! Apparently Szasz either did not take Hegel into account or saw him through Popper's lens. Hegel was a real historicist, not an extreme one like Marx, but a moderate one, and thus not the least bit vulnerable to Popper's attack.

In a sense, it is unfortunate that Popper influenced Szasz. In fact, it is difficult to imagine Popper having a beneficial effect on anyone except another dogmatic inductionist who indefatigably argues against speculative philosophy, rationalism, and even (sometimes) common sense. Granted that Szasz himself and many profound, open-minded thinkers are also inductionists, still they generally show greater respect than Popper does for other points of view, at least at first. Most of Popper's positions are based on either misunderstandings, shallow readings, or perhaps even deliberate distortions of his predecessors. For example, his well-known "subjectivist blunder" argument against what he calls the "bucket theory" (Popper, 1975, pp. vii, 2) of knowledge—that is, the idea of Thomas Aquinas, in *Quaestiones Disputatae de Veritate*, Q. 2, Art. 3, Arg. 19 (1952), that "*nihil est in intellectu quod non sit prius in sensu*" ["nothing is in the intellect which is not first in the senses"]; which came to be commonly quoted as "*nihil est in intellectu quod non prius fuerit in sensu*" ["nothing is in the intellect which was not first in the senses"]; which Locke developed in subtle and far-reaching ways; and to which Leibniz, in *Nouveax Essais sur l'Entendement Humain*, Book II, Chapter 1, § 2 (1951, p. 409), added "*excipe nisi ipse intellectus*" ["except the intellect itself"]—is based on a misrepresentation of Locke and an apparent ignorance of Leibniz. Popper relies much too much for his knowledge of the history of philosophy on Bertrand Russell's *History of Western Philosophy* (1945), which Russell wrote tongue-in-cheek and which has been thoroughly discredited as a serious source of information about anything except Russell's own frame of mind. Sometimes Popper's mistakes in the history of philosophy are defensible and excusable, but sometimes they are so horribly inaccurate that they invite contempt. For example, Popper's view of Hegel is not consistent with any viable interpretation of Hegel. Popper (1975, p. 125) believes that, for Hegel, the universe exercises tyrannical and absolute control over the individual, who has no power and no creativity. It is odd to affiliate such an allegation of absolutism with one of relativism—yet Popper (1975, p. 126) calls Hegel a "relativist" too!

The logical empiricism and semiology of Hans Reichenbach, the positivism of Richard von Mises (Ludwig's brother), and the operationalism of Percy W. Bridgman and Albert Einstein all inform Szasz's investigative method. Even more so, echoes of early twentieth-century British linguistic analysis, particularly that of Russell, pervade the text, as Szasz seeks to understand how language, or the way that certain concepts are expressed, has contributed toward what he considers the perversion of psychiatry and the medicalization of psychology. In rejecting Freud's view of the relation between physical and psychological phenomena, Szasz accepts Russell's reduction of apparently worldly differences to differences in "modes of representation or language" (Szasz, 1972, p. 94). Yet Szasz denies Russell's—and by implication also Wittgenstein's—assertion that the chief purpose of language is to convey facts (Russell, 1974, p. x). Such a purpose, writes Szasz, applies only to "the language of science, mathematics, and logic" and not to "sign-using behaviour encountered in many other situations" (Szasz, 1972, p. 128). This is a narrow interpretation—or perhaps a misinterpretation—of Russell and Wittgenstein, who each recognize and respect figurative, symbolic, and, at least in the case of Wittgenstein, even mystical uses of language. Russell correctly identifies Wittgenstein's goal in the *Tractatus*: to explore the possibility of creating a "logically perfect language," that is, one which "has rules of syntax which prevent nonsense" (Russell, 1974, p. x). Such a goal is indeed most fruitfully pursued with regard to fact-conveying language only, but Russell's and Wittgenstein's comprehensive view of language in general is still broader than Szasz indicates. Russell says that "we use language with the intention of meaning something by it" (Russell, 1974, p. ix), and such meaning may be anything at all, as long as the language conveys it as accurately as possible in accordance with the logic of language. Wittgenstein expresses a similar idea in § 4 and § 4.001 of the *Tractatus*: "A thought is a meaningful sentence. The totality of sentences is language."[1] Even if, as Wittgenstein famously says, "The world is all that is the case" (§ 1) and "The world is the totality of facts" (§ 1.1) (1974, pp. 6–7), these facts may still be expressed obliquely, allusively, poetically, or metaphorically, with no necessary offense to either logic or language.

Szasz's main use of Russell is to segue into a favorable and extended appropriation of the work of Susanne Langer. In what is probably the book's most significant philosophical contribution, Chapter 7, "Hysteria as Communication," Szasz states explicitly that he intends to implement her program to produce a systematic understanding of non-discursive signs and non-linguistic expressions. The thesis of Langer's Chapter 5, "Language," in *Philosophy in a New Key* is that only humans are capable of language, because, unlike other animals, only humans are capable of creating, understanding, and using connotative, multivalent, or subtly allusive symbols, rather than merely indicating meanings with signs or signals, which apes and all kinds of "lower" animals

---

[1] Wittgenstein, 1974, p. 34: "Der Gedanke ist der sinnvolle Satz. Die Gesamtheit der Sätze ist die Sprache." (My translation)

can readily do (Langer, 1957, p. 105). Moreover, language is necessarily a social crea-tion; humans isolated from other humans do not learn language (Langer, 1957, p. 108). The reciprocity of human interaction is what engenders human communication on the genuinely linguistic (i.e., symbolic), not merely semiotic, level. These are themes that were first developed in Ernst Cassirer's monumental three-volume *Philosophy of Symbolic Forms* (1955–7),[2] and Langer gratefully and conspicuously acknowledges her debt to Cassirer. Thus, since Langer's Chapter 5 seems to be the part of her magnum opus that influenced Szasz's Chapter 7 the most, we could say that the real influence on Szasz here is, transitively, Cassirer. Moreover, since *Philosophy in a New Key* is a book about the philosophy of art, and even more specifically, about the philosophy of music, and since the more generally conceived *Philosophy of Symbolic Forms* laid the ground-work for Langer's book, Szasz might have done well to consult Cassirer as well, partic-ularly Chapters 2 and 3 of Volume 1, *Language*, and all of Volume 2, *Mythical Thought*.

Szasz's concern in his Chapter 7 is not linguistic denotation, but non-discursive communication. The forms that interest him here are what Langer calls "presenta-tional," as opposed to "discursive." For Langer, discursive and presentational forms are both part of language. Even though the presentational is "lower than the discursive" because it does not involve words, their difference is only "formal"; both are required for "articulate conceptual thinking," and the presentational is often semantically richer than the discursive (Langer, 1957, pp. 102-3, 110). It is this rich semantics of, for ex-ample, "body language" that Szasz seeks to explore. He approves and develops her primary thesis: "Meaning has both a logical and a psychological aspect" (Langer, 1957, p. 53), and finds common ground with her claim that "recognition of presentational symbolism as a normal and prevalent vehicle of meaning widens our conception of rationality far beyond the traditional boundaries, yet never breaks faith with logic in the strictest sense" (Langer, 1957, p. 97).

Szasz also approves and develops Langer's attacks on Freud. They agree that Freud is too quick to label deviations from the prevailing psychosocial "norm" as sick, neu-rotic, or harmful, and too slow to call them creative, constructive, or beneficial. Langer even claims that Freudian psychology cannot explain "artistic excellence" (Langer, 1957, p. 207). In comparing the symbolization processes, symbolic functions, and symbolized meanings of mathematical logic and Freudian psychology, respectively, she suggests that, despite the fact that both logic and psychology "preoccupy and in-spire our philosophical age" (Langer, 1957, p. 22), the two really have nothing to do with each other and derive "from entirely different interests" (Langer, 1957, p. 23), so that it would be a mistake to use the word "symbol" in either context without recognizing this equivocation. She implies that Freud's theories of dreams, symbols, etc., which are, after all, empirical and falsifiable, not deductive, import too much un-warranted or overly standardized logic into his interpretations of particular psycho-logical observations, and that this intrusion vitiates his science. In other words, he is guilty of the fallacy of hasty generalization (converse accident). She argues that Freud's

---

[2] A fourth volume, *The Metaphysics of Symbolic Forms*, was added posthumously, compiled by a team of scholars led by John Michael Krois in the 1990s, from Cassirer's manuscripts of the 1920s.

dream theories "do not fit the scientific picture of the mind's growth and function at all" (Langer, 1957, p. 38). Szasz (1972, p. 171) would agree with her that the human appropriation and use of psychological symbols is highly individualized and in no way related to any kind of quantifiable, deductive, or overarching logic.

Langer criticizes Freud even more sharply on the issue of genetic psychology: that is, the science that studies the "genesis," growth, and evolution of the mind's (and/ or the brain's) capacities for thought, imagination, language, etc. She observes that both common sense and the science of genetic psychology agree that art is "play" and "luxury," but asserts to the contrary that this widely-accepted view is false and that art is actually serious business, an indication of genius, and an essential component of true humanity (Langer, 1957, p. 37). Art always involves manipulating symbols and creating *ex nihilo* new and more deeply significant symbols, which are sophisticated activities far beyond mere play, closer to necessities for achieving full human integrity than to luxuries for those who have either already achieved this integrity by other means or who do not care whether they ever achieve it by any means. Genetic psychology, as conceived by Freud and others, depends upon animal studies and upon a mechanistic, behavioristic, or even deterministic outlook which favors physiology over less tangible aspects of the whole human being (e.g., the use of symbols) (Langer, 1957, pp. 28-9), and shortchanges human integrity, reducing full human consciousness to the single aspect of mind or thinking (Langer, 1957, pp. 27, 38). Langer rejects any investigative method which extrapolates from animal psychology to draw conclusions about human psychology (Langer, 1957, p. 39). In so doing, she identifies two general types of theories about what properly constitutes humanity from a psychological point of view: (1) the human is "the highest animal," whose "supreme desires" arise internally from the naturally human "supreme mind"; (2) the human is an ordinary, low, or perhaps even the "lowest" animal, whose higher aspirations arise from some sort of "admixture," which may or may not be, in the case of religious symbols and tendencies, "otherworldly" (Langer, 1957, p. 39), or, in the case of Freudian sexual symbols, perversions, or neuroses, thisworldly.

To interpret humans in the same terms or by the same criteria with which biologists interpret amoebas, jellyfish, or even apes does injustice to the uniquely human ability to express and continuously reinvent ourselves verbally, linguistically, rationally, artistically, symbolically, etc. (Langer, 1957, pp. 28, 32-3). Just as Aristotle defines the human as a "rational animal," Cassirer defines the human as *animal symbolicum*, the "symbolizing animal" (Cassirer, 1970, pp. 25-6). For Cassirer, insofar as it is the ability to symbolize which separates humans from all other animals, humans are the only animals capable of creating myths, which must perforce be composed of symbols (Luft, 1984). Again we see that what Szasz acknowledges as having taken from Langer, she had first taken from Cassirer, whom Szasz does not explicitly acknowledge.

Cassirer and Szasz share a negative assessment of Freud's genetic psychology grounded in sexual instinct (Cassirer, 1970, p. 21). Szasz employs Langer to challenge Freud's fundamental thesis that humans would prefer to remain in childhood, indulging only in simple animal gratification and aimless play, but breaking out of childhood, albeit reluctantly, only because of culturally conditioned sexual drive (Szasz, 1972, pp. 1701). Szasz proposes instead that humans have a natural urge to learn and that they regress to childhood when their learning is stifled (e.g., by religious doctrines or social taboos) (Szasz, 1972, pp. 171–2). He amends Langer's (i.e., Cassirer's) "basic thesis" of the human need "for symbolization and symbolic expression" in two ways, by asserting: (1) "a primary . . . irreducible . . . need for object contact and human relationships"; and (2) "that the notions of objects, symbols, rules, and roles are intimately connected, so that [human] growth towards personal identity and integrity on the one hand, and towards social tolerance and decreasing need for group narcissism on the other, go hand in hand with increasing sophistication in regard to the understanding and use of symbols, rules, roles, and games" (Szasz, 1972, p. 171).

Oddly enough, one of the strongest apparent influences on *The Myth of Mental Illness* is someone whom Szasz does not name there—Søren Kierkegaard—insofar as the long discussion of indirect communication in the "Hysteria as Communication" chapter is stamped throughout with Kierkegaardian content. The whole idea of indirect communication is quintessentially Kierkegaardian; it is associated with him as intimately as the idea of absolute universal forms is associated with Plato. Kierkegaard, in the persona of his pseudonym Anti-Climacus, writes that indirect communication occurs in either of two ways: (1) reducing the communicator to nothing, "then incessantly composing qualitative opposites into unity" (Kierkegaard, 2004, p. 117); or (2) the personality of communicator intruding upon the message and providing a mysterious but significant relationship to it (Kierkegaard, 2004, pp. 117–19). In other words, in the first case, the receiver, listener, reader, etc., constantly strives to resolve the presented contradictions while the communicator, in the background, never attempts to denote anything, but only to present more numerous and more perplexing contradictions; but in the second case, the receiver, etc., is stymied between the communicator, in the foreground, and whatever oblique message is hidden by or in the communicator's personality. Szasz, in partial agreement, claims that "referential ambiguity allows one to make indirect communications intentionally, by employing expressions known to be interpretable in more than one way. It is precisely that some types of communications have *multiple meanings* that make them suitable as methods of indirect communication."[3]

3.3 *Insanity: The Idea and its Consequences*

The second of Szasz's three main books continues the theme of the first, but aims to be more specific, more scholarly, and more fully documented. Yet just a peek at its index, bibliography, and notes reveals a breadth of citations that borders on eclecticism. If there seems to be minimal systematic connection among his references, then the burden would be on Szasz to show, provide, or even invent this connection—and he fails at this task. From Blackstone's commentaries to Isaiah Berlin's essays to Beethoven's letters to Hobbes's dogmatism to Charles Sanders Peirce's pragmatism to Mark Twain's epigrams, it may almost seem as if Szasz is reaching for support wherever he can get it. But the fact is that he does not *need* the support of previous thinkers. Having redefined "illness" categorically in terms of only physical lesions, he feels confident that he can build his entire theory on that alone. While he appreciates, for

---

[3] Szasz, 1972, p. 142; original italics. With regard to hysteria, cf. pp. 141–51.

instance, that the ancient Greeks in general and Plato in the *Phaedrus* in particular associated "madness" with "inspiration" and "illumination" rather than with "illness," he does not need them to the extent that Hume needed Locke and Bacon upon which to build his empiricism, that Wolff needed Leibniz upon which to build his overarching systematic metaphysics, or that Kant needed Hume to awaken him from "dogmatic slumber" (Kant, 1950, p. 8). Szasz builds his theory on his own foundations, not on foundations laid by others. He is not a "dwarf standing on the shoulders of giants."[4] When, for example, he uses Hobbes to his advantage, he interpolates, but not unjustly, and glosses over his disagreements with Hobbes (e.g., on the issue of free will).

In this book, at least, Szasz relies to quite a large extent on the assertive individualism of Hobbes, especially Hobbes's idea—basic to social contract theory—that the government may not legitimately take away the individual's rights unless the individual has first freely empowered the government to do so under certain circumstances following due process. Despite saying in Chapter 16 of *Leviathan* that "children, fools, and madmen" may be remanded to guardians,[5] Hobbes is nevertheless clear that anyone who for any reason is judged to be "mad" does not, on that account, naturally forfeit any individual human rights, nor ought, on that account, to have these rights forcibly curtailed without due process (Szasz, 1972, pp. 219–20). Szasz's central argument against involuntary commitment is partially grounded in Hobbes's theory of madness and its social manifestations (Laor, 1984). Szasz finds little to quarrel with Hobbes's description and categorization of various types, causes, and aspects of madness.[6] He cites Hobbes to support his arguments that crime is not disease (Szasz, 1997, p. 104); that involuntary, dangerous, or futile psychiatric interventions ought not to exist (Szasz, 1997, p. 126); that metaphors ought to be recognized as such and not taken literally (Szasz, 1997, pp. 138–9, 145, 321); that we ought to adopt a naturalistic, common-sense view of miracles, supernatural events, fantastical doctrines, and unusual theories (Szasz, 1997, p. 185); that individuals owe it to themselves and to society to develop deliberative skills, circumspect outlooks, and strength of character (Szasz, 1997, p. 272); and that many people seek to be slaves of religion, the state, or some other abstract master which will absolve them of having to think for themselves (Szasz, 1997, p. 302). However, Hobbes's claim in Chapter 27 that "only children and madmen are excused from offenses against the law natural" (Hobbes, 1972, p. 345) would support the insanity defense in law, which Szasz vigorously opposes.

Szasz relates nearly all of what he uses of Hobbes to Chapter 47 of *Leviathan* (Hobbes, 1972, pp. 704–15). Szasz's attraction to this chapter is obvious, since Hobbes's topic here is one of Szasz's favorites: *Cui bono?*—the question of who benefits from a certain action, a certain social structure, a certain political stance, a certain worldview, etc. (Szasz, 1997, pp. 295–6, 358). What Szasz seems primarily to have taken from

---

[4] Saying of Bernard of Chartres (twelfth century), "Pigmaei gigantum humeris impositi plusquam ipsi gigantes vident," made current in the Anglophone world by Robert Burton (1577–1640) in *The Anatomy of Melancholy* and by Isaac Newton (1643–1727) in his letter to Robert Hooke of February 15, 1676.

[5] Hobbes, 1972, p. 219. I have modernized spelling in all quotations from Hobbes.

[6] Hobbes, 1972, pp. 139–147, especially p. 140; Szasz, 1997, p. 65.

Hobbes and elevated to central prominence is this idea of *Cui bono?*. Yet Szasz might have done well to examine Hobbes more thoroughly, and especially Chapter 13 on the natural human condition and Chapter 21 on liberty (Hobbes, 1972, pp. 183–8, 261– 74). If he had done so, then he might have realized just how antithetical Hobbesianism is to Szasz's libertarianism. Szasz indeed tries to make Hobbes into a proto-libertarian, but in so doing he ignores that Hobbes is in fact a monarchist, an authoritarian, and a mechanist. For Hobbes, the very notion that there might be such a faculty as free will is absurd (Chapter 5). He limits the possibilities of liberty and freedom to the motion of living physical bodies (Chapters 14 and 21). His mechanistic view of humanity holds that people are each individual selfish machines, without free will, but with natural and insatiable greed, lust, avarice, envy, and spite. But Szasz is an unabashed believer in human free will. Moreover, he takes the real existence of free will as a plain fact which anyone can understand and which does not require any sophisticated research or edu- cation to discern (Szasz, 1997, p. 232). In this he seems close to the viewpoint that Kant expressed in *Groundwork of the Metaphysics of Morals*, although he does not cite Kant on this issue or appear to notice the similarity.

All libertarians are driven by self-interest; yet there are two general camps of libertarians, which I would call the egoistic and the altruistic. The former, whose paradigms would be Stirner, Ayn Rand, and Murray Rothbard, believe in freedom for themselves alone, identify self-interest with selfishness, do not care whether an- yone else is free or not, and expect others to watch out for themselves and to get their freedom if and only if they can. Their motto could be "I'll fight for mine. Stop me if you can. Getting yours is your problem." The latter, whose paradigm would perhaps be Bernard de Mandeville, believe that the freedom of one enhances the freedom of all, deny that self-interest is necessarily selfish, strive to foster the common good, and expect the freedom of the individual to be socioeconomically beneficial. Their motto is either "Private vice, public virtue" or "Private greed, public benefit." The former seem not to care about the common good at all, and their theories seem to contain little be- yond ulteriorly motivated justifications of crass, heartless, unmitigated selfishness; but the latter show a genuine concern for society, and sincerely believe that giving each in- dividual free rein to exercise natural free will to the greatest possible extent is a positive good for society as a whole. Hobbes writes that in nature, without government, human life is "solitary, poor, nasty, brutish, and short" (Hobbes, 1972, p. 186) (Chapter 13). Egoistic libertarians would be at home in this world, but altruistic libertarians would prefer to try to build a world through individual liberty in which life is "communal, rich, pleasant, civilized, and long." Szasz seems most naturally to belong to the latter camp. What Hobbes calls the "war of all against all" (Hobbes, 1983, p. 34) in *De Cive* and the "war of every man against every man" (Hobbes, 1972, pp. 185, 188, 196) or the "war of every one against every one" (Hobbes, 1972, p. 185) in Chapters 13 and 14 of *Leviathan* may well be a Stirnerian/Randian paradise, but it is the opposite of what Hobbes wants, and if Szasz feels any affinity with Stirner or Rand, then, *ipso facto*, to that extent he is removed from Hobbes.

For Hobbes, humans are naturally wicked, selfish, and vile. They have a natural de- sire for personal power (Chapter 11), sometimes manifest as greed or covetousness (Chapters 6 and 10), so that whoever acquires great wealth is on that account honored, even by those who have been thereby impoverished (Chapter 10), and even if these impoverished people are thereby "displeased" (Hobbes, 1972, p. 123) (Chapter 6). Such is the nature of jealousy. The poor gladly play the game of the rich, even though they are destined—with few widely separated individual exceptions—to continue as losers. Jealousy, envy, and perverse hope spur them to keep playing this game, without even trying to change the rules. The game, whose rules, if any, are set by the strongest or richest members of communities, occasionally expands into war, which "consisteth not in actual fighting; but in the known disposition thereto" (Hobbes, 1972, p. 186). Hobbes, although an advocate for the powerful, especially the monarch, whom he holds inviolable and above the law, is no friend of the rich, as he writes in Chapter 27: ". . . to rob a poor man, is a greater crime, than to rob a rich man; because 'tis to the poor a more sensible damage" (Hobbes, 1972, p. 352). From the nineteen laws of nature that Hobbes enumerates regarding war and peace (Chapters 14 and 15), we readily infer that the rich are the natural targets of the poor, the "haves" of the "have-nots," but not the powerful of the weak.

Even though humans are by nature warlike, Hobbes's first and second laws of nature are that they should seek peace (Chapter 14) (Hobbes, 1972, p. 190). Hence they form communities and, eventually, states or commonwealths, even though there is no intrinsic or positive value in community, and even though the state or commonwealth is a contrivance, a means to an end, a necessary evil, an "artificial man" led by and embodied in a single human, the monarch, to whom citizens pledge blind obedience and surrender portions of their natural but dangerous liberty in exchange for commensurate portions of security, stability, and peace. Toward this end alone, people associate in durable political groups, not because these groups are good in themselves, but because they may be used to promote selfish interests. Yet Hobbes contradicts himself on this very point, as he writes glowingly of culture, art, literature, navigation, architecture, science, etc. (Chapter 13), none of which, in their pure form, serve private or selfish interests, but only the common good. He eventually argues that the common good cannot be established, protected, or ensured without a strong central government to inject fear into the heart of every citizen (Hobbes, 1998, p. 71; 1972, pp. 226, 296, 427).

Hobbes limits commonwealths or forms of government to only three: (1) monarchy or tyranny, (2) democracy, and (3) aristocracy or oligarchy (Hobbes, 1972, pp. 239–40, 245). The monarchy or autocratic state is an "artificial man" (Hobbes, 1972, pp. 81, 217–18, 220, 247) (Introduction, Chapters 16 and 19), a contrivance designed, not to create genuine peace, but to impose the semblance of peace (i.e., tranquility under force and fear).

Szasz, it seems, would disagree with most of this. The Hobbesian commonwealth is the "artificial man," Leviathan, but, because Hobbes himself is a monarchist, it is actually the individual human sovereign, typically the king, in whom the commonwealth is "personated" (Chapter 16), who is the "artificial man" (Hobbes, 1972, p. 247), the "mortal God" (Hobbes, 1972, p. 227), "the essence of the commonwealth" (Hobbes, 1972, p. 228), who cannot be accused, judged, or punished by any other person or entity (Chapter 20) (Hobbes, 1972, p. 252). In other words, the pessimistic Hobbes advocates precisely the type of absolute sociopolitical control that Szasz detests. Hobbes does not approve of the "divine right of kings" theory promulgated by his contemporary Charles I; he believes that kings are legitimate only by contract with their subjects, the citizens of the commonwealth. However, insofar as he sees the king as the personification of the commonwealth, he would surely have approved of the "L'état c'est moi" attitude of Louis XIV. Hobbes is quite clear in Chapter 13 that people need "a common power to keep them all in awe" (Hobbes, 1972, p. 185)—an idea which is anathema to Szasz. Hobbes believes, as the linchpin of his political philosophy, that the best form of government is the strongly centralized state; Szasz regularly and characteristically argues against the state's control of individual lives and against centralized power. Hobbes is very willing for the individual to give up quite a lot of personal liberty—which he defines negatively in Chapter 14 as "the absence of external impediments" (Hobbes, 1972, p. 189), in Chapter 21 as "the absence of opposition" (Hobbes, 1972, p. 261), and positively in Chapter 21 as "the sovereign power of life" (Hobbes, 1972, p. 264)—in order, by contract with the sovereign power of the "artificial man," the commonwealth, the modern hierarchical state, to acquire quite a lot of security and peace; but Szasz is not nearly so willing. Chapter 15 shows that, in the state of nature, the war of all against all, with "all men having right to all things" (Hobbes, 1972, p. 202), and where "every man is presumed to do all things in order to his own benefit" (Hobbes, 1972, 213), the concept of justice is meaningless. Only in a contractually established state can justice exist (Hobbes, 1972, p. 202). But for Szasz, justice is tantamount to liberty itself.

Interestingly, although Szasz and Hobbes disagree about the necessity and desirability of the autocratic power of the state, they agree about the undesirability of similar power exercised by the Church. For both thinkers, ecclesiastical or religious authority soon degenerates into irrational theocracy, which systematically works against natural human freedom, aspirations, and growth. Hobbes expects his sovereign to acquire and maintain power through contract with citizens under the auspices of God—not from church authorities—and to exhibit Christian values. In other words, for Hobbes, the ideal monarch would be one who has internalized the best Christian ethics and who sincerely lives by this heartfelt code, regardless of whatever the Church might say. In his time, Hobbes had to be very careful not to offend either the Church of England or any of the other strong Protestant faiths in Great Britain; but he could—and did—quite easily attack the Roman Catholic Church without fear for his life, person, or freedom. Yet it is just as easy for us today to infer that his criticisms of Roman Catholicism could also be true of any centralized ecclesiastical polity (e.g., the Anglican Communion), and that his accusations against the autocratic leader of any such hierarchy (e.g., the Pope) could likewise apply to the Archbishop of Canterbury. Hobbes is explicitly critical of officious bishops in general, implying their arrogance and asking of their actions: *Cui bono?* (Hobbes, 1972, p. 182; Szasz, 1997, p. 358). The Church's power over the state benefits only the Church leaders, not the rank and file of believers, not the state or its citizens, and certainly not Christian principles. Szasz writes:

> Warfare and forceful subjugation are the traditional methods for enforcing new rules. These methods, however, are useful only for the strong. The weak must rely on more subtle techniques of persuasion . . . Christianity and psychoanalysis among them. (Szasz, 1972, p. 184)

By separating Church and State, religion was deprived of its power to abuse the individual, and the State was deprived of one of its major justifications for the use of force. The upshot was a quantum leap toward greater individual liberty such as the world had never seen. By separating Psychiatry and the State, we would do the same for our age. (Szasz, 1997, p. 314)

3.4 *Fatal Freedom: The Ethics and Politics of Suicide*

Is Szasz a moral philosopher (i.e., an ethicist, an axiologist) or a theorist of the value of actions or of individual or social morality? For Szasz, there is only one way to understand ethics, either medical ethics or ethics in general, and that is by asking, with Hobbes, the classic Roman question: *Cui bono?* Whom will this action benefit? If it benefits primarily either the individual moral agent who initiates it or a goal which this individual knowingly supports, then fine. But if it benefits someone or something else, which the initiating individual moral agent either opposes, does not support, does not recognize, does not know about, or cannot avoid, then we must regard it with suspicion, and with a view toward possibly, eventually condemning it as anti-individual, anti-freedom, or anti-autonomy. For example, Szasz writes that suicide "is our ultimate, fatal freedom . . . For a long time, suicide was the business of the Church and the priest. Now it is the business of the State and the doctor. Eventually we will make it our own business, regardless of what the Bible or the Constitution or Medicine supposedly tells us about it" (Szasz, 1999). That is, since control over one's own life is the supreme individual freedom, we must wrest this prerogative from these other entities and return it to the individual. To allow external forces to exercise such a large degree of restriction of individual freedom certainly does not benefit the individual and—arguably—does not benefit these external hegemonies either. Any such argument, for Szasz, would be along the lines of asserting that any restriction on individual freedom does commensurate damage to the body politic or to society at large.

Szasz's philosophy of suicide is a key aspect of his thought. It is the topic not only of *Fatal Freedom* but also of *Suicide Prohibition: The Shame of Medicine* (Szasz, 2011), the widely reprinted "The Ethics of Suicide" (Szasz, 1971), and several other articles and book chapters. On this issue he seems to have been most keenly influenced by the Roman Stoics and Camus. He agrees with the Stoics that suicide is a question for each individual alone to decide, without influence or coercion from any external agent; and with Camus that the decision whether or not to live is the key decision in anyone's life. He names Donne, Hume, Voltaire, Goethe, and Schopenhauer as his allies and praises Hume for his "modern, secular-libertarian argument against religious and legal interference with suicide" (Szasz, 2002, p. 14). Pursuing these themes further in *Suicide Prohibition*, Szasz sees suicide as the ultimate act of free will and closely follows Nietzsche in this (Luft, 2013). In the context of medicine, especially for terminally ill or horribly suffering patients who would like to exercise a "right to die" on their own terms, Szasz believes that the suicide of a patient could involve a method such as the voluntary stopping of eating and drinking (VSED), because that would be entirely the decision of the patient; but could not legitimately involve physician-assisted suicide

(PAS), because the physician is an autonomous agent in juxtaposition to the patient, not the moral equivalent of Brutus's slave, who was essentially just a non-autonomous extension of Brutus and whom Brutus ordered to hold the sword while he, Brutus, ran onto it. Thus Szasz holds that PAS is murder, because helping to kill the patient, even if in accord with the patient's wishes, is ultimately the physician's decision, not the patient's.

Some have argued that Szasz is a Cartesian dualist (Richards, 2014). This ascription is ill-informed and ill-advised. Mind/body dualisms in general, and Cartesian dualism in particular, need to be theisms so that: (1) God can provide the sustenance and maintenance that the immaterial soul, spirit, *res cogitans*, or whatever we choose to call it, requires but that the material world can never provide; and (2) God can provide some sort of effective connection between *res cogitans* and *res extensa*, perhaps in the form of a magic pineal gland (as Descartes himself believed). But Szasz is no theist. Therefore, any mind/body dualism would be inconsistent with his philosophy. Moreover, Szasz scarcely ever mentions Descartes and seems to have only a superficial knowledge of his work.

If Szasz is not a theist, is he then a materialist or an atheist? That would be difficult to pin down with precision, but, given his frequent and energetic assertions of his distrust of (and perhaps even contempt for) organized religion, to attribute atheist tendencies to him would not be far-fetched. He is too assertive and self-confident to be merely agnostic. His affinity for Hobbes suggests that he may have a mechanistic model of humanity, insofar as Hobbes sees humans as selfish machines who seek only to satisfy themselves as individuals and who, toward that goal alone, enter into community with others. Szasz's passages on Christian oppression—for example, "the beliefs and practices of Christianity are best suited for slaves" (Szasz, 1972, p. 183)—could have been written by Nietzsche. Nor is he less critical of other religious traditions. Yet the God(s) whom he criticizes and dismisses throughout his corpus are only the positive, anthropomorphic deities of organized religion(s), not the transcendent God of the philosophers (e.g., the Eckhartian Godhead, the Tillichian ground of being, or even the Hegelian absolute). In any case, God does not figure prominently in Szasz's thought, as it does in, for instance, that of Plato, Descartes, Spinoza, Leibniz, or Whitehead, none of whom seem to have had much influence on him.

References

Cassirer, Ernst. 1955–7. *Philosophy of Symbolic Forms*. New Haven: Yale University Press.

Cassirer, Ernst. 1970. *An Essay on Man: An Introduction to a Philosophy of Human Culture [1944]*. New Haven: Yale University Press.

Engel-Jánosi, Friedrich. 1944. *The Growth of German Historicism*. Baltimore: Johns Hopkins Press.

Hobbes, Thomas. 1972. *Leviathan*, edited by C.B. Macpherson. Harmondsworth: Penguin.

Hobbes, Thomas. 1983. *De Cive: The English Version*, edited by Howard Warrender. Oxford: Clarendon.

Hobbes, Thomas. 1998. *On the Citizen*, edited by Richard Tuck and Michael Silverthorne. Cambridge: Cambridge University Press.

Kant, Immanuel. 1950. *Prolegomena to Any Future Metaphysics*, translated by Lewis White Beck. Indianapolis: Bobbs-Merrill.

Kierkegaard, Søren. 2004. T*raining in Christianity and the Edifying Discourse Which Accompanied It*, translated by Walter Lowrie, edited by John F. Thornton and Susan B. Varenne. New York: Random House.

Langer, Susanne K. 1957. *Philosophy in a New Key: A Study in the Symbolism of Reason, Rite, and Art*, 3rd edn. Cambridge: Mass.: Harvard University Press.

Laor, Nathaniel. 1984. "Hobbesian Principles in Szasz's Writings." *Clio Medica* **19**: 32–9.

Leibniz, Gottfried Wilhelm Freiherr von. 1951. *Selections*, edited by Philip P. Wiener. New York: Charles Scribner's Sons.

Luft, Eric v.d. 1984. "Cassirer's Dialectic of the Mythical Consciousness." *Reports on Philosophy (Krakow)* **8**: 3–13.

Luft, Eric v.d. 2001. "Thomas Szasz, M.D.: Philosopher, Psychiatrist, Libertarian." *Alumni Journal, published by the SUNY Upstate/Syracuse Medical Alumni Association* (Summer): 9–12.

Luft, Eric v.d. 2013. *The Value of Suicide*. Part II, Chapter 5, "Disharmony in Dualism"; Part IV, Chapter 2, "Suicide in Medical Contexts." North Syracuse, New York: Gegensatz Press.

Nietzsche, Friedrich. 1980. *Sämtliche Werke: Kritische Studienausgabe*, edited by Giorgio Colli and Mazzino Montinari. Vol. **4**, *Also Sprach Zarathustra*. Berlin: de Gruyter.

Popper, Karl R. 1975. *Objective Knowledge: An Evolutionary Approach*. Oxford: Clarendon.

Richards, Christina. 2014. "Of Cocaine and Scaffold Bars: A Critique of The Myth of Mental Illness by Thomas Szasz." *Existential Analysis* **25** (1): 66–78.

Russell, Bertrand. 1945. *A History of Western Philosophy*. New York: Simon and Schuster.

Russell, Bertrand. 1974. "Introduction." In *Tractatus Logico-Philosophicus/Logisch-philosophische Abhandlung*, Ludwig Wittgenstein, translated by D.F. Pears and B.F. McGuinness. London: Routledge & Kegan Paul.

Szasz, Thomas S. 1970. The Manufacture of Madness: A Comparative Study of the Inquisition and the Mental Health Movement. New York: Harper & Row.

Szasz, Thomas S. 1971. "The Ethics of Suicide." *Antioch Review* **31**, 1 (Spring): 7–17.

Szasz, Thomas S. 1972. *The Myth of Mental Illness: Foundations of a Theory of Personal Conduct*. London: Paladin.

Szasz, Thomas S. 1984. *The Therapeutic State: Psychiatry in the Mirror of Current Events*. Buffalo: Prometheus.

Szasz, Thomas S. 1997. *Insanity: The Idea and its Consequences*, 2nd edn. Syracuse: Syracuse University Press.

Szasz, Thomas S. 1999. "Suicide as a Moral Issue: Who Should Control When and How We Die?" *The Freeman: Ideas on Liberty* **49** (7) (July): 41–2.

Szasz, Thomas S. 2002. *Fatal Freedom: The Ethics and Politics of Suicide (with a New Preface)*. Syracuse: Syracuse University Press.

Szasz, Thomas S. 2011. *Suicide Prohibition: The Shame of Medicine*. Syracuse: Syracuse University Press.

Thomas Aquinas. 1952. *Questiones Disputatae de Veritate: Truth*, translated by Robert W. Mulligan. Chicago: Henry Regnery Company. Accessed April 9, 2018. <dhspriory.org/thomas/QDdeVer2.htm#3>

Vatz, Richard E., and Lee S. Weinberg (eds). 1983. *Thomas Szasz: Primary Values and Major Contentions*. Buffalo: Prometheus.

Wittgenstein, Ludwig. 1974. *Tractatus Logico-Philosophicus/Logisch-philosophische Abhandlung*, translated by D.F. Pears and B.F. McGuinness. London: Routledge & Kegan Paul.

Chapter 4

Conceptual models of normative content in mental disorders

John Z. Sadler

4.1 Introduction

When I was a nerdy teenager in small-town Indiana in the 1960s, my parents indulged me with a membership to the *Psychology Today* Book Club, which featured monthly releases of both popular and scholarly books in psychology from authors such as Abraham Maslow, Masters and Johnson, Rollo May, and—you guessed it— Thomas Szasz. I read *The Myth of Mental Illness* (1961) when I was in high school, and I thought this book was the coolest thing this side of Frank Zappa. With maturity, I recognized the depth and complexity of Szasz's work, his phenomenal influence in the mental health field and Western culture, and I appreciated the persistent ethical problems in psychiatry which occupied him over his lifetime. Szasz was, without doubt, a major contributor to my personal and professional identity, and this chapter is a deeply felt "thank you" to a man whom I barely met, yet feel I have known for most of my life.

4.2 Vice-laden mental disorders

I would like to address the concept of mental disorder from a different direction than I or others have done previously. However, many readers will recognize ideas, especially from Szasz. My prior work (Sadler 1997, 2002, 2005, 2013) has described many ways in which concepts of mental disorder are "value-laden"—that is, harboring meanings which require value judgments: values defined as attitudes or dispositions which are action-guiding and praiseworthy or blameworthy. In this sense, all mental disorders—indeed, all diseases—are *value-laden* concepts in that they imply, at minimum, a set of social judgments involving the desirability of the phenomenon being considered as a "disease." For instance, a myocardial infarction (MI) is something that most everyone does not want to have (that is, MIs are disvalued). Similarly, having schizophrenia is something many people do not want, and a few do want (that is, schizophrenia has value or disvalue attached to it), and having schizophrenia alters one's disposition to act. Fulford (1989) notes that diseases are generally bad things to have, and the problem with mental disorders, as he points out, is that not everyone agrees about whether this or that mental disorder is a bad thing to have. Szasz, of course, believed that mental illnesses were not diseases in a strict sense, and subsequently was explicitly opposed to what he saw as an illegitimate social control function of psychiatry (Szasz, 1961).

One question that drives this chapter is the question of what *kind* of values are entailed in our concepts of mental disorder. Philosophers have long distinguished different kinds of values: aesthetic values applying to concepts of beauty or artistic appreciation, epistemic values in appraising knowledge claims, ethical values in right/wrong judgements, among others. There are also varieties of values in medical discourses (Sadler, 1997). In the more recent DSM categories and criteria (APA 1994, 2000, 2013) we read of disease-related values—concepts like disability, impairment, injury, distress, and dysfunction. These disease-related values are morally neutral; we typically do not attribute moral rightness or wrongness to these concepts, which we can define without appeal to moral values. For instance, "disability" is a failure of one or more normal capabilities of people. But typically we do not consider people who are immoral as "disabled"—and the same goes for impairment and dysfunction. Importantly, the value-ladenness of disease concepts typically refers to social norms, as implied in the foregoing concepts of disability, impairment, injury, and dysfunction, all of which are meaningful in reference to societal expectations of "functioning" as a person. Social norms, however, can and do change. Thus, what might have been judged socially as an impairment in one historical or cultural moment or context, may not be at another historicocultural moment. For example, consider the reversal of homosexuality as a mental disorder in the 1978 second edition of DSM-II (APA, 1968) and the progressive "professional normalizing" of homosexuality since then.

However, another set of values emerge with closer scrutiny of DSM categories—ones associated with wrongful, immoral, or criminal conduct. I call these kinds of values "vice concepts," because they are defined and understood as wrongful, immoral, or criminal. More precisely, they cannot be defined without "wrongfulness" meanings; doing so would lose the full contemporary meaning of the diagnostic term. For example, each of the four A categories of the diagnostic criteria for DSM-5 conduct disorder reveals that their meaning entails some sort of immoral or criminal conduct: "aggression to people or animals," "destruction of property," "deceitfulness or theft," and "serious violations of rules" (APA 2013, pp. 469–70). Something like conduct disorder, then, is "vice-laden" because its definition and criteria entail wrongful or criminal concepts like deceitfulness, aggression, destruction, etc. (Sadler, 2014). Examination of a number of other DSM categories will also reveal vice-laden concepts and criteria: for example, antisocial personality disorder, pedophilia, intermittent explosive disorder (Sadler, 2008, 2013). In contrast, categories like major depressive disorder, panic disorder, and schizophrenia, among others, are defined and value-laden with medical traditional values like distress, disability, impairment, injury, and dysfunction. The key point here is not the particulars of the criteria; the point is that some, but not all, DSM categories are vice-laden in my technical sense. Here are a few examples of vice-laden terms from DSM-5 diagnostic criteria (APA, 2013):

Intermittent Explosive Disorder: Criterion A.2. ". . . damage or destruction of property and/or physical assault . . . physical injury against animals or other individuals."

Conduct Disorder: Criterion A.11. "Often lies . . . 'cons' others."

Kleptomania: Criterion A. ". . . steal[ing] objects that are not needed."
Borderline Personality Disorder: Criterion A.8. ". . . difficulty controlling anger."
Narcissistic Personality Disorder: Criterion A.6. ". . . interpersonally exploitative."
Exhibitionistic Disorder: Criterion A. ". . . exposure of one's genitals."

A key element in my recent scholarship cited here and elsewhere is that having vice-laden categories of psychopathology is a problem for psychiatry, and more broadly, a social problem for all of us (Sadler, 2008, 2013). Let me sketch the problems that vice-laden categories pose to psychiatry, the mental-health community, and society.

4.3 Psychiatry and mental health in a police role

About sixty years ago, Szasz began writing about the problem of psychiatry functioning as a fourth arm of the sociopolitical regulation of deviance: the other three arms being education, religion, and the criminal justice system (Szasz, 1961). As a medical discipline, Szasz believed that it was inappropriate for physicians to impose "treatment" on individuals who were merely idiosyncratic in behavior and belief, and were not infringing upon others. If such individuals *were* infringing upon others, for Szasz, they warranted criminal justice interventions. Moreover, because Szasz was convinced that *all* mental illnesses are merely metaphorical diseases (i.e., not genuine diseases with a defined pathophysiology), mental disorders which are largely, or even significantly, defined as involving wrongful and criminal conduct would be even more offensive to Szasz's sense of the role of medicine and physicians as healers. In short, physicians are healers, not police or agents of social-deviance control. He was also concerned about the potential for abuse of psychiatric power, given the relatively few legal constraints on coercive seclusion and treatment. These ideas are, or will be, familiar to all readers of this volume.

These concerns are still legitimate today. Psychiatry has significant nonmedical power over the fates of people involved with criminal or immoral deviance, and much of this power is inscribed formally in psychiatry's diagnostic categories in the form of vice-laden mental disorders.

4.4 Erosion of medical morality

Pellegrino (1999), among others, has commented upon the crucial role of "medical morality" in physicians' identity. The primary purposes or goals of medicine, in Pellegrino's straightforward view (1999, pp. 55–7), are to help, heal, care, and cure people. This simple fourfold schema of medical morality not only constitutes the purposes of medicine but also generates its ethical or moral core, reinforced concretely in the Hippocratic oath and codes of medical ethics forward. Having vice-laden mental disorders confounds medical morality with other, nonmedical, social welfare concerns: specifically, reducing crime and promoting virtuous, law-abiding citizens. Of course, these social welfare concerns are crucial in themselves, but in the setting of health care, reducing crime and promoting virtue generally lie outside the bounds of medical morality and have significant other implications, as will be discussed here.

4.5 **Public wariness of psychiatry and mental health**

Mental-health literacy research has indicated that large portions (in some cases, the majority) of the public distrust psychiatrists, psychiatric treatments, and the mental health system in general (Angermeyer and Dietrich, 2006; Gulliver et al., 2010; Jorm, 2012; Pescosolido, 2013; Phelan et al., 2000). The reasons for this public distrust are complex and cannot be reviewed here. However, one can only wonder about the contribution of vice-laden mental disorders and the police function of psychiatry, on the one hand, and public wariness of the field, on the other. ("Police function" here refers to psychiatrists' regulation of any social deviance, vicious or non-vicious—from homelessness to disruptive public ranting to frank criminal offending.) How many psychiatrists have been told by members of the public that they fear being "locked up"? Psychiatry's police function, diagnostically authorized by vice-laden mental disorders, may well be a cause for public fear of the field.

4.6 **Mixed messages and stigma**

The American Psychiatric Association (APA), among others, has gone to extraordinary efforts to address the stigma of mental illness and to present mental illnesses as "brain diseases" (Corrigan and Watson, 2004), publicly campaigning that mental disorders are diseases like any other (Malla et al., 2015). Yet the plain facts, as demonstrated by our diagnostic classifications, are that mental disorders are not diseases like any other. Some mental illnesses are like diseases (e.g., Alzheimer's dementia), but others are like immorality, bad character, and criminality (e.g., antisocial personality disorder), and still others embody elements of both disease and immorality (e.g., pedophilic disorder and intermittent explosive disorder). Diseases in internal medicine, injuries in surgery, and impairments in rehabilitation medicine do not include immoral, wrongful, or criminal conduct in their diagnostic signs and symptoms. However, many mental-disorder categories in psychiatry do. This practice can send a public message that mental illnesses are what morally bad people have, reinforcing stigmatizing attitudes toward the mentally ill and the centuries-old ideas that the mentally ill have character defects, are dangerous, and are morally deficient. The history of the stigma of madness is long and persistent (Fabrega, 1990, 1991). Vice-laden mental disorders perpetuate stigma, fears, avoidance, and discrimination.

4.7 **Incoherent and inchoate social welfare policies and services**

A single individual can qualify for a number of social welfare policies and institutions in the U.S. (Frank and Glied, 2006; Rothman, 2017). Consider, for example, an intellectually disabled, psychotic, seventeen-year-old criminal offender. This individual could qualify for the mental health system, the juvenile courts, the juvenile criminal justice system, and the intellectual disability system. If this person is homeless, one can add housing and related services to the social needs list. Similarly, adults with severe mental disorders disproportionately occupy jails and prisons (Stanford, 2014). Mentally ill individuals often end up incarcerated because of the failure of adequate mental health and substance abuse care, housing, rehabilitation, and vocational opportunities. Too often they move around from system to system, patching up one or other of their social welfare concerns, but rarely obtaining coherent and coordinated care (Frank and Glied, 2006; Morrissey and Goldman, 1984). Our patients, especially those with vice-laden disorders, elicit little in the way of political sympathy for reform (Hartwell, 2004) and even innovative, effective programs fail because of inadequate funding and other resources (Smith et al., 2009). At the same time, because of poor community resources, mentally ill individuals, with and without criminal records, routinely enter and re-enter hospital care, sociologically termed the "revolving door" (Rubinow, 2014) and amplified through related social injustices such as poverty, discrimination, and racism (U.S. DHHS, 2012).

Our bungled social welfare policies and institutions are *simultaneously intrusive* (through involuntary seclusion and treatment laws and a punishment-oriented criminal justice system) and *neglectful* (through complex qualification criteria for social welfare services, insufficient funding, insufficient services and resources, complex and exclusionary policies for treatment eligibility—such as insurance/no insurance, age constraints, severity constraints, etc.—and a general failure to coordinate and integrate services). Many people migrate from social welfare institution to institution, receiving partial services at best, redundant services often, and sometimes no care at all—with the thousands of incarcerated mentally ill being the most recently reviled example. Few receive the comprehensive multisystem care which the evidence base supports (Torrey et al., 2015) and which other Western democratic societies routinely offer as coherent, cradle-to-grave, social welfare services (Blekesaune and Quadagno, 2003; NationMaster, 2018; Saraceno and Saxena, 2002). Most tragic is that our system deincentivizes ill people to seek mental health care, including the minority who are at risk to act out criminally.

Of course, the causes of this lamentable state of affairs are complex. I offer the problem of vice-laden mental disorders as only one component, though one that I believe is crucial in impact because it structures our social thinking. The problem of confounding mental illness with immoral and wrongful conduct affects how clinicians, the public, service users, and policymakers think. Importantly, how we think shapes how we develop social policies.

With these problems in mind, I now turn to the implicit, sometimes explicit, conceptual models that have been applied to the problem of the relationship between mental disorders and immoral and criminal conduct.

4.8 Four models of the vice/mental disorder relationship

If we are to think more clearly about the roles of vice and mental illness in social welfare efforts, a first step is to sketch how we think about them now. Perhaps, more accurately, we should sketch the *assumptions* about the vice/mental disorder relationship (VMDR) now. Once we understand our implicit, taken-for-granted ways of thinking, then we may conceive new ways to understand the relationships between vice and mental illness.

Only in the past twenty years have philosophers of psychiatry begun to recognize, analyze, and reflect upon the significance of the built-in values that are assumed in categories and criteria of mental disorders. The idea of value-ladenness of mental disorders, and in particular the significance of particular *kinds* of values, is still a new idea. No wonder then that the VMDR is taken for granted in mainstream psychiatry. The value of the philosophy of psychiatry to social problems is its ability to expose and illuminate the taken-for-granted assumptions which underlie social policy. The assumptions then can be examined "under the clear light of day" and evaluated for social reform or action.

Four conceptual models of the VMDR, with their accompanying assumptions, shape our everyday thinking and action. These four accounts are not comprehensive or encompassing, and variations on these models are common. Rather, these models address four practical tropes which are intended to serve as heuristic tools in thinking about the VMDR. They can be tested against our everyday experience in working with the mentally ill and with people who do wrong things. The accounts represent social tropes that manifest in our thinking about the relationship between vice and mental illness, and carry a range of metaphysical assumptions about the nature of reality and being human. They are relatively agnostic about how to engage practically with vice and mental illness; rather, as metaphysical assumptions, they precondition our thinking and thus constrain our approaches to the practical social challenges posed by vice and mental illness.

The four conceptual models are (1) the *coincidental* account, (2) the *moralization* account, (3) the *medicalization* account, and (4) the *mixed* account. As presupposed tropes, they do not necessarily represent any particular individual's or school's thought; however, they do depict a range of heuristic assumptions about the VMDR. Also, as heuristics, in the consideration of individual cases or contexts, one or more of these accounts may be operative—so in practice these conceptual models may overlap in their applications and relevance, as illustrated in the following.

4.8.1 **The coincidental account**

This approach makes the assumption that, most of the time, wrongful, immoral, and criminal conduct is independent of mental disorders. That is, vicious behaviors are often, perhaps usually, causally marginal or independent of any mental disorder the person might have. For example, a person with hypertension may rob banks, or be a law-abiding bank teller. Hypertension is causally irrelevant to moral conduct or lack thereof. Similarly, the bank robber may have panic disorder, as may the bank teller, but having a panic disorder is irrelevant to lawbreaking or law-abiding behavior. Being an outlaw and having panic disorder are *coincidental*.

While these kinds of coincidental relationships may be common across the universe of immoral actions or criminal offenses and people with mental illnesses, there are, of course, exceptions to the coincidental correspondence of immoral conduct and psychopathology. Consider the fictional mobster Tony Soprano. His panic attacks may be causally related to his criminal conduct, but are more likely a *consequence* of his criminal conduct rather than a cause of it. Under DSM diagnostic guidelines, Soprano's lawbreaking is irrelevant to the diagnosis and clinical features of the condition. So, in this sense, as a defining diagnostic feature of panic disorder in the DSMs, Soprano's criminality is irrelevant and coincidental, in the same way as his being Italian or overweight are coincidental to the diagnostic core concept of panic disorder.

Antisocial or immoral conduct can be coincidental with other disorders as well. Consider the delirium syndrome, which is commonly associated with combative behavior; but such behavior is not even mentioned in the diagnostic criteria for DSM-5 delirium (APA, 2013). Similar claims could be made for schizophrenia, bipolar disorder, major depressive disorder, and others. In summary, people who act immorally or criminally get sick too, and the correspondence between their illness and their misconduct may be, and often is, a coincidence.

4.8.2 **The moralization account**

This account holds that social deviance that infringes upon others (e.g., crime or moral misconduct like lying, marital infidelity, racism) should be defined and addressed within the nonmedical domains of social welfare (e.g., educational, religious, criminal justice systems and institutions). Under the moralization account, these "other-infringing" behaviors have no role in definitions of disease and mental disorders. An advocate for a pure "moralization" account views illness behavior and moral transgressions of various kinds as independent, even ontologically distinct, categories of experience and personal conduct. Such an advocate would consider antisocial thoughts and behaviors as unfortunate, but non-essential, clinical features of a core disorder characterized by medical (dis)values of disability, dysfunction, injury, or distress. A moralization advocate would want to expunge vice-laden criteria and categories from the DSMs as an inappropriate confounding of illness or disease with other-infringing social deviance (i.e., crime and immorality).

This account approximates that of Szasz (1961), though some aspects of his view of the VMDR would be distinctive and more radical. Szasz would argue that the whole DSM confounds disease with *mores* of personal conduct; mental disorders are only metaphorical diseases, and therefore focus on human "problems in living" that span those addressed by the educational, religious, and criminal justice systems. To the degree that the human problems described in the DSM could be aided by counselors with or without medical training, so be it, as long as the clients consent and freely participate. But it would again be an error, in Szasz's view, to call such counseling on problems in living "psychotherapy," because therapy is something that physicians and other healers offer and deliver to people with diseases proper (Szasz, 1978). For Szasz, offering therapy for criminality or depression makes as much sense as offering therapy for unemployment, being lonely, or being poor. He would reject both vice-laden and non-vice-laden mental disorders, because all mental disorders are only metaphors for diseases. But what Szasz shares with the moralization account is a Western, post-Enlightenment, metaphysical view that human nature has distinct domains of health, on the one hand, and the moral domain of right and wrong, on the other (Porter, 2004). Social institutions should respect these domains and not corrupt them by treating them as similar, interchangeable, or continuous.

4.8.3 **The medicalization account**

The medicalization account is a counterpoint to the moralization account. It holds that social deviance of an immoral or criminal kind does not substantively differ from social deviance associated with the signs and symptoms of disease, mental disorders, or psychopathology. Both of these kinds of undesired human experiences and behaviors are subject to biomedical or scientific understanding, explanation, and, aspirationally, control (Conrad, 2007; Sadler et al., 2009). The medicalization advocate rejects the idea that illness and wrongful thought and conduct are somehow metaphysically distinct; rather, both are simply varieties of human nature, experiences, and behaviors which can be elucidated causally and potentially predicted as well as manipulated by science and technology.

Perhaps the closest actual example of the medicalization account is contained within self-described neurocriminologist Adrian Raine's work. In a series of books and extensive research articles (Glenn and Raine, 2014; Raine, 1993, 2002, 2014), Raine's research program has built a case that criminal conduct has a relevant biology and that criminal behavior represents a multilevel and causally determined event, as does any other human biosocial behavior. While his primary scientific focus is on neuroscientific or biological explanations of criminal deviance, in terms of policy and intervention he embraces psychosocial concepts and approaches. From his own website: "We take a biopsychosocial perspective to our investigation of antisocial behavior in which our end-goal is to integrate social, psychological, and environmental processes with neurobiological approaches to better understand antisocial behavior" (Raine, 2018).

A second example of a medicalization account is transhumanism. Recently, scholars of transhumanism (i.e., an ideology of human enhancement through technology) and so-called "virtue engineering" or "moral enhancement" have advocated an implementation of applied neuroscience and genetics which would address the neurogenetic causes of antisocial or immoral conduct and develop interventions which would permit the engineering of people to be more virtuous, or at least, less immoral or criminal (Jotterand, 2011; Persson and Savulescu, 2008, 2012; Savulescu and Kahane, 2009). This thread of scholarship has not focused primarily on the scientific mechanisms or techniques of virtue engineering or moral enhancement, but rather on the ethics and social desirability of such developments and the manipulations of such mechanisms, when and if they are developed.

For clarity, an advocate of the medicalization account does not necessarily require explicitly *medical* interventions, with their associated medical morality, to be applied to criminal offenders or even to ordinary immoral conduct like lying, conniving, cheating, etc. Rather, the medicalization advocate embraces the idea that wrongful and criminal conduct can be understood, explained, and manipulated as classical disease states are understood, explained, and manipulated (i.e., by scientific research). In this sense, the medicalization account, as sketched here, reflects an endeavor to develop biopsychosocial scientific explanations of various kinds of misconduct, being agnostic about the appropriate social agents or institutions which might manipulate or intervene in such misconduct. This interventive neutrality then permits a variety of interventive responses to the scientific explanations of vice (technically defined here as varieties of immoral and criminal misconduct). Medicalization advocates come in different "brands"—so to speak—as we will see in the following.

4.8.4 **The mixed account**

The mixed account, with little surprise here, mixes elements of the aforementioned three accounts. I claim that the mixed account is the dominant way of thinking in Western mental health care and theorizing. One need not look too far in mental health theory and social practice to find strong evidence of the mixed account of the VMDR. There are many examples.

Perhaps a first step is to understand the historical origins of the mixed account, to serve as both an example and a context-setting. The history of modern psychiatry is laden with examples of confounds between the seemingly strict distinction between the medical and the moral. In the post-Enlightenment era, the psychological realm of the moral was delegated to the emerging Western common and criminal law, the principles and early practices of which emerged from Holy Roman Empire morality and prescriptive doctrine (Sadler, 2013; Porter, 2004; Makari, 2016). The then-emerging natural sciences, medicine, and later, psychiatry, developed alliances with post-Enlightenment values of rationality, skepticism, empiricism, and investments in the methods of knowledge emerging from modern science. This partial alliance with modern science and scientific causality was tempered with older loyalties to Abrahamic religious morality. The Abrahamic metaphysics articulated in the Middle Ages later played into psychiatry through loyalty to metaphysical concepts like individual responsibility (from the Church's requirements for salvation), deserts (one gets what one deserves), and free will, undergirding the idea of individual, personal responsibility for actions. Perhaps most importantly, in the post-Enlightenment era the psychological domain of morality was retained by religion and assimilated by the emerging common and criminal law, while the other psychological domains or "faculties" were embraced by medicine, with cognition, affection (emotion), and conation (motivation) (Radden, 1994; Porter, 2004) being fundamental to medical psychiatry.

At first, psychiatry was dominated by non-moral disorders; psychopathology was a manifestation of alterations in cognition, affection, and conation, and was characterized by classical categories like mania, delirium, melancholia, dementia, etc., which still prevail today through new iterations in the DSMs. Morality was independent. The realm of the sinful and immoral, along with the emerging concepts of crime and criminality (e.g., "other-infringing" social deviance), was left to the Church, law, and education (Kelly, 1999; Plucknett, 2010). But psychiatry had tremendous difficulty in sealing off the moral from the rest of psychology and its derivative, psychopathology, because the stubborn appearance of social deviance did not quite fit into a strict medical-moral distinction. These included eighteenth- and nineteenth-century categories like homicidal insanity, monomanias like kleptomania, erotomania, and pyromania, sexual deviations, and the emerging contemporary concept of psychopathy, which became largely defined in terms of remorseless antisocial conduct (Goldstein, 2001; Irvine, 2005; Cleckley, 1941). Not until the late twentieth century did wide interest in understanding normal and pathological moral capabilities develop, leading to modern philosophy and scientific psychology and neuroscience developing an interest in "moral" psychology (Sinnott-Armstrong, 2008a,b,c; Patrick, 2006).

But problems with psychological morality were always there, whether philosophy, medicine, or science cared or not. The metaphysical split between Church and law, on the one hand, and science, medicine, and psychiatry, on the other, set the metaphysical stage for the difficulties which I have described as vice-laden mental disorders. Nineteenth-century vice-laden mental disorders like homicidal insanity, kleptomania, and pyromania were described by Jean-Étienne Esquirol and like-minded colleagues because they believed that psychopathology could invade the moral domain and that "forensic psychiatrists" were necessary to demonstrate to juries that an otherwise coherent murderer, firesetter, or thief could be mad (Goldstein, 2001; Sadler, 2015). Contemporaneously, Christian psychiatrists in the U.S. (from the colonial period forward) resisted the concept of sickness in the mind, because the soul (or mind) was immortal and eternal, and therefore could not be diseased. "Mental" illness was rather a corruption of the body and brain (Porter, 2002, 2004).

This historical and metaphysical tension between morality as distinct from psychology, freely chosen, and personally responsible, and morality as complex a multicausal entity as any other, is played out today in myriad ways. One popular domain in the philosophy of psychiatry is the debate about personality disorders as moral versus bioscientific or biomedical concepts (Charland 2006, 2010; Zachar and Potter, 2010a,b). Another is the role, in addiction, of blame, or personal responsibility, versus the view that addiction is a biopsychosocially determined condition devoid of moral content (Pickard, 2011; Fingarette, 1988). Another example of the vice versus mental illness confound is the insanity defense.

The insanity defense has always been controversial (Robinson, 1996), since it reflects the vivid contradictions between implicit versions of the medicalization account (e.g., the defendant should be excused because his behavior was sick or complex—causally determined) and the moralization account (e.g., the defendant should be convicted and punished because he is individually responsible for the criminal offense). As Stephen Morse points out, even the disciplines of psychiatry and clinical psychology move fluidly between these two metaphysical standpoints, to their chagrin and confusion: "When one asks about human action, 'Why did she do that?' two distinct types of answers may therefore be given. The reason-giving explanation accounts for human behavior as a product of intentions that arise from the desires and beliefs of the agent. The second type of explanation treats human behavior as simply one more bit of the phenomena of the universe, subject to the same natural, physical laws that explain all phenomena" (Morse, 1998, p. 338).

Translating this insight into my own terms, mental health clinicians offer understandings of vicious conduct in terms of Abrahamic medieval religious metaphysics (i.e., a "moralization account" utilizing the assumptions of free will, personal responsibility, and deserts for wrong actions) as well as in terms of scientific complex multicausality (i.e., a "medicalization account," where human actions are assumed to be net products of causal vectors and constraints). No one should be surprised that the insanity defense is controversial; it rubs our noses in an unresolved, high-stakes conflict in Western culture.

Paradoxically, Western culture is simultaneously comfortable and conflicted with the medicalization and moralization accounts. A telling example is the post-DSM-III category of pedophilia, where an individual has the desire or compulsion to molest children sexually. The simultaneous comfort and conflict is publicly exemplified by the APA: "An adult who engages in sexual activity with a child is performing a criminal and immoral act and this is never considered normal or socially acceptable behavior. Darrel A. Regier, M.D., M.P.H., Director, American Psychiatric Association's Division of Research states, 'there are no plans or processes set up that would lead to the removal of the Paraphilias from their consideration as legitimate mental disorders'" (APA, 2003).

An implication here is that pedophilia is both a legitimate crime and a legitimate mental disorder, and psychiatrists share police and healer functions. I will not flesh out the context which provoked Regier's response, other than there was public and professional concern about an alleged consideration of removing pedophilia from the DSM as a mental disorder—as implied by his statement. Pedophilia, in this context, is both medicalized and moralized: a truly "mixed" account of the VMDR.

My final example of the predominance of the mixed account is mental health literacy research (Jorm, 2012; Angermeier and Dietrich, 2006; Gulliver et al., 2010; Pescosolido, 2013) which focuses on, among other things, public attitudes to, as well as understandings of, mental illness. Among the most robust findings of this international research on public attitudes and beliefs is that, depending upon the study, large minorities, or the majority, of the public continue to believe that mental illness is the person's fault, as well as an illness (Phelan et al., 2000, Pescosolido, 2013); that people delay or do not seek treatment because of shame, distrust of mental health professionals, or fear of being "locked up" (Gulliver et al., 2010; Wang et al., 2007); and that mentally ill people are much more dangerous than they in fact are (Phelan et al., 2000; Pescosolido, 2013). In stark contrast, people with broken legs, myocardial infarctions, or hypertension are not feared by the public as dangerous, nor viewed as immoral simply because of their illnesses!

4.9 Social application of the accounts

Here, I consider a few of the social implications and possibilities for "reform" in view of these heuristic conceptual models.

The mixed account predominates in psychiatry as well as the public sphere. The mixed account predominates, in part, because of the tensions between the two post-Enlightenment positions assumed by medicine and psychiatry, on one side, and law and religion, on the other. The widely maintained assumptions around free will, individual responsibility, and deserts persist in contemporary criminal law and contemporary Abrahamic religious traditions. On the other hand, complex multicausal science harbors its own metaphysical assumptions about a deterministic, structural, and comprehensible universe, where, incidentally, concepts like free will and personal responsibility are problematic at best, and absurdities at worst (Kane, 2011). Psychiatry spans both worlds, just as Morse (1998) describes. A continuation of the mixed account is likely, and it will perpetuate social problems. Indeed, a continuation of the mixed account may lead to its own expansion, as complex multicausal science explains more and more moral phenomena, and as more and more wrongful conduct is "medicalized" as illness.

However, under the various accounts here described, we could imagine social agents or institutions which could implement a range of interventions for misconduct (broadly conceived). Advocates of an account could differentiate into various social roles, framing various social actions, and reflecting various sets of overlapping social values and sociopolitical causal vectors. We can consider briefly a few applications, and very briefly some social implications, starting from the standpoint of the medicalization account.

4.9.1 Psychiatric moral expansionism

This variety of medicalization expands the domain of psychiatry to incorporate progressively more "disorders" of, or involving, moral conduct, especially as the interventions ("treatments") are developed under biopsychosocial mechanisms. We could call this practice *psychiatric moral expansionism* (PME). Under PME, the current list of mental disorders with vice-laden concepts or criteria would expand, correspondent to the development of mechanisms of vice-laden behavior syndromes. Thus PME would shift the equilibrium between the models in favor of medicalization, but with persisting elements of the mixed account. Instead of being rejected as inappropriate to medical morality, vices (i.e., particular criminal behaviors and immoralities) would progressively be understood as other kinds of disease, and the sciences of mental health could tend to engulf the social problems of antisocial behavior and crime. We can see the recent interest in the neuroscience and genetics of psychopathy (Sinnott-Armstrong, 2008b) as a tangible expression of a PME trend. Raine's aforementioned research program, if implemented into mainstream clinical practice, would be a second example of PME.

PME poses puzzling implications, several of which have already been mentioned in consideration of today's VMDR confounds of vice and illness. One implication could be the expanse, and expense, of broader technoscientific solutions to crime and misconduct, which has up to the present been the domain of social sciences like criminology and political science. We can speculate how the public would respond to the further medicalization of crime or the political liberalization of crime intervention, away from punishment and toward the embracing of new technologies of criminal rehabilitation, whether medical or nonmedical.

4.9.2 Psychiatric moral exclusionism

In contrast to the medicalization trope of psychiatric moral expansionism, we could consider *psychiatric moral exclusionism* (PMEx). Practices emerging from this standpoint, which shifts the social equilibrium away from the mixed model toward the moralization model, would intend to draw strict boundaries between wrongful thought or conduct and disease or illness. One PMEx possibility would be of Szasz "winning" the social argument and mental illnesses being dispensed with altogether, and those with bona fide biomedical disease credentials being absorbed into neurology or other medical specialties—the "death" of psychiatry as we know it, and the rise of a neurobiology-dominant discipline of "clinical neuroscience" (Reynolds et al., 2009). Those conditions without such bona fide credentials would be relegated to other professional and nonprofessional fields like social work, pastoral care, counseling (not clinical), psychology, and various kinds of alternative help.

More likely, in my view (but still unlikely), would be a conscientious effort by organized psychiatry to address vice-laden disorders, and either give them bona fide disease status or drop them from classifications of psychopathology. This might well be motivated by conscientious psychiatrists who are truly discomforted by the erosion of medical morality in policing misconduct, and who believe that vice concepts do not belong in medical categories or practices.

4.9.3 Interventional criminology

A third possibility, complementary to the prior possibility of eliminating vice concepts from psychiatry, might be the development of professional practitioners who are experts in interventions and the rehabilitation of wrongdoers: imagine a profession of "interventional criminology." Interventional criminologists would develop, test, and refine biopsychosocial programs to help reform criminal and moral offenders.

Much more could be speculated upon if the problem of vice-laden mental disorders were to be given serious social attention. An obvious set of normative questions arise about what model or approaches to the VMDR *should* be applied, and why. However, these questions require, at the minimum, an article of their own.

References

American Psychiatric Association (APA). 1968. *Diagnostic and Statistical Manual of Mental Disorders [DSM-II]*, 2nd edn. Washington, D.C.: American Psychiatric Association.

American Psychiatric Association (APA). 1980. *Diagnostic and Statistical Manual of Mental Disorders [DSM-III]*, 3rd edn. Washington, D.C.: American Psychiatric Association.

American Psychiatric Association (APA). 1994. *Diagnostic and Statistical Manual of Mental Disorders [DSM-IV]*, 4th edn. Washington, D.C.: American Psychiatric Association.

American Psychiatric Association (APA). 2000. *Diagnostic and Statistical Manual of Mental Disorders [DSM-IV]*, revised 4th edn. Washington, D.C.: American Psychiatric Association.

American Psychiatric Association (APA). 2003. *American Psychiatric Association Statement: Diagnostic Criteria for Pedophilia*. (June 17). Accessed April 12, 2018. <web.archive.org/web/20070629090023/http://www.psych.org/news_room/press_releases/diagnosticcriteriapedophilia.pdf>.

American Psychiatric Association (APA). 2013. *Diagnostic and Statistical Manual of Mental Disorders [DSM-5]*, 5th edn. Arlington, Virginia: American Psychiatric Association.

Angermeyer, Matthias C., and Sandra Dietrich. 2006. "Public Beliefs About and Attitudes Toward People with Mental Illness: A Review of Population Studies." *Acta Psychiatrica Scandinavica* **113** (3): 163–79.

Blekesaune, Morten, and Jill Quadagno. 2003. "Public Attitudes Toward Welfare State Policies: A Comparative Analysis of 24 Nations." *European Sociological Review* **19** (5) (December): 415–27.

Charland, Louis C. 2006. "The Moral Nature of the Cluster B Personality Disorders." *Journal of Personality Disorders* **20** (2): 119–28.

Charland, Louis C. 2010. "Medical or Moral Kinds? Moving Beyond a False Dichotomy." *Philosophy, Psychiatry, and Psychology* **17** (2) (June): 119–25.

Cleckley, Hervey Milton. 1941. *The Mask of Sanity: An Attempt to Reinterpret the So-Called Psychopathic Personality*. St. Louis: Mosby.

Conrad, Peter. 2007. *The Medicalization of Society: On the Transformation of Human Conditions into Treatable Disorders*. Baltimore: Johns Hopkins University Press.

Corrigan, Patrick W., and Amy C. Watson. 2004. "At Issue: Stop the Stigma: Call Mental Illness a Brain Disease." *Schizophrenia Bulletin* **30** (3): 477–9.

Fabrega, Horacio. 1990. "Psychiatric Stigma in the Classical and Medieval Period: A Review of the Literature." *Comprehensive Psychiatry* **31** (4) (July–August): 289–306.

Fabrega, Horacio. 1991. "The Culture and History of Psychiatric Stigma in Early Modern and Modern Western Societies: A Review of Recent Literature." *Comprehensive Psychiatry* **32** (2) (March–April): 97–119.

Fingarette, Herbert. 1988. *Heavy Drinking: The Myth of Alcoholism as a Disease*. Berkeley: University of California Press.

Frank, Richard G., and Sherry A. Glied. 2006. *Better but Not Well: Mental Health Policy in the United States Since 1950*. Baltimore: Johns Hopkins University Press.

Fulford, K.W.M. 1989. *Moral Theory and Medical Practice*. Cambridge: Cambridge University Press.

Glenn, Andrea L., and Adrian Raine. 2014. "Neurocriminology: Implications for the Punishment, Prediction, and Prevention of Criminal Behaviour." *Nature Reviews Neuroscience* **15** (1): 54–63.

Goldstein, Jan E. 2001. *Console and Classify: The French Psychiatric Profession in the Nineteenth Century*, revised edn. Chicago: University of Chicago Press.

Gulliver, Amelia, Kathleen M. Griffiths, and Helen Christensen. 2010. "Perceived Barriers and Facilitators to Mental Health Help-Seeking in Young People: A Systematic Review." *BMC Psychiatry* **10**: 113. Accessed April 17, 2018. <bmcpsychiatry.biomedcentral.com/articles/10.1186/1471-244X-10-113>

Hartwell, Stephanie. 2004. "Triple Stigma: Persons with Mental Illness and Substance Abuse Problems in the Criminal Justice System." *Criminal Justice Policy Review* **15** (1): 84–99.

Irvine, Janice M. 2005. *Disorders of Desire: Sexuality and Gender in Modern American Sexology*, revised edn. Philadelphia: Temple University Press.

Jorm, Anthony F. 2012. "Mental Health Literacy: Empowering the Community to Take Action for Better Mental Health." *American Psychologist* **67** (3): 231–43.

Jotterand, Fabrice. 2011. "'Virtue Engineering' and Moral Agency: Will Post-Humans Still Need the Virtues?" *AJOB Neuroscience* **2** (4) (October): 3–9.

Kane, Robert (ed.). 2011. *The Oxford Handbook of Free Will*, 2nd edn. Oxford: Oxford University Press.

Kelly, John Maurice. 1999. *A Short History of Western Legal Theory*. Oxford: Oxford University Press.

Makari, George. 2016. *Soul Machine: The Invention of the Modern Mind*. New York: W.W. Norton.

Malla, Ashok, Ridha Joober, and Amparo Garcia. 2015. "'Mental Illness is Like any Other Medical Illness': A Critical Examination of the Statement and its Impact on Patient Care and Society." *Journal of Psychiatry and Neuroscience* **40** (3) (May): 147–50.

Morrissey, Joseph P., and **Howard H. Goldman**. 1984. "Cycles of Reform in the Care of the Chronically Mentally Ill." *Psychiatric Services* **35** (8) (August): 785–93.

Morse, Stephen J. 1998. "Excusing and the New Excuse Defenses: A Legal and Conceptual Review." *Crime and Justice* **23**: 329–406.

NationMaster. 2018. "Economy: Social Welfare Spending: % of GDP: Excluding Education: Countries Compared." Accessed April 19, 2018. <www.nationmaster. com/country-info/stats/Economy/Social-welfare-spending/%3E-%25-of-GDP/ Excluding-education>

Patrick, Christopher J. (ed.). 2006. Handbook of Psychopathy. New York: Guilford.

Pellegrino, Edmund D. 1999. "The Goals and Ends of Medicine: How are They to be Defined?" In *The Goals of Medicine: The Forgotten Issues in Health Care Reform*, edited by Mark J. Hanson and Daniel Callahan, pp. 55–68. Washington, D.C.: Georgetown University Press.

Persson, Ingmar, and Julian Savulescu. 2008. "The Perils of Cognitive Enhancement and the Urgent Imperative to Enhance the Moral Character of Humanity." *Journal of Applied Philosophy* **25** (3): 162–77.

Persson, Ingmar, and Julian Savulescu. 2012. *Unfit for the Future: The Need for Moral Enhancement*. Oxford: Oxford University Press.

Pescosolido, Bernice A. 2013. "The Public Stigma of Mental Illness: What Do We Think; What Do We Know; What Can We Prove?" *Journal of Health and Social Behavior* **54** (1): 1–21.

Phelan, Jo C., Bruce G. Link, et al. 2000. "Public Conceptions of Mental Illness in 1950 and 1996: What Is Mental Illness and Is It to Be Feared?" *Journal of Health and Social Behavior* **41** (2): 188–207.

Pickard, Hanna. 2011. "Responsibility Without Blame: Empathy and the Effective Treatment of Personality Disorder." *Philosophy, Psychiatry, and Psychology* **18** (3): 209–24.

Plucknett, Theodore F.T. 2010. *A Concise History of the Common Law*, 5th edn. Indianapolis: Liberty Fund.

Porter, Roy. 2002. *Madness: A Brief History*. Oxford: Oxford University Press.

Porter, Roy. 2004. *Flesh in the Age of Reason*. New York: W.W. Norton.

Radden, Jennifer H. 1994. "Recent Criticism of Psychiatric Nosology: A Review." *Philosophy, Psychiatry, and Psychology* **1** (3) (September): 193–200.

Raine, Adrian. 1993. *The Psychopathology of Crime: Criminal Behavior as a Clinical Disorder*. New York: Elsevier.

Raine, Adrian. 2002. "Biosocial Studies of Antisocial and Violent Behavior in Children and Adults: A Review." *Journal of Abnormal Child Psychology* **30** (4) (August): 311–26.

Raine, Adrian. 2014. *The Anatomy of Violence: The Biological Roots of Crime*. New York: Vintage.

Raine, Adrian. 2018. "Adrian Raine: Richard Perry University Professor, Departments of Criminology, Psychiatry, and Psychology." Accessed April 19, 2018. <crim.sas.upenn.edu/ people/adrian-raine>

Reynolds III, Charles F., David A. Lewis, Thomas Detre, et al. J. 2009. "The Future of Psychiatry as Clinical Neuroscience." *Academic Medicine* **84** (4) (April): 446–50.

Robinson, Daniel N. 1996. *Wild Beasts and Idle Humours: The Insanity Defense from Antiquity to the Present*. Cambridge, Mass.: Harvard University Press.

Rothman, David J. 2017. *Conscience and Convenience: The Asylum and Its Alternatives in Progressive America*, revised edn. New York: Routledge.

Rubinow, David R. 2014. "Out of Sight, Out of Mind: Mental Illness Behind Bars." *American Journal of Psychiatry* **171** (10) (October): 1021–44.

Sadler, John Z. 1997. "Recognizing Values: A Descriptive-Causal Method for Medical/Scientific Discourses." *Journal of Medicine and Philosophy* **22** (6) (December): 541–65.

Sadler, John Z. (ed.). 2002. *Descriptions and Prescriptions: Values, Mental Disorders, and the DSMs*. Baltimore: Johns Hopkins University Press.

Sadler, John Z. 2005. *Values and Psychiatric Diagnosis*. Oxford: Oxford University Press.

Sadler, John Z. 2008. "Vice and the Diagnostic Classification of Mental Disorders: A Philosophical Case Conference." *Philosophy, Psychiatry, and Psychology* **15** (1): 1–17.

Sadler, John Z. 2013. "Vice and Mental Disorders." In *Oxford Handbook of the Philosophy of Psychiatry*, edited by K.W.M. Fulford et al., pp. 450–79. Oxford: Oxford University Press.

Sadler, John Z. 2014. "Conduct Disorder as a Vice-Laden Diagnostic Concept." In *Diagnostic Dilemmas in Child and Adolescent Psychiatry: Philosophical Perspectives*, edited by Christian Perring and Lloyd A. Wells, pp. 166–81. Oxford: Oxford University Press.

Sadler, John Z. 2015. "The Crippling Legacy of Monomanias in DSM-5." In *The DSM-5 in Perspective: Philosophical Reflections on the Psychiatric Babel*, edited by Steeves Demazeux and Patrick Singy, pp. 141–55. Dordrecht: Springer.

Sadler, John Z., Fabrice Jotterand, et al. 2009. "Can Medicalization Be Good? Situating Medicalization Within Bioethics." *Theoretical Medicine and Bioethics* **30** (6): 411–25.

Saraceno, Benedetto, and Shekhar Saxena. 2002. "Mental Health Resources in the World: Results from Project Atlas of the WHO." *World Psychiatry* **1** (1): 40–4.

Savulescu, Julian, and Guy Kahane. 2009. "The Moral Obligation to Create Children with the Best Chance of the Best Life." *Bioethics* **23** (5): 274–90.

Sinnott-Armstrong, Walter (ed.). 2008a. *Moral Psychology: Vol. 1, The Evolution of Morality: Adaptations and Innateness*. Cambridge, Mass.: MIT Press.

Sinnott-Armstrong, Walter (ed.). 2008b. *Moral Psychology: Vol. 2, The Cognitive Science of Morality: Intuition and Diversity*. Cambridge, Mass.: MIT Press.

Sinnott-Armstrong, Walter (ed.). 2008c. *Moral Psychology: Vol. 3, The Neuroscience of Morality: Emotion, Brain Disorders, and Development*. Cambridge, Mass.: MIT Press.

Smith, Paula, Paul Gendreau, and Kristin Swartz. 2009. "Validating the Principles of Effective Intervention: A Systematic Review of the Contributions of Meta-Analysis in the Field of Corrections." *Victims and Offenders* **4** (2): 148–69.

Stanford Law School Three Strikes Project. 2014. "When Did Prisons Become Acceptable Mental Healthcare Facilities?" Accessed April 15, 2018. <law.stanford.edu/wp-content/uploads/sites/default/files/child-page/632655/doc/slspublic/Report_v12.pdf>

Szasz, Thomas S. 1961. *The Myth of Mental Illness. Foundations of a Theory of Personal Conduct*. New York: Hoeber-Harper.

Szasz, Thomas S. 1978. *The Myth of Psychotherapy: Mental Healing as Religion, Rhetoric, and Repression*. Garden City, New York: Doubleday Anchor.

Torrey, E. Fuller, D.J. Jaffe, Jeffrey L. Geller, and Richard Lamb. 2015. Fraud, Waste and Excess Profits: The Fate of Money Intended to Treat People with Serious Mental Illness. Accessed April 12, 2018. <mentalillnesspolicy.org/wp-content/uploads/wastereport.pdf>

U.S. Department of Health and Human Services (DHHS), Agency for Healthcare Research and Quality (AHRQ). 2012. *National Healthcare Disparities Report*. Accessed April 11, 2018. <archive.ahrq.gov/research/findings/nhqrdr/nhdr12/index.html>

Wang, Philip S., et al. 2007. "Delay and Failure in Treatment Seeking After First Onset of Mental Disorders in the World Health Organization's World Mental Health Survey Initiative." *World Psychiatry* **6** (3) (October): 177–85.

Zachar, Peter, and **Nancy Nyquist Potter**. 2010a. "Personality Disorders: Moral or Medical Kinds—or Both?" *Philosophy, Psychiatry, and Psychology* **17** (2) (June): 101–7.

Zachar, Peter, and **Nancy Nyquist Potter**. 2010b. "Valid Moral Appraisals and Valid Personality Disorders." *Philosophy, Psychiatry, and Psychology* **17** (2) (June): 131–42.

Part II

The concept of mental illness

Chapter 5

Szasz, suicide, and medical ethics

George J. Annas

5.1 Introduction

Ever since the U.S.-sponsored trial of the Nazi doctors at Nuremberg, where psychiatrist Leo Alexander was the primary medical consultant to the prosecution, psychiatrists have played a prominent role in medical ethics. Perhaps the best-known ethicist-psychiatrist is Jay Katz, a scholar of the Holocaust and an expert on informed consent and human experimentation. Others include Willard Gaylin, co-founder of the Hastings Center (the first bioethics think tank) in 1969; Michael Grodin, a bioethicist, Holocaust scholar, and teacher for more than four decades; Paul S. Appelbaum, a leading scholar on competence; and Robert Jay Lifton, the leading scholar on atrocities and their prevention. Szasz did not think of himself as primarily a medical ethicist, but he fits comfortably among this group. This is because psychiatry and Szasz are at the center of bioethical debates on autonomy, coercion, normality, responsibility, and the role of the physician who works for the state. In this chapter, I focus on one particular bioethical controversy that has dominated discussion for almost fifty years: the "right to die," also known as the right to commit suicide with a physician's assistance, usually simply called either "physician-assisted suicide" or "PAS."

In one of his books on suicide, *Fatal Freedom*, Szasz observes: "Never before have people been so overwrought about suicide as we are" (Szasz, 2002, p. 113). He made this observation, and wrote this book, shortly after the U.S. Supreme Court issued its two unanimous rulings that there is no constitutional right to commit suicide or to have PAS. Just before those rulings, Oregon had become the first state to "legalize" PAS by providing physicians who followed certain rituals with legal immunity for supplying their terminally ill patients with lethal drug prescriptions. Szasz was, not suprisingly, adamantly against medicalizing suicide by designating physicians, especially psychiatrists, as gatekeepers to suicide: "It is an evasion fatal to freedom" (Szasz, 2002, p. xv). He was, he wrote, for "unassisted suicide." As he put it in 1978 (just after the Karen Ann Quinlan case): "I believe a person, every person, is a moral agent. That comes before everything else. Individual self-determination is, in my view, more important than health, than medical care, than psychiatric treatment" (Szasz, 2011, chapter 1, no. 3). He argued that people should be at liberty to kill themselves, but that this liberty did not imply a "right" to assistance or to the agreement of anyone else or of the state. Szasz also objected to medicalizing suicide, and thereafter legalizing it by granting physicians legal immunity for prescribing lethal drugs to their suicidal patients with the intent that they use these drugs to kill themselves. Szasz centrally argued that we cannot sensibly even discuss suicide if we cannot name it—and we cannot. We consistently use language to obfuscate rather than to clarify the actions we approve of. We want, for example, to call "self-killing" almost anything else, from "self-deliverance" to "self-determination" with the physician's blessing and "aid," "aid-in-dying," "death with dignity," and even simply "alleviating suffering."

In this chapter, I summarize current law, apply Szasz's arguments to the law, and finally suggest that Szasz is right to oppose increasing the power of physicians by granting them legal immunity for writing lethal drug prescriptions. More tangentially, I also suggest that we may need more discussion before eliminating current drug prescription requirements altogether.

5.2 **The "right" to suicide**

Two basic strategies have been employed by those who believe that physicians should be able to prescribe lethal drugs for their terminally ill or suicidal patients: pursuit of a new constitutional right to empower patients, and passage of new state laws to empower physicians. Bioethicists have been deeply involved in both. The first strategy, which was largely based on the model that abortion proponents used successfully in the late 1960s and early 1970s, suffered a lethal blow in 1997 when the Supreme Court ruled unanimously in two cases that there is no such constitutional right. The second strategy has been the primary one since then, and is based on the Oregon law first adopted by ballot initiative in 1994, and in California by legislation in 2015.

When the PAS cases came before the Supreme Court, observers were unsure as to how the Court would rule. In retrospect, the cases were easy for the Court, which, while split on some of the reasoning, decided unanimously in each case that there was no constitutional right to PAS by drug prescription. The arguments in the two cases before the Court both concerned the reach of the Fourteenth Amendment. In the first case, a group of physicians and patients argued that the due process clause of the Fourteenth Amendment required that the Court recognize this right and forbid Washington State from applying their criminal laws to PAS by drug prescription. In the second case, a group of physicians led by Timothy Quill argued that if New York patients had a right to refuse treatment and die, forbidding those who did not need treatment to continue to live from obtaining lethal drugs to end their lives was a violation of the equal protection clause of the Fourteenth Amendment (Annas, 1996). As the Supreme Court's two opinions illustrate, both of these arguments, each of which had been accepted by different U.S. Courts of Appeals, are extremely weak.

The substantive due process argument put forward in the case from Washington is that the liberty protected by the due process clause of the Fourteenth Amendment includes "a right to commit suicide which itself includes a right to assistance in doing so" (Washington v. Glucksberg, 1997, at 703). The Court has two established methods of defining a new constitutional right: Either the right must be "deeply rooted in this nation's history and tradition" (Washington v. Glucksberg, 1997, at 721) or it must be "fundamental to ordered liberty" (Duncan v. Louisiana, 1968, at 181). A quick review of U.S. history by the Court reveals no historic tradition of treating suicide as a fundamental right, rather it has always been treated as a "grievous, though nonfelonious, wrong" (Washington v. Glucksberg,

1997, at 714). The right to refuse treatment is deeply rooted in American history. As to ordered liberty, the Court found the relevant interest of individuals to be protected by the right to refuse treatment (and not in the suggested right to assistance with suicide). Given these conclusions, Washington merely had to demonstrate that it had a "rational basis" for prohibiting assisted suicide for the Court to uphold their law against it. The Court determined that Washington could demonstrate any number of legitimate state interests that provided a rational basis for their law, including preserving human life, preventing suicide, protecting the ethics of the medical profession, protecting vulnerable groups from abuses, and preventing a slippery slope leading to involuntary killing (Washington v. Glucksberg, 521 U.S. 702 [1997]). It should be underlined, however, that the Court was not objecting to individuals making up their own minds to refuse treatment, even if that refusal ended in death. The Court, for example, specifically approved of "terminal seda-tion," a procedure they described as ending tube feeding and putting the patient into a coma (to end suffering), even if this would lead to the patient's death. As a justification, the Court adopted the Catholic Church's "double effect" principle which permits doing a good act with the knowledge that a bad effect (e.g., death) may flow from it, as long as the main motivation is to alleviate suffering.

The equal protection case from New York was even easier for the justices. New York's argument was that removing a life-sustaining technology such as dialysis or a ventilator to produce death could not be legally distinguished from providing a terminally ill patient with a lethal drug, so that permitting the first while denying the second violated the equal protection of laws. The Court simply disagreed with framing the facts this way, finding that the two situations were different and that all patients were treated the same under existing law. In the Court's words: "Everyone, regardless of physical condition, is entitled, if competent, to refuse unwanted lifesaving medical treatment; no one is permitted to assist a suicide" (Vacco v. Quill, 1997, at 793). The Court went further, noting that the distinction between the two acts (withdrawing treatment and assisting in a suicide) is "a distinction widely recognized and endorsed in the medical profession and in our legal traditions" (Vacco v. Quill, 1997, at 800).

The Court did, nonetheless, underline that even though there is no constitutional right to physician assistance with suicide, if individual states want to authorize their licensed physicians to assist in the suicides of their competent patients by prescribing drug overdoses, the constitution does not prohibit states from so doing. Put another way, the powers to regulate the practice of medicine and to outlaw assisted suicide are state powers, not federal powers (Annas, 1997). States have the legal power to enact and enforce PAS legislation. The bioethics debate about what states and physicians *should* do continues. The major continuing controversy is about the proper role of the physician. Should physicians be held to act only in their patients' best interests with their patients' informed consent, or should physicians be able to call upon the power of the state to prescribe or withhold drugs from their patients as the physicians see fit?

5.3 **State legislation**

In 1991, voters in Washington defeated Initiative 119, which would have author-ized PAS and voluntary euthanasia, both of which were included under the term "physician aid-in-dying." The following year, California voters rejected a similar measure, Proposition 161, that defined physician "aid-in-dying" as "a medical procedure that will terminate the life of the qualified patient in a painless, humane and dignified manner whether administered by the physician at the patient's choice or direction or whether the physician provides means to the patient for self-administration" (California, 1992, § 2525.2 k). Both measures received about 46 percent of the vote.

Two years later, in 1994, Oregon voters, learning from this experience, narrowed and adopted their own "death with dignity" law. The law did not cover active physician killing (euthanasia), but applied only to PAS. Specifically, physicians were granted legal immunity from civil or criminal penalties for writing prescriptions for lethal drugs for any patient suffering from a terminal illness "who has voluntarily expressed his or her wish to die" and has made "a written request for medication for the purpose of ending his or her life in a humane and dignified manner" (Oregon, 1994, § 127.805 s.2.01). The request must be in writing, witnessed, and completed over no less than a fifteen-day period. No physician is required to write a prescription for lethal drugs, but those that do and follow the provisions of the new law are "immune" not only from civil and criminal liability, but also from any professional disciplinary action. The physician may also be present when the patient takes the drug to end his or her life (Annas, 1994).

The 2015 California law, which was adopted by the state legislature and signed by the governor, is essentially identical to the Oregon law, with only a few notable differences. The first is its title: the "End of Life Option Act." Second, the drugs prescribed to end a person's life are labeled "aid-in-dying drugs." An additional form (completed after the fifteen-day waiting period) called "the final attestation form" is to be filled out within forty-eight hours of self-administering the aid-in-dying drug. This form includes the line "I make this decision to ingest the aid-in-dying drug to end my life in a humane and dignified manner" (California, 2015, § 443.11). The form must be placed in the deceased's medical record. Presence at the suicide is also clarified. Individuals "may, without civil or criminal liability, assist the qualified individual by preparing the aid-in-dying drug so long as the person does not assist the qualified person in ingesting the aid-in-dying drug" (California, 2015, § 443.14.a).

The California law passed primarily because of a lobbying effort led by Brittany Maynard, a twenty-nine-year-old who was dying of brain cancer. She moved from California to Oregon, to end her life with drugs, because she believed that no physician would help her to obtain the lethal drugs she wanted in California. She made a powerful six-minute video for the advocacy group Compassion & Choices, urging the California legislature to adopt Oregon's law (Brittany Maynard Legislative Testimony, 2015). She presented a very compelling argument, and became nationally known as a spokesperson for PAS. She described her position in *People* magazine: "I don't want to die, but I am dying . . . My [cancer] is going to kill me and it's a terrible, terrible way to die. So to be able to die with my family with me, to have control of my own mind, which I would stand to lose—to go with dignity is less terrifying. When I look into both options I have to die, I feel this is far more humane" (Egan et al., 2014). Her husband, Dan Diaz, was with her at the end: "By late afternoon 'she just knew it was time,' Diaz says. 'She was tired of the pain, the discomfort, the suffering, the seizures.

Even that small one that morning was a reminder of how sick she really was.' Breaking open the capsules of secobarbital and mixing the drug with water, she drank it in their bedroom, talking and joking to keep everyone at ease. 'Within five minutes she was asleep,' Diaz says. 'And within 30 minutes, her breathing slowed to the point where she passed away. She was surrounded by the people she loved, and her passing was peaceful'" (Egan, 2015).

Brittany's story was very similar to that of Diane—another young, white, dying cancer patient who feared a painful and prolonged death (Quill, 1991). Diane's story initiated the PAS debate in the medical literature, and Quill was also the lead petitioner in the Supreme Court's suicide case from New York. As Steven Miles and Allison August note, attempting to rescue young, white women is a trope that runs through "right to die" cases, from Karen Quinlan, to Nancy Cruzan, and later, to Terri Schiavo (Miles and August, 1990). Who could object to trying to help any of these young women either by authorizing terminating treatment or by "legalizing" PAS? The short answer, I think, is that there are no good reasons to limit the right to refuse treatment of competent adults (exercised either directly or through their surrogates), but there are many good reasons to object to PAS (and, of course, suicide by proxy is simply not possible). Before I suggest my own reasons for opposing the Oregon/California PAS model, I will summarize Szasz's broader critique of these state laws.

5.4 **Szasz on physician-assisted suicide**

Szasz's central objection to providing immunity to physicians for lethal drug prescriptions is that legal immunity increases the power of physicians over patients, when what we should be doing is increasing the liberty of patients. As he put it simply: "Legalizing PAS gives more control to physicians, not to patients" (Szasz, 2002, p. 118). In Szasz's analysis, patient autonomy is synonymous with patient liberty; it is about what the individual can do by him or herself, without the assistance or concurrence of anyone else. Autonomy (liberty) is (or should be) a characteristic of the individual alone "without calling for specific performance by any other party" (Szasz, 2002, p. 113). The term "right," on the other hand, "is other-directed . . . lodging a 'rightful' claim against others or the State, for example, to payment for services rendered as contractually agreed upon" (Szasz, 2002, p. 113). The "right to die" in his view is an example: Patients are not free to commit suicide on their own. Physicians are the gatekeepers to assisted suicide, and a physician's permission is needed to get access to the lethal drugs. Suicide assistance by drug overdose becomes a part of the practice of medicine. This means that physicians determine which suicides are medically appropriate and which should be prevented, by institutionalization if necessary. The ability to call on the state to coerce the patient is one which Szasz has always argued is illegitimate, and PAS is just a special case of his broader critique. As he puts it, the focus of his critique of PAS is the state-supported "power of the psychiatrist, exemplified by the paradigmatic psychiatric procedures of civil commitment and the insanity defense-and-disposition" (Szasz, 2004, p. 295). As he would argue, people should be at liberty to kill themselves, but this liberty does not imply or necessitate the state conferring a "right" to suicide or a "right to die."

The power to prescribe lethal medication (or not) is closely related to the psychiatrist's power to commit a patient (e.g., for being suicidal and thus a danger to one's self). In Szasz's words: "I maintain that our longing for doctors to give us lethal drugs betokens our desire to evade responsibility for giving such drugs to ourselves, and that so long as we are more interested in investing doctors with the right to kill than in reclaiming our own right to drugs, our discourse about rights and drugs is destined to remain empty, meaningless chatter" (Szasz, 1996, p. 154). Szasz asserts that it is "a basic moral wrong for a physician, *qua physician*, to kill a patient or anyone else and call it 'euthanasia'" (Szasz, 1996, p. 154, original italics). He opposes the right to PAS because he supports the right to "physician-unassisted suicide" (Szasz, 2002, pp. 71, 76), regards advocates of PAS as anti-libertarian, and believes that both PAS and coerced suicide prevention epitomize the fruits of statist medicine.

So that people would be able to make their own choices, Szasz has proposed what he labels "pharmacological autonomy" (1996, p. 150): the freedom of individuals to make their own choices about which drugs to take—a freedom "similar to the freedom we enjoy vis-à-vis food or religion" (1996, p. 150). In his book on access to drugs, he returns to the subject of suicide: "Deprived of drugs useful for committing suicide, we nevertheless continue to cling to the hope of receiving the drugs we need to die a painless death when we are terminally ill. The result is that we now seriously entertain the preposterous idea of giving doctors and judges the right to kill us" (1996, pp. 150–51). "Preposterous" may seem a strong adjective in this context, but Szasz means it. He goes on to argue that the logic of PAS leads to the "appalling conclusion" (1996, p. 151) that it is better to have "euthanasia, mercifully administered by 'ethical' doctors" (1996, p. 151) under the authority of the state (a practice of totalitarian governments) than it is to have "a free market in drugs" (1996, p. 151). In so doing, Szasz argues (persuasively I think) that we "expect a grand alliance between medicine and the state to solve our existential tasks of living and dying for us" (1996, p. 151). Of course, even if one thinks that family members should not be prosecuted for aiding a competent family member's death, with the patient's insistence, this does not mean that physicians must or should be used by the state to assist in their patients' suicides.

Americans, on the other hand, at least in Oregon and California, have come to accept state-sanctioned PAS, but only, I think, by naming it something else. Suicide is widely seen as an avoidable human tragedy and suicide prevention as a major public health problem, with more than 800,000 suicides worldwide per year. Szasz has no problem with non-coercive suicide prevention programs or with psychiatrists who counsel their patients against committing suicide. Where he draws the line is at using the state's power to force treatment or to confine the person against their will to attempt to prevent suicide. More to the point in this context is that the PAS law drafters want to assure the public that no real suicide is going on—only merciful pain control at the end of life. That is why the phrase "physician-assisted suicide" does not appear in either of the PAS laws. Instead, Oregon adopts the phrase "death with dignity," and California, the rhetoric of choice, as in "end of life option." Dignity and choice are, of course, highly valued by society, and it is not surprising that these terms are preferred over the word "suicide." More surprising, perhaps, is that although both laws legally protect physicians who assist in suicide, they limit the method to drug overdoses and the population "qualified" for suicide to those who are terminally ill with less than six months to live (a qualification to be determined by the physician). Neither of these limits have any constitutional or ethical justification. Finally, it is worth noting that although the claim is patient rights, in fact the procedures required by the law make the process of obtaining and taking drugs much slower, more bureaucratic, and burdensome to the patient, as well as less private and less accountable.

Even more telling to me is that the Court, in ruling on the suicide cases, did not explicitly acknowledge that it has never been illegal to prescribe pain medication that competent, terminally ill patients *might* use to commit suicide, so long as the physician's intent in providing the drugs was to foster the patient's well-being by giving them more control over their lives and that the drugs themselves had an independent, legitimate medical use (Annas, 2006b). A legitimate medical use would include such things as pain control, sleeping assistance, or alleviating a wide variety of suffering. Szasz might disagree (I do not think so), but such a prescription can legitimately be seen as suicide prevention rather than assistance in suicide. This is, for example, how I would characterize Quill's prescription of pain medications (which could also be used to commit suicide) to his patient Diane. Diane was able to live longer (and commit suicide later) than she would have because she had the comfort of knowing that whenever her life became intolerable to her, she could end it by consuming an overdose of the pain medications. Of equal interest, neither of the Appellate Court decisions that were appealed to the Supreme Court could point to even one case of a physician ever being criminally prosecuted for the drug-prescribing conduct they approved of. Both courts would have been on much stronger legal and ethical grounds had they simply acknowledged that intent matters in the criminal law and that prescriptions written under the narrow circumstances contemplated in the Oregon and California laws are not assisted suicide by definition (Annas, 1994, p. 1243).

5.5 Is physician-assisted suicide like abortion?

It has been suggested that Szasz should have seen PAS as the mirror image of abortion: both capable of self-administration, but much safer and effective if done by a physician. I think that Szasz is right to dismiss this analogy, and this is why.

When my colleagues Leonard Glantz, Wendy Mariner, and I wrote a brief to the Supreme Court on behalf of bioethics professors regarding the two PAS cases, we made two major arguments. The first was that there is no constitutional right to either suicide or assisted suicide. Rather, the constitutional right at issue is the right to refuse treatment. The second argument was aimed at protecting the abortion right. Specifically, we argued that rejecting a constitutional right to physician assistance in suicide did *not* entail rejecting a constitutional right of pregnant women to terminate a pregnancy, because these two actions are fundamentally different. To summarize the abortion argument, we made four points: (1) the abortion right is based on the woman's interest in her own life, health, and future, none of which are at issue in PAS; (2) unlike PAS, the population the abortion right applies to is easily identified (i.e., every pregnant woman), and there are no vague qualifiers like "the terminally ill"; (3) unlike abortion, PAS is not a medical procedure (and there is no principled way to distinguish among methods of suicide), so to request assistance in suicide is not a personal *medical* decision; and (4) regulating PAS would require intrusions into the physician-patient relationship that have not been permitted in the abortion context (Brief, 1996).

It is probably unsurprising that I continue to believe that these arguments are correct, and remain content that the Court did not see its rejection of PAS as an opportunity to re-examine its abortion jurisprudence. Nonetheless, after reading Szasz again, I think the analogy can be made sharper by comparing PAS to birth control, specifically to contraception by drugs. In this case, we could argue that there is a parallel between "death control" and "birth control" insofar as prescription drugs are used to prevent conception at the beginning of life and to accomplish suicide at life's end. It can be argued that the only way women can gain control over their own lives is through access to safe and effective methods of contraception, just as it can be argued that at some point people may need drugs to kill themselves as their only method to control pain and suffering. But even this analogy is shaky at both ends. There is no "birth control"; what is being controlled is conception (hence "contraception"), but the term "conception control" is too clunky. Likewise, suicide will bring an end to pain, and so may be considered "pain control," but it is overly dramatic to equate suicide with "death control," something we have almost as little control over as we had over our own births. Seemingly, no matter how we try to face the facts that humans are born and die, we inevitably wind up oversimplifying the terms that we adopt at the beginning and end of life to make our actions seem more reasonable and ethical.

5.6 Is Szasz's position on physician-assisted suicide right?

Ethicists Margaret Battin and Ryan Spellecy, strong supporters of the Oregon and California laws, insist that Szasz either misunderstands or is purposely misleading in his position on PAS, and believe that he went wrong in rejecting the abortion analogy. They especially object to Szasz's claim that people can kill themselves without the assistance of a physician who is an expert in drug overdoses. They argue, for example, that even Socrates needed the assistance of his jailer to determine how much poison he should drink to assure death. They argue further that even under Szasz's legalized drug regime, it would still be necessary to seek advice about what drug to take, and in what dose, and that there are no other satisfactory sources of information other than physicians (Battin and Spellecy, 2004). The use of family and friends, they believe, could produce abuse and coercion.

Szasz himself wrote a response to their critique. His central point was that their major objection to his proposal is also the major objection to their (Oregon and California) regime of PAS. Their core objection is that the "patient" might take the wrong combination of drugs and survive with severe mental impairments. But, as Szasz says: "This is also true for physician-prescribed barbiturates: they too may be taken incorrectly or vomited with undesirable results. What Battin and Spellecy are saying here is that they are concerned *lest patients try to kill themselves and fail*" (Szasz, 2004, p. 299, original italics). Szasz continues by noting that, if this is the problem, then the only solution is euthanasia, which he calls "physician-assisted execution" (Szasz, 2004, p. 299). This is where we began the history of state laws, with Washington rejecting a ballot initiative that covered not only PAS but lethal injection by physicians as well.

Szasz has the upper hand here. There is a constitutional (and ethical) right to refuse any medical intervention. There is also a legal right for physicians to prescribe medications to patients for legitimate medical purposes (e.g., pain, sleep), risking, but not intending, that their patients use these drugs to end their lives. Szasz and I agree that it is a mistake to pass state immunity statutes that increase the power of physicians over patients, granting physicians legal immunity which they do not need (as a matter of law) and should not want (as a matter of ethics). The drug legalization argument is more difficult. Nonetheless, in the suicide context, there is little evidence that people who want to kill themselves, especially terminally ill patients, cannot get access to the drugs they want to use to end their lives. In any event, this issue is much broader than the question of assisted suicide, and should be debated—as I think Szasz would agree—in a broader societal context.

The treatment of hunger-striking prisoners at Guantanamo Bay Prison, an extreme situation for sure, is nonetheless a worthwhile illustration of the dangers of state medicine. More than one hundred prisoners at Guantanamo have been on hunger strikes at various times since 2002. All these hunger strikes since 2005 have been met with force-feeding regimes, usually by nasal IVs administered by medics while the competent, refusing prisoner was in a restraint chair (Annas, 2006a). The official medical rationale was that the prisoners were suicidal and were engaged in "self-harm," so that the physicians were obligated to "save their lives" by force if necessary. This is a powerful illustration of what Szasz would characterize as an abuse of power by physicians at the behest of the state, and a fundamental violation of medical ethics principles. It is also the inevitable result of the state using physicians for their own purposes, and also played out in post-9/11 torture regimes in which physicians were used to make sure torture victims would survive the CIA's torture tactics (Annas and Crosby, 2015). Better to keep the state's physicians away from punishment and torture; and best never to provide physicians involved in the punishment, torture, or deaths of their "patients," including by suicide, with legal immunity for their actions.

References

Annas, George J. 1994. "Death by Prescription: The Oregon Initiative." *New England Journal of Medicine* **331**: 1240–3.

Annas, George J. 1996. "The Promised End: Constitutional Aspects of Physician-Assisted Suicide." *New England Journal of Medicine* **335**: 683–8.

Annas, George J. 1997. "The Bell Tolls for a Constitutional Right to Physician-Assisted Suicide." *New England Journal of Medicine* **337**: 1098–103.

Annas, George J. 2006a. "Hunger Strikes at Guantanamo: Medical Ethics and Human Rights in a 'Legal Black Hole.'" *New England Journal of Medicine* **355**: 1377–82.

Annas, George J. 2006b. "Controlled Substances, and Physician-Assisted Suicide: Elephants in Mouseholes." *New England Journal of Medicine* **354**: 1079–84.

Annas, George J., and Sondra S. Crosby. 2015. "Post-9/11 Torture at CIA 'Black Sites': Physicians and Lawyers Working Together." *New England Journal of Medicine* **372**: 2279–81.

Battin, Margaret P., and Ryan Spellecy. 2004. "What Kind of Freedom? Szasz's Misleading Perception of Physician-Assisted Suicide." In *Szasz Under Fire: The Psychiatric Abolitionist Faces His Critics*, edited by Jeffrey Schaler, pp. 277–90. Chicago: Open Court Publishing Co.

Brief for Bioethics Professors *Amicus Curiae* Supporting Petitioners, Vacco v. Quill, and Washington v. Glucksberg (No. 95-1858 and No. 96-110) in the Supreme Court of the United States. 1996. (November 12).

Brittany Maynard Legislative Testimony. 2015. (March 30). Accessed April 7, 2018. <www.youtube.com/watch?v=Mi8AP_EhM94>

California. 1992. Death with Dignity Act (Proposition 161).

California. 2015. End of Life Option Act. Assembly Bill No. 15, Approved by Governor. (October 5). Accessed April 7, 2018. <leginfo.legislature.ca.gov/faces/billNavClient.xhtml?bill_id=201520162AB15>

Duncan v. Louisiana. 1968. 391 U.S. 145, 164.

Egan, Nicole Weisensee. 2015. "Brittany Maynard's Husband: 'I Think About Her Every Day.'" *People* **83** (4) (January 26): 60–4.

Egan, Nicole Weisensee, Tara Fowler, and Caitlin Keating. 2014. "Cancer Patient Brittany Maynard: Ending My Life—My Way." *People* **82** (18) (October 27): 64–9.

Miles, Steven H., and Allison August. 1990. "Courts, Gender, and 'the Right to Die.'" *Journal of Law, Medicine, and Ethics* **18** (1–2) (Spring–Summer): 85–95.

Oregon. 1994. Death With Dignity Act.

Quill, Timothy E. 1991. "Death and Dignity: A Case of Individualized Decision Making." *New England Journal of Medicine* **324**: 691–4.

Szasz, Thomas S. 1996. *Our Right to Drugs: The Case for a Free Market*. Syracuse: Syracuse University Press.

Szasz, Thomas S. 2002. *Fatal Freedom: The Ethics and Politics of Suicide*. Syracuse: Syracuse University Press.

Szasz, Thomas S. 2004. "Reply to Battin and Spellecy." In *Szasz Under Fire: The Psychiatric Abolitionist Faces His Critics*, edited by Jeffrey Schaler, pp. 291–300. Chicago: Open Court Publishing Co.

Szasz, Thomas S. 2011. *The Szasz Quotationary: The Wit and Wisdom of Thomas Szasz*, edited by Leonard Roy Frank. Accessed April 7, 2018. <www.amazon.com/Szasz-Quotationary-Thomas-ebook/dp/B005N261VM>

Vacco v. Quill. 1997. 521 U.S. 793.

Washington v. Glucksberg. 1997. 521 U.S. 702.

Chapter 6

Agency, mental illness, and psychiatry: A response to Thomas Szasz

Robert W. Daly

6.1 Introduction

This chapter has two aims: The first is to draw attention to Szasz's understanding of persons as agents, as human beings capable of human action, of activity insofar as it is authored by a person on the basis of knowledge and choice, including knowledge of what is best, or good, or right, or ethical—or moral. The second aim is to offer a critique of his use of the term "agency" in interpreting the phenomena of mental illness and the establishment of psychiatry as a medical specialty—topics of great interest and import to him and to us. While Szasz's investigations of human agency, mental illness, and psychiatry have been completed, the questions that concerned him remain.

6.2 Exposition—persons as agents

Szasz's concept of persons as agents is presumed or explicitly informs many of his assertions about mental illness, psychiatry, and related legal matters. In my judgment, his preeminent contribution to psychiatry is his insistence on the importance of agency and its exercise in the discernment of mental illness, and for the problems associated with aiding those who suffer this condition.

I am not the first to appreciate Szasz's concern with persons as agents and with what is ethical. For example, I commend to your attention the introductory text edited by Richard Vatz and Lee S. Weinberg (1983), which publishes critical articles by Michael S. Moore, Ronald Pies, C.G. Schoenfeld, and others, and replies by Szasz. More recently, thanks to Jeffrey Schaler, we have *Szasz Under Fire* (2004). In it, essays by R.E. Kendell, K.W.M. Fulford, H. Tristram Engelhardt, Ronald Pies, and others, together with Szasz's replies, are of immediate interest to those concerned with agency and responsibility in psychiatric theory and practice. I also note the work of Ronald Leifer (1969, 2013), who has for many years made creative use of Szasz's corpus in his studies of psychiatry, psychotherapy, the Buddhist tradition, and the human condition.

6.2.1 **Some typical comments by Szasz about agency, responsibility, and freedom**

On agency

"As philosophers have always emphasized, what distinguishes us as human beings from other living things is that we *act*. The idea of the person as moral agent thus presupposes and includes the idea of intentionality. But what, exactly, does it mean to assert that we act? It means realizing that our life in inherently, inexorable, social. We act in the double sense that we behave and perform" (Szasz, 1987, p. 222). "I shall approach the subject of the analytic relationship from a broad psychosocial base viewing man as a *person* who uses signs, follows rules, and plays games—not as an *organism* that has instincts and needs or as a patient who has a disease" (Szasz, 1965, p. 3).[1] While he acknowledges that persons have "personalities," Szasz writes:

> The distinction between happening and action is crucial to my argument . . . throughout this book. I have suggested that, in general, we view physicochemical disorders of the body . . . as happenings; and that we view so-called mental illnesses or psychiatric disorders . . . as actions. Sometimes the line of demarcation between happening and action is not clear. The point at which a passively incurred event becomes transformed into a role-playing situation, provided that the person affected is neurologically intact, will depend on his own attitude toward his human condition . . . [that is] . . . whether he is hopeful or dejected, oriented toward active mastery or passive endurance. (Szasz, 1974, p. 154)

On autonomy

"It is freedom to develop one's self—to increase one's knowledge, improve one's skills, and achieve responsibility for one's conduct. And it is freedom to lead one's own life, to choose among alternative courses of action so long as no injury to others results" (Szasz, 1965, p. 22).

On intentionality

"Although we regard some human actions as obviously intentional and some bodily movements as clearly unintentional, the meaning of the terms *intentional* and *unintentional* is often vague and uncertain, open to different interpretations. This terminological opacity is characteristic of our entire vocabulary for describing and explaining human behavior. It applies also to words such as *deliberate, voluntary* and *conscious*, and their antonyms; and it reflects our pervasive ambivalence about human existence" (Szasz, 1987, p. 216).

On responsibility

Writing about the analytic relationship, Szasz observes that "although the analyst tries to help his client, he does not 'take care of him.' The patient takes care of himself . . . he is 'expected to recover,' not in any medical or psychopathological sense, but in a purely

---

[1] It is essential that the reader recognizes the importance of this procedural rule depicting the "analytic relationship," a rule that is foundational for understanding Szasz's view of mental illness and of psychiatry—a rule to which I shall later return.

moral sense, by learning more about himself and by assuming greater responsibility for his conduct. He learns that only self-knowledge and responsible commitment and action can set him free" (Szasz, 1965, p. 24). The goal of psychoanalysis is to preserve and expand the patient's autonomy when he or she is in a "quandary" (Szasz, 1965, p. 191) by "effecting a translation from the language of excuses into the language of responsibility" (Szasz, 1965, p. 203).

On freedom and lack of freedom

Under the title "The Psychiatric Symptom as Restriction of Freedom," Szasz informs us that the "symptoms" of hysterical paralyses, phobias, obsessions and compulsions, hypochondriasis, and schizophrenia, *as espoused by the patient*, "denote ideas, feelings, inclinations, and actions that are considered undesirable, involuntary, or alien" or "inappropriate" (Szasz, 1965, p. 13) and entail a claim by the patient that he or she suffers "an essential restriction of . . . freedom to engage in conduct available to others similarly situated in his society . . . the expression of loss of control or freedom . . . something he cannot help doing or feeling or as something he must do" (Szasz, 1965, p. 14).

Further: "We must keep in mind that personal conduct is also a form of communication and, as communication, is always qualified as free and voluntary or unfree and involuntary. The possession or lack of freedom of one person has a crucial effect on the degree of liberty of those people with whom he associates. Hence, the concept of liberty is bound to play a significant role in psychiatry and psychotherapy" (Szasz, 1965, p. 16). "The kind of *personal* freedom that psychoanalysis promises can have meaning only for persons who enjoy a large measure of economic, political, and social freedom" (Szasz, 1965, p. 28). "A person is free only when he knows the circumstances under which he will be penalized; he can maintain his liberty by not engaging in acts that are prohibited" (Szasz, 1965, p. 148). "Indeed, we can understand another person only in proportion to our willingness to restrain ourselves from dominating him or submitting to him" (Szasz, 1965, p. 149). "In sum, if the therapist truly desires to liberate the patient, to help him become *personally free* he must arrange a therapeutic situation where such freedom can develop and flourish" (Szasz, 1965, p. 150, original italics). Analogously, the founders of the United States wanted "to make it possible for people to be *politically free*" (Szasz, 1965, p. 150, original italics).

6.2.2 **A deeper look at Szasz's views on agency**

To achieve a richer view of Szasz's views on agency, consider his concern with ethics, his recognition of the difficulties of making practical judgments regarding agency *in actual cases*, and his preference for a very important but limited concept of persons as agents.

Like most people, Szasz recognized that actions are not only voluntary—"you" or "I" or "we" know that we are doing them—they are also very commonly *problematic* regarding what it is best, or good, or right to do. That is, they are of "ethical" interest. Giorgio Agamben has expressed the general orientation toward ethics I find espoused by Szasz:

> The fact that must constitute the point of departure for any discourse on ethics is that there is no essence, no historical or spiritual vocation, no biological destiny that humans must enact or realize. This is the only reason why something like an ethics can exist, because it is clear that if humans were or had to be this or that substance, this or that destiny, no ethical experience would be possible—there would be only tasks to be done . . . There is [however] in effect something that humans are and have to be, but this something is not an essence nor properly a thing. *It is the simple fact of one's own existence as possibility or potentiality.* But precisely because of this things become complicated; precisely because of this ethics becomes effective. (Agamben, 1993, p. 43)

It is with this sense of ethics that Szasz speaks of freedom, in its many guises and disguises, as self-determination, self-realization, self-control, and as personal liberty to do as one will;[2] and of the problems of reasonably and responsibly exercising one's freedom as an agent—in keeping with the law and restricted by the moral norm of not harming others while exercising one's capacity as an agent.

Szasz was well aware of the difficulties of making practical judgments about the nature of someone's activities. He held that the meaning of distinctions such as intentional/unintentional, voluntary/involuntary, free/unfree, used in appraising and interpreting human activities, may be clear in theory. However, he also observed that the use of these terms in the judging of human activities and experiences *in actual cases* can be "vague and uncertain, open to different interpretations" (see Szasz on intentionality in Section 6.2.1). In his early papers, Szasz clearly presumed these ideas, yet as time progressed, he offered little discussion of these matters relative to the loss of agential capacity manifested in "symptoms."

I take the following summary to be consistent with Szasz's view of "agency": An action is not activity that simply "happens." Nor is an action properly called an "event"— as if there were no agent who authored it (Macmurray, 1999, pp. 148–64). A person is known as an *agent* and that person's activities are *action(s)* insofar as a person's activities, in relation to others and "all the furniture of the universe," are authored by that person on the basis of his or her knowledge and choice, and to the extent that an activity is *intended* by that person. Choice, based on knowledge, is the power to perform or not perform an act; an act being the exercise of freedom, the capacity to determine the future through action (Macmurray, 1999, p. 134).

To illustrate, consider an elaborate collective action—a jury reaching a verdict at the conclusion of a trial. Such activity entails many elements: *knowledge* of the motives, desires, interests, projects, abilities, and circumstances of the persons engaged in the proceedings; the identification of *considerations* that bear on authorized verdicts; *deliberation* regarding these matters; *judgment* regarding a verdict that is just; and *reasons* for their *decision* in the case. Activity as action by an individual in a different setting might be exhibited in scoring the winning goal in the final soccer game of the World Cup. In both cases, persons are *responsible for* their conduct, and *accountable to* others for their actions. "Responsibility" for action is predicated of persons as agents. This

---

[2] Szasz was familiar with the studies of freedom conducted by Mortimer Adler (1958) and his associates at the University of Chicago and at the Institute for Philosophical Research in San Francisco (personal communication).

means that agential *responsibility* is not correctly ascribed to a person's "genes," "brain," "ego," "personal dispositions," "unconscious forces," or "social influences," *insofar* as an activity is considered an "action" of a person as agent.

By contrast, the movements marking a grand mal seizure displayed by a member of the jury or the soccer player would be a clear instance of activities that were not actions. A seizure is an activity that is "involuntary," "unfree," or an "event," that is, an activity that is not an action of a person as agent, not an activity for which he or she as an agent is immediately responsible.

The *questions* raised and answers provided by Szasz about persons, mental illness, psychiatry, medicine, and law employ or presume this lexicon and grammar. This language and associated concepts must be of interest to those who disagree with his *answers* to questions about mental illness and psychiatry.

6.3 Critique of Szasz's use of the word "agency"

For those who value aspects of Szasz's work, agreeing with some features and disagreeing with others, it is difficult to identify a beginning point for discussion of his work. The problem is to discern a relatively clear point of departure, a *that about which Szasz and his critics are speaking*, albeit in different ways. One needs to identify a relevant and uncontested state of affairs that is not disputed by any of the parties. There is such a point of departure. Szasz and his commentators all affirm the suffering exhibited by persons who are commonly perceived as and called "mentally ill." They also acknowledge the facts regarding the actual activities (or lack of activities) of such persons. For example, Ralph Slovenko cites the following passage by Szasz (2001): "When I say that mental illness is not an illness I do not deny the reality of the behaviors to which the term points, or the existence of the people who exhibit them, the suffering the denominated patients may experience, or the problems they cause for their families. I merely classify the phenomena people call 'mental illnesses' differently than do those who think they are diseases" (Slovenko, 2004, p. 140). In short, the occasions and reality of "symptoms" (see Szasz on freedom and lack of freedom in Section 6.2.1) are not, generally speaking, in dispute. What is in dispute is the perception, naming, classifying, understanding, and meaning of those symptoms—and the practices that follow from differing interpretations.

How did Szasz characterize "the symptoms," "the behavior," and "the suffering" of persons who exhibit the phenomena? How, in consequence of this characterization and other findings, did he depict psychiatry? Szasz asserted that symptoms are the marks of "problems in living," the wrong or otherwise deficient use of a person's capacity for action. In his view, even disabling problems are manifestations of bad habits acquired in the course of life. With the exception of symptoms that mark diseases of the brain (see Szasz on agency in Section 6.2.1), symptoms are ethical problems pertaining to *the best or right exercise of a person's agential powers,* problems of knowing how to use one's capacity for action to lead a life, or a good life. In the language of conditions, symptoms are manifestations of *states of ignorance* or misguided practical judgments by a person regarding how to specify and achieve a good life, accompanied by learned habits of disability. They are, in some way, the wrong exercise of a person's agential powers, a failure of right reason, a problem for which the sufferer, as agent, is ulti-mately, prospectively at least, responsible. For example, Szasz writes: "I prefer to view hallucinations as a type of disowned self-conversation: the 'voices' the patient allegedly hears are his own thoughts. And I prefer to view delusions as stubborn errors or lies, that the patient is not interested in correcting" (Szasz, 2004, pp. 54–5).

According to Szasz, what is needed (if sought by the agent) is a special educa-tional response to the patient's exotic problem of ignorance. As there is no organ-ismic disordering to be understood, explained, or treated, it is an error to interpret the person's story, suffering, experiences, language, and other activities as a form of *ill health*. So it is a mistake to constitute psychiatry as a specialty of medicine. According to Szasz's critics—for example, Pies (1979, 2004), Fulford (1989, Chapter 1), Kendell (2004)—this account of "symptoms" and of psychiatry is not adequate for most of the occasions that arouse its use. Why?

These authors have another intuition about the symptoms, suffering, and disa-bility exhibited by people who are said to be "mentally ill." In their view, even when symptoms are apprehended as misguided actions, they *also present themselves as events*, as *something that is happening to* the person as agent, not just something that one does, did, or failed to do out of ignorance. Insofar as the symptoms are events, they are not determined by the agent, but in some other or additional way. These authors hold, therefore, that we cannot appeal in a straightforward or simple way only to an agent's knowledge, potential knowledge, misguided reasons, intentions, or choices, in order to aid such a person. Further, in keeping with their intuition, these critics do not agree with Szasz's claim that in all circumstances it is only the patient's judgment that matters in the perception of symptoms and disorder. For these commentators and for these reasons, the sufferer is a person who is disordered, undergoing an illness or disease (Pies, 1979, 2004; Kendell, 2004). The symptoms are signs of *"action-failure"* (Fulford, 1989, Chapters 7 and 8).

Enduring symptoms, which to some important extent are perceived as events, "stand in the place of action." When and where action is expected by a person as agent, the sufferer finds, or others find, behavior (i.e., activity without choice grounded in knowledge) and experiences without intelligible references to either the sufferer's own knowledge or others' knowledge of the sufferer. What is perceived and differentiated in these circumstances is organismic disordering of the behavioral and experiential foundations of *the capacity for action,* not simply puzzles about best conduct or the right exercise of that capacity (Daly, 1991, 2013).

The remainder of this critique is concerned with the ideas and the arrangement of the ideas that inform the common intuitions of these and other critics.

With the question of how to apprehend the behavior, experience, or suffering of an agent before us, I turn to a lexicon, grammar, and set of ideas that are rejected, excluded, or ambiguous in Szasz's texts. The near absence of these ideas and of their place in understanding agency, and in apprehending the phenomenology of "mental illness" in relationship to agency, give rise to some of the difficulties encountered by those who value Szasz's scholarship and observations, but who disagree, in part or altogether, with Szasz's interpretation of the state of affairs in question. The presence and utilization of these ideas, *in addition to* the traditional lexicon of agency, can make perceiving the phenomena of mental illness an immensely more difficult task in both theory and practice than either the exclusive application of the traditional lexicon of agency or the exclusive use of the perception of the person as a human organism. These concepts, as they pertain to agency, mental illness, and psychiatry are as follows:

a. The "condition" or "state" of a person as agent.

b. The "person as an organism," "health," "ill health."

c. "Personality," "sanity," and "diminution of sanity."

d. "Psychiatry" as a "medical specialty."

With these concepts in mind, I shall argue that *insofar as* the "symptoms" and "restriction of freedom" exhibited by a person who is said to be "mentally ill" are perceived as *events that happen when manifestations of agency are reasonably expected*, symptoms reveal a kind of undesirable, pathological, organismic condition of that person as agent. As such, it is a problem with one's distinctly human *organismic equipment* for living a life, a state not determined by the agent, but in some other way. Symptoms reveal a diminution of a person's *sanity*, of a kind of human health, that is, of the behavioral and experiential foundations of *the capacity for* action. Diminutions of sanity are not characteristically or simply problems with the *use* or *best exercise* of that equipment.

This construction of the state of affairs in question (the suffering, symptoms, and restriction of freedom of those who are called "mentally ill"), and the effort to restore particular persons to sanity, grounds the claim that psychiatry is a specialty of medicine.

In the brief analyses that follow, I will emphasize the manner in which these concepts pertain to individual persons as agents, and are related to and coincidental with questions about the best exercise of a person's agential powers. My approach is not intended to obscure nor to deflect questions relative to the exercise of agential capacity, or to defend or reject any particular practices or theories of etiology now favored by psychiatrists. This alternative depiction of the state of affairs in question *does not* simplify or resolve many of the conceptual, clinical, legal, scientific, ethical, or social problems experienced by psychiatrists, their organizations, or their patients. However, it does reveal, to some extent, why there are so many difficulties in and about psychiatry and why certain difficulties prove to be intractable in theory, and are resolved (if they are resolved) only in practice.

6.3.1 The condition or state of a person as agent

In this text, the term "condition" refers to how things stand for a while with respect to some person or other entity. Actions can bring about a condition, or a condition can influence or shape an action. A condition or set of conditions may be necessary for an action to be performed. But a condition per se is not the name of an action or of an event. Rather, it refers to a state of being of a human person.

While there are as many conditions as our projects require, of interest here are conditions predicated of individual persons with regard to our capacity to act. Because we must, or desire to, act in certain ways to be alive, or live, or live well, we also desire to have *the capacity* to act in certain ways. Two vignettes illustrate the difference between actions and conditions understood as states of being relative to the capacity for action.

The first vignette borrows from the language of games (as Szasz often did), and concerns the game of hockey. When my leg or hockey stick is broken or my skates are not sharp, I cannot play the game of hockey very well, or even at all, no matter how well-trained and experienced a player I am. The same holds true when the compressor to make the ice breaks down. These untoward conditions are problems *for*—but not *of*—the game of hockey.

The second vignette concerns the act of digging a trench. Imagine that I am digging a trench with a shovel and having difficulty realizing my intention in keeping with some norm of efficacy or efficiency. Is it because I am using the wrong shovel? Or is it because I do not know how to use the shovel? Or is it that the handle of the shovel is broken, or the earth I am trying to move is such that I need a different kind of tool to dig this trench? Or is it because I am having back pain? Whatever it is *will* count as an undesirable condition relative to my capacity to dig a trench, and so to my intention to dig the trench relative to some good I am trying to achieve. So will conditions that are favorable to digging the trench well (e.g., strength, skill, determination, soft ground).

We give names to desirable states of individual persons that underwrite or enhance our powers of action to achieve our aims. We admire some states with which people are endowed (e.g., great vision). We honor and admire persons when they have gone to great lengths to successfully acquire practical skills or reflective knowledge valued by a community of agents. Conversely, we attend to and name undesirable conditions (e.g., back pain) that impede or limit our capacity for action.

Problems concerning the best, or right, or reasonable exercise of agential powers in the conduct of life are ubiquitous. So too are problematic conditions of persons as agents, that is, problems with the development, excellence, diminution, distortion, loss, or lack of human agential powers per se.

A person can encounter many undesirable conditions relative to his or her capacity to act (with *equipment* for living a life), to which attention, and the attention of others, is directed: conditions that pertain to one's *opportunities* to act (e.g., conditions of living or working that are not safe); or a condition in which one lacks essential resources; or in a personal relationship—a misunderstanding or enmity; or of injustice in a community—conditions that one cannot rectify alone. Other conditions pertain to one's *ability* to act: for example, a state of *ignorance* (of French in France, or of civil engineering when designing roads) or conditions of *ill health* (an injury, great pain, deformation, illness, or malnutrition) that impede a person's ability to secure his or her "prudential interests" (Margolis, 1976, p. 252). Conditions are also distinguished in relation to one another in different ways, depending on our aims. Different conditions may be predicated of a person at the same time (e.g., one may be young, impoverished, but learned).

In short, there are many occasions when we attend to the condition of a person, because conditions pertaining to abilities and opportunities enhance or impede the actions we can perform, and so, *in those ways, a person's capacity for action informs and constitutes a feature of that person's agency.*

6.3.2 **The person as an organism; health and ill health**

Attention to the condition of a person as agent is typically aroused relative to various norms for action in typical situations or for creative actions in unique circumstances. In both cases, we want a person to be *able to*, and to *have an opportunity to*, do what is expected, required, or desired. One important set of conditions pertaining to a person's capacity for action, assumes, for good reasons, that human persons as agents are persons who are also human organisms.

Human persons exist as particular individuals living lives as human agents in re-lation to other human agents and to all that is. To exist as a human agent necessarily implies one's existence as a particular, living, human organism. *There are no actions by any human person without a complex organismic foundation for those actions.* The idea of a person as agent must therefore contain, reveal, and acknowledge a concept of a particular person as a particular human organism. This acknowledgment can generate a tension in theory as well as practice, namely, how to relate our concept of a person as an agent and to our concept of that same person as an organism. This tension can be the source of ambiguities, ironies, indeterminacies, puzzles, and conflicts when making judgments about persons and about their activities as agents.

While there are many reasons for such tensions, one reason is that the person as an organism and the organismic conditions of persons are not known or characterized in the traditional lexicon and grammar (knowledge, reasons, judgment, intention, movement determined by knowledge and choice, etc.) which are used to depict a person as an agent. The organismic conditions of a person are instead characterized by terms which refer to a vast number of physical, biological (including psycholog-ical), cultural, and social factors and processes, which we do not compose, develop, or author.

With regard to the organismic foundations of a person's capacity for action, we speak (as noted) of abilities and opportunities. As to the origins of the *ability* to act, we refer to *acquirements*—what comes about as a result of how a particular human life is lived: for example, what has been experienced and learned, what has happened, or what has been done that, as agent, one is not aware of; acquisitions that operate, not as knowledge, but organismically (e.g., as conditioned responses, habits, dispositions); and motives of which we are not aware. Ability to act is also composed of *endowments*—what is given (e.g., one's genes), essential in underwriting the development of life as human: for example, one's particular (as well as general) form, age, gender, stage of life; the composition of cells and their elements that constitute organs; systems of organs with processes that sustain vital functions such as respiration, circulation, digestion, elimination, reproduction, and mentation.

The idea of "personality" espoused here assumes that no behavior or experience, whether ordered or disordered, integrated or disintegrated, with the traditional features of agency, "stands in isolation." All are elements of personal individuality as a whole, regardless of how they come about (e.g., past experience and actions; the synthesis of proteins, toxins, degenerations, etc.). Any factor that enters into the determination, shaping or otherwise influencing (immediately or remotely) the behavioral and experiential foundations of agency, can shape personal individuality and so be relevant to our understanding of sanity and its diminutions. Whether such factors do *in fact* shape personality is a matter of empirical demonstration (Rapaport, 1960, pp. 39–72; Daly, 1991, pp. 380-4).

With regard to *opportunities* to act, we recall that a person is agent, or acts, *in relation to* the other; that is, to that which is apprehended as not-the-self (Macmurray, 1999, Chapter 5). One's capacity to act is shaped not only by abilities facilitated and constrained in their development by the actions of others and natural events, but also by the enduring and incidental features of the world in which a person seeks to realize his or her intentions. So with respect to describing the organismic foundations of the capacity for action, it is imperative to identify and name the organismic features of the *opportunity* to act as well as the circumstances in which one is acted upon. So we recognize the organismically relevant features and dynamics of the natural world, of interpersonal relationships, of culture and community, society, political economy, and the historical epoch in which relationships are composed and recomposed as the agent and the other change in the course of time.

We refer then, in this general way, to this dynamic, complex, developing, and organized (or disorganized) array of factors, arranged in different ways in various conditions, as the *organismic foundations* of the capacity (or lack thereof) of a person for action. We distinguish these foundations in theory and practice from other foundations of agency: for example, knowledge, or skill in using knowledge to decide what to do in living a life. We specify, as we discern them, the various states or conditions of an organismic type that enhance or impede a person's capacity for action.

Agency, construed in terms of a person's knowledge, reasons, choices, intentions, and movements as authored by the person, is underwritten by the organismic foundations of agency, even when we acknowledge that some of these foundations (e.g., habits) are themselves shaped by the person's actions or lack thereof. We typically invoke the concepts and language of organism in the service of our concerns about agency. At the same time, the idea of the person as an organism is necessary for a more complete portrait of the person as an agent.

The possibility of agency and of its exercise depends throughout its entire range on the constitution and functioning of persons as particular human organisms. A person's condition as an organism shapes or influences. and to some extent determines. the capacities of the person as agent; that is, it may enhance or limit the agent's capacity to know and to chose well in, and by means of action in, relationships with other persons—even if it is often difficult or impossible to specify exactly how, when, or why organismic processes, states, and the habitats in which persons live underwrite a person's capacity for action.

Szasz, for the most part, set aside organismic considerations in his texts (see Szasz on agency in Section 6.2.1), or, when he did include them, as when he spoke of personal individuality, did not view them in an organismic context. This is one of the reasons that he had little to say about health and ill health.

Health and ill health

"Health" and "ill health" are terms used to value (as well as specify) organismic states of persons as desirable or undesirable, good or poor, ordered or disordered—relative to a person's ability to act with an intention to secure some good in relation to someone or something, in some context or habitat.

In clear cases, we say a person is in "good health" when the organismic foundations of action enable a person, by means of his or her action, to secure his or her prudential interests. Similarly, when a person is unable (or is likely to become unable) to secure those interests because of a diminution of his or her organismic capacity for action, we say that person is in "ill health." Insofar as an organismic state imperils the capacity to secure one's prudential interests, we designate that state as "pathological," implying a strong sense of "undesirable." Canguilhem rightly says: "The doctor is called by the patient. It is the echo of this pathetic call which qualifies as pathological all the sciences which medical technology uses to aid life" (Canguilhem, 2007, p. 226).

No matter what we believe about how states of health and ill health arise, it is, above all, the advent or fear of ill health that brings organismic features of life and living to our attention. The organismic foundations of agency are, by stipulation, excluded from Szasz's depiction of "symptoms." In keeping with a two-substance view of human beings (as "body" and "mind"), the ideas of the holistic "organismic foundations of agency," "health," and "ill health" are assigned by Szasz, not to persons as agents, but to "the body" (one way, in theory, to construe and organize the organismic foundations of action), and, in terms of practice, to "neurology."

6.3.3 Sanity, diminution of sanity, personality

Persons and societies of persons distinguish kinds of ill health (e.g., sickness, injury, pain, deformation, malnutrition), that is, undesirable organismic states or disorders that in clear cases diminish or imperil the capacity of a person as agent to secure his or her prudential interests.

Recall that Szasz wrote that psychiatric symptoms "denote ideas, feelings, inclinations, and actions that are considered undesirable, involuntary, or alien" or "inappropriate" (Szasz, 1965, p. 13). All such symptoms "entail an essential restriction of the patient's freedom to engage in conduct available to others similarly situated in his society" (Szasz, 1965, p. 14). Examples of these symptoms include hysterical paralyses, phobias, obsessions, compulsions, hypochondriasis, and schizophrenia. "The common element in these and other so-called psychiatric symptoms is the expression of loss of control or freedom" (Szasz, 1965, p. 14). "The possession or lack of freedom of one person has a crucial effect on the degree of liberty of those people with whom he associates. Hence, the concept of liberty is bound to play a significant role in psychiatry and psychotherapy" (Szasz, 1965, p. 16).

Szasz contends that "symptoms" are best interpreted, named, and responded to as signs of "problems in living," from which people are to recover "in a purely moral sense" (Szasz, 1965, p. 24): problems more akin to ethical problems than to problems of health. Perceiving or construing such state of affairs as diminished organismic capacity for action or as ill health is, at best, a category mistake. At worst, it is a myth that generates unwarranted and pernicious social and legal practices. In Szasz's view, the idea of "sanity" is a "fatuity" (Szasz, 1987, p. 232).

I agree with Szasz that the phenomena typically called "mental illnesses" are not illnesses, though not for the same reasons. In my view, the states of agents which we are seeking to characterize are not illnesses in the same sense that injuries are not illnesses. An injury is not an illness. It is another form of ill health, another kind of organismic impairment of the ability to act. Diminutions of sanity are yet another kind of ill health, neither illness or injury—though admitting of analogies and disanalogies to both.

Furthermore, the symptoms are not "mental" if by this designation we imply that they are disorders of the "mind" as contrasted with the "body." "Mind" and "body" are not the names of entities or existents, but rules for attending to persons in one way rather than another. *Human persons*, not minds or bodies, enjoy health or suffer ill health (Kendell, 2004, p. 41) even if attending to persons and speaking in this way can have legitimate uses. According to Szasz, the phenomena of persons under consideration are human behavior and experience, human suffering, and practical problems for the sufferer and for others. As the *recognition of these phenomena* is not grounded by or correlated with, findings of an anatomical abnormality of "the body," these phenomena are not to be apprehended as illnesses or diseases or problems of health. This view has been credibly contested on clinical, historical, and philosophical grounds by scholars such as Pies and Kendell. Hence, Szasz's mythologizing of mental illness is a "philosophical position" which "underpins all Szasz's subsequent arguments and is, in my view, profoundly mistaken. Neither minds nor bodies suffer from diseases. Only people (or, in a wider context, organisms) do" (Kendell, 2004, p. 41).

States of health and ill health are assigned to living human beings. But, in a strict sense, with regard to sanity and its diminution, only persons deemed agents or capable of agency (however immature or postmature) are eligible for attributions of sanity or judged to suffer diminutions of that state (Daly, 2013, pp. 6–10). I find the inclusion and use of the lexicon, grammars, and concepts of the "condition of sanity" as a kind of "health" and of the "diminution of sanity" as a kind of "ill health" to be essential for a complete depiction of the phenomena in question, most specifically insofar as they are perceived as events that happen and diminish agency.

In contrast to Szasz, I find the practical judgment that a person is "sane"—a judgment about the organismic state of an agent—affirms that the organized and dynamic array of organismic factors (whatever their type or origin), manifested in the experience and behavior of a person *as agent* (known collectively and variously as "the personality of an agent"), are sufficiently integrated with that person's knowledge to *enable* him or her to author actions in relation to others that (at a minimum) permit that person to secure his or her basic interests. Reaching a judgment that an agent is sane, in either a lay or a medical context, will include consideration, not only of formal qualities of "mental" processes or functions (e.g., perceiving, thinking, remembering, feeling), but also of *what* is perceived, remembered, thought, felt—or not—relative to the integration of personality with the agent's knowledge and choices. The same may be said about appraisals of other activities (experiences, behavior, or actions) in reaching such judgments. Psychiatry addresses the activities of persons in terms of the integration (or lack thereof) of a person's behavior and experience with respect to that person's capacity as agent to secure, through action, his or her prudential interests, and to secure those interests relative to having a life, even a good life.

Problems in living (i.e., problems about the best exercise of agential powers) may be factors in precipitating many kinds of ill health, including diminutions of sanity. Being in a state of diminished sanity also generates problems in living for the person who suffers such a condition, as well as for others. As Szasz notes, others have difficulty performing consistently with their norms and desires that presume the sanity of the person whose sanity is now diminished (see Szasz on freedom and lack of freedom in Section 6.2.1).

6.3.4 Psychiatry as a medical specialty

Because, for Szasz, symptoms are manifestations of ethical problems, it is an error to interpret people's stories, sufferings, and symptoms as forms of ill health and to constitute psychiatry as a specialty of medicine. Since, in his view, this error is not recognized, but perpetuated, he views psychiatry as a social device by which the state gains extralegal control of persons (a crime, of sorts, against humanity). Psychiatry, whatever else it may be, should not, in Szasz's view, be organized in theory or in practice as a *medical* specialty.

At its best, psychiatry is a form of secular spiritual guidance. Spiritual direction, whether religious or secular, insofar as it addresses the question of how best to conduct a life, presumes the sanity of those who seek guidance. The manifestations of mental illness signal a problem of acquired ignorance for which an educational remedy is needed, and not a problem of health for which a treatment should be provided.

Of course, many commentators disagree with Szasz's view of psychiatry. In their view, something "organismic" has happened, and is happening, that has disintegrated or disorganized the behavioral and experiential foundations of a person's capacity to act, thereby limiting what he or she can or cannot do. There is a problem with his or her equipment for acting, not just with the question of how best to use that equipment. While bearing in mind the agent's challenges, they assert that psychiatry is, or ought to be, a specialty of medicine.

The initial symptoms of a diminution of sanity are defined by "the cry and suffering of the patient," which point to a pathological organismic disability with respect to agential capacity—no matter what else those symptoms point to. It is for this reason that persons are first judged and designated as being in a state of ill health. In this way, the disordered condition of a person with "mental illness" is no different from that of persons in other organismic states that are experienced and apprehended as pathological (i.e., sickness, injury, malnourishment, deformation, or pain). Many, though not all, of these other forms of ill health originate, at least in part, in either ignorance or the wrong exercise of agential powers; for example, failure to seek appropriate care when one is disabled by pain and sickness, or to follow preventive or therapeutic measures, or persisting in habits and practices known to lead to organismic infirmities. But these states are not, for these reasons, designated or considered to be problems of education, even when education can play a prominent role in their treatment.

Like persons who suffer from other forms of ill health, those who experience diminutions of sanity (as already noted) precipitate an urgency—a kind of urgency that recurs—which generates practices for recognizing this mode of suffering and responding to it. What psychiatrists share and value (or ought to share and value) with other physicians is the regular enactment of the practical intention to recognize states of ill health and to restore to health those persons who suffer organismic disorders. That is the reason why psychiatry can and should be counted as a *medical* specialty— for the same general reason why any medical specialty can lay claim to that status. In virtue of this common aim, psychiatrists are reasonably counted as members of a distinctive class of professional healers who operate (whether well or poorly) within (and in part *define*) the contemporary social institution of clinical medicine.

What makes psychiatry different from other specialties is the principle in terms of which psychiatrists' work is distinguished from that of general physicians and other clinical specialists. Practitioners of psychiatry are physicians who respond to various states of affairs when it is correctly judged that a person as agent is suffering from an undesirable organismic condition, a form of ill health manifested in that person's behavior and experience. Their aim is (or should be) to restore individual agents to sanity and thereby to their full powers as agents, insofar as that is possible. It is for this reason that, in psychiatry, the organismic capacity for action is depicted as the "personality" of the agent. Of necessity, the materials of which we are composed underwrite, in certain ways, the possibility of personal individuality—and so of the behavioral and experiential foundations of agency. In the service of restoring the sanity of an agent when it is diminished, the burden and the privilege of the clinical psychiatrist, together with the patient, is to discern and amend for the better (insofar as possible) the organismic factors constituting the behavioral and experiential foundations of the agent's capacity for action. Thus, the psychiatrist will employ *in practice* a concept of persons as agents that reveals (or should reveal) a robust idea of human agency: a concept that *includes*, not *excludes*, an organismic view of personality *and* the traditional view of agency—an achievement that is the singular mark of the successful clinical psychiatrist. There are significant differences between the principles of clinical psychiatry and those of neurology (Daly, 2013).

This understanding of the aim and ideal of psychiatric practice as a medical specialty is credible even if psychiatry exhibits many features that are *not* analogous to those of other branches of clinical medicine; disanalogies that Szasz recounted at length. Yet such observations do not count as good reasons for asserting that psychiatry is not qualified to be a medical specialty.

Disanalogies among specialties abound. None of the historically emergent specialties are alike in every respect, either with regard to the sorts of patients to whom they minister, the kinds of health they seek to restore, or to the particular ends, means, and principles which they embody. For example, some physicians are concerned with the health and ill health of special populations (e.g., children); some with the elaboration of certain techniques (e.g., radiology). Many are associated with particular clinical

venues (e.g., hospitalists); others with organizations or institutions that are not primarily concerned with restoring and maintaining health (e.g., courts, prisons, the armed
forces, health insurance companies). Moreover, different specialists are educated, organized, and compensated in different ways, and exhibit a host of variable relations
with the vicissitudes of markets, the law, and civil society.

Nor must we disavow all of psychiatry as a medical specialty because some of its
well-known features pose questions and practical difficulties. For example, psychiatry
as a *singular* medical specialty is difficult to characterize with precision and clarity,
given the heterogeneous array of disorders and alleged disorders with which patients
and psychiatrists contend, the many factors to be considered when making practical
judgments about the personalities of agents, and the diverse organizational and legal
environments (private offices, public outpatient clinics, public and private hospitals,
the ER, various wards, etc.) in which these judgments are made. The difficulties are
compounded by the fact that:

Psychiatrists can disagree about diagnoses (kinds of diminutions of sanity) and about
the correct form of treatment of various kinds of disordered states.

Some psychiatrists, freely, controversially, though in keeping with the law and in relation to the authority of judges, engage in the process of involuntary civil commitment and other legal proceedings within the criminal justice system pertaining to
disordered persons.

The clinical jurisdictions and disciplines of psychiatry overlap those of other medical specialties (e.g., neurology), and those of other professions (e.g., clinical psychology and social work).

The practices of psychiatrists, at times, display similarities to practices beyond the distinctive scope of medicine—those of spiritual guides, and of teachers who instruct
us on how life should be lived.

Even if we grant the veracity of these claims, there is no compelling reason to believe
that psychiatry can amount to anything more or less than a mechanism of social control, or, that it properly has, as its principal aim, the discernment of the best exercise
of right reason. Its practitioners have, or should have, a credible, persistent, sufficiently
valuable, and distinctive intention: to restore to sanity, persons as agents.

In sum, I discern no compelling reason to dismiss psychiatry as a medical
specialty.

6.4 **Conclusion**

It is the clarity, consistency, energy, and scholarship with which Szasz presents his
ideas about agency, mental illness, and psychiatry that challenge others to discover
the reasons why they agree with him or believe him in error. It is, in part, because of
his work that others and I have been inspired to refine our ideas about agency and action, health, and ill health, sanity and its diminution, and the cultural and institutional
foundations of psychiatry and medicine.

Szasz does a service to clinical psychiatry and to psychoanalysis by insisting on
the import of agency and action in understanding the activities of the persons who

participate in these institutions. The utility and coherence of that contribution is constrained by the organismic-free concepts of human agency informing that service.

Acknowledgments

The author thanks John Patrick Daly, Ph.D., Ronald Pies, M.D., Paul W. Prescott, Ph.D., and Kendra Winkelstein, J.D. for their suggestions regarding the preparation of this chapter.

References

Adler, Mortimer. 1958. *The Idea of Freedom: A Dialectical Examination of the Conceptions of Freedom*. Garden City, New York: Doubleday.

Agamben, Giorgio. 1993. *The Coming Community*, translated by Michael Hardt. Minneapolis: University of Minnesota Press.

Canguilhem, Georges. 2007. *The Normal and the Pathological*, translated by Carolyn R. Faucett and Robert S. Cohen. New York: Zone Books.

Daly, Robert W. 1991. "A Theory of Madness." *Psychiatry* **54** (4) (November): 368–85.

Daly, Robert W. 2013. "'Sanity' and the Origins of Psychiatry." *Association for the Advancement of Philosophy and Psychiatry Bulletin* **20** (1): 2–17.

Fulford, K.W.M. 1989. *Moral Theory and Medical Practice*. Cambridge: Cambridge University Press.

Kendell, R.E. 2004. "The Myth of Mental Illness." In *Szasz Under Fire*, edited by Jeffrey Schaler, pp. 29–48. Chicago: Open Court.

Leifer, Ronald. 1969. *In the Name of Mental Health: The Social Functions of Psychiatry*. New York: Science House.

Leifer, Ronald. 2013. *Engagements with the World: Emotions and Human Nature*. Bloomington, Indiana: Xlibris.

Macmurray, John. 1999. *The Self as Agent*. Amherst, New York: Humanity.

Margolis, Joseph. 1976. "The Concept of Disease." *Journal of Medicine and Philosophy* **1** (3) (September): 238–55.

Pies, Ronald. 1979. "On Myths and Countermyths: More on Szaszian Fallacies." *Archives of General Psychiatry* **36** (2) (February): 139–44.

Pies, Ronald. 2004. "Moving Beyond the 'Myth' of Mental Illness." In *Szasz Under Fire*, edited by Jeffrey Schaler, pp. 327–53. Chicago: Open Court.

Rapaport, David. 1960. *The Structure of Psychoanalytic Theory: A Systematizing Attempt*. New York: International Universities Press.

Schaler, Jeffrey (ed.). 2004. *Szasz Under Fire: The Psychiatric Abolitionist Faces His Critics*. Chicago: Open Court.

Slovenko, Ralph. 2004. "On Thomas Szasz, the Meaning of Mental Illness, and the Therapeutic State: A Critique." In *Szasz Under Fire*, edited by Jeffrey Schaler, pp. 139–58. Chicago: Open Court.

Szasz, Thomas S. 1965. *The Ethics of Psychoanalysis: The Theory and Method of Autonomous Psychotherapy*. New York: Basic Books.

Szasz, Thomas S. 1974. *The Myth of Mental Illness: Foundations of a Theory of Personal Conduct*, revised edn. New York: Harper & Row.

Szasz, Thomas S. 1987. *Insanity: The Idea and its Consequences*. New York: John Wiley & Sons.

Szasz, Thomas S. 2001. *Pharmacracy: Medicine and Politics in America*. Westport, Conn.: Praeger.

Szasz, Thomas S. 2004. "Reply to Kendell." In *Szasz Under Fire*, edited by Jeffrey Schaler, pp. 49–55. Chicago: Open Court.

Vatz, Richard E., and Lee S. Weinberg (eds.). 1983. *Thomas Szasz: Primary Values and Major Contentions*. Buffalo: Prometheus.

Chapter 7

Taking Szasz seriously—and his critics, too: Thesis, antithesis, and a values-based synthesis

K.W.M. Fulford

7.1 Introduction

As the author of *The Myth of Mental Illness* (1960, 1961), Tom Szasz attracted applause and criticism in equal measure. He was applauded by opponents of medical psychiatry for advancing the thesis that mental illnesses are defined by evaluative norms and hence are outside the scope of biomedical science. Mental health issues, so the opponents of psychiatry believe, are best dealt with by social and psychological rather than biological interventions. But Szasz, for the same reason, has been criticized by proponents of biomedical psychiatry. Arguing antithetically to Szasz that mental illnesses are no different in any material respect from bodily illnesses, his critics accused him of excluding patients from clinical care. An obituary in the *Lancet,* reflecting this antithetical view, cited with approval Paul Appelbaum's and Thomas Gutheil's (1979) dismissal of Szasz as putting patients at risk of "rotting with their rights on" (Williams and Caplan, 2012).

In this chapter, I outline a third way of responding to Szasz's myth that knits together thesis and antithesis in a new values-based synthesis. The chapter is in two main sections: The first builds on the story of a real (though biographically disguised) person to establish the new synthesis. The second outlines how the new synthesis is being applied in psychiatry and in bodily medicine. The term "bodily medicine" is used here to mark the distinction between, on the one hand, areas of medicine like cardiology and gastroenterology, and, on the other, psychiatry. The term has many cognates ("general medicine," "internal medicine," and so forth). All of them imply (as Szasz and many of his critics generally imply) that "bodily" and "mental" are disjunctives.

I conclude with a brief personal anecdote about Tom Szasz.

7.2 Establishing a new values-based synthesis

In this section, I outline how taking the Szasz of *The Myth of Mental Illness* and his critics equally seriously leads, via philosophical value theory, to a new approach to working with complex and conflicting values in health care called values-based practice (VBP).

Philosophical value theory is an application of the "Oxford School" of ordinary language analytic philosophy to the language of values (Hare, 1952). The method adopted here, correspondingly, will be that of ordinary language philosophy. What this amounts to, for present purposes, is a focus on the "medium not the message": to proceed by close attention to language use, to the words and phrases actually used, rather than by direct engagement with the arguments as such.

J.L. Austin (1956–1957) exemplified this approach in his exploration of ordinary language usage in legal cases. Here, I begin not with a legal case, but with the story of a real (though biographically disguised) person, whom I will call Simon, and an exploration of ordinary usage as exemplified by two major psychiatric diagnostic classifications: the World Health Organization's (1992) International Classification of Diseases (ICD), and DSM-V (2013). ICD and DSM, as will be seen, turn out to provide very different ways of understanding Simon's story. It is these different understandings that lead, by way of philosophical value theory, to a values-based synthesis between Szsaz and his critics.

7.2.1 **Simon's story**

Simon was a forty-year-old, Black, senior American lawyer, from a middle-class, Baptist family. Before the onset of his symptoms, he reported sporadic, relatively unremarkable, psychic experiences. These had led him to seek the guidance of a professional "seer," with whom he occasionally consulted on major life events and decisions.

Around four years before the first interview, his hitherto successful career was threatened by legal action from his colleagues. Although he claimed to be innocent, mounting a defense would be expensive and hazardous. He responded to this crisis by praying at a small altar that he set up in his front room. After an emotional evening's outpouring, he discovered that the candle wax had left a "seal" (or "sun") on several consecutive pages of his Bible, covering certain letters and words. He described his experiences thus: "I got up and I saw the seal that was in my father's Bible and I called X and I said, you know, 'something remarkable is going on over here.' I think the beauty of it was the specificity by which the sun burned through. It was . . . in my mind, a clever play on words." Although the marked words and letters had no explicit meaning, Simon interpreted this event as a direct communication from God, which signified that he had a special purpose or mission.

From this time on, Simon received a complex series of "revelations," largely conveyed through the images left in melted candle wax. He carried photos of these, which left most observers unimpressed, but were, for him, clearly representations of biblical symbols, particularly from the Book of Revelation, (the bull, the twenty-four elders, the ark of the covenant, etc.). They signified: "I am the living son of David . . . and I'm also a relative of Ishmael, and . . . of Joseph." He was also the "captain of the guard of Israel." He found this role carried awesome responsibilities: "Sometimes I'm saying— O my God, why did you choose me, and there's no answer to that." His special status had the effect of "increasing my own inward sense, wisdom, understanding, and endurance" which would "allow me to do whatever is required in terms of bringing whatever message it is that God wants me to bring."

He expressed these beliefs with full conviction: "The truths that are up in that room are the truths that have been spoken of for 4000 years." When confronted with skepticism, he commented: "I don't get upset, because I know within myself, what I know."

Simon's story, although open to competing interpretations (Jackson and Fulford, 1997), is typical of the kind of story with which psychiatrists might be faced clinically. In the language of psychiatry, Simon is readily understood as suffering from a psychotic mental illness. The beliefs he derived from his wax "seals" are "delusional perceptions" as defined by standardized diagnostic schedules such as the Present State Examination (PSE) (Wing et al., 1974, symptom 82, pp. 172–3). Delusional perceptions in most psychiatric diagnostic manuals, including ICD (WHO, 1992), are, in turn, diagnostic of schizophrenia (or a related functional or even organic psychotic illness). Such an interpretation is, of course, open to challenge; and Simon's story, as it continued, does indeed challenge this interpretation.

Simon was empowered by his experiences and decided to take on his accusers. His "revelations," moreover, guided him in how to proceed with his court case. Just how this worked is impossible to say. Perhaps he was subconsciously tapping into his own knowledge as a lawyer. At all events, the guidance was effective. He won his case, seeing off his accusers as racially motivated competitors. His legal practice prospered. He made a great deal of money. He used this to set up a trust fund for the study, not of psychotic illness, but of religious experience.

Again, there are different ways in which the positive outcome of Simon's story might be understood. But sticking with the language of psychiatry, Simon has what many might think is an unlikely ally for his own understanding of his experience as religious rather pathological: DSM-V (APA, 2013). DSM is similar to ICD in the significance which it attaches to delusional perceptions (covered by DSM's Criterion A). However, DSM differs from ICD in requiring, for a diagnosis of psychotic mental illness, an additional "criterion of clinical significance." This "Criterion B," as it is called, for schizophrenia runs thus: "For a significant portion of the time since the onset of the disturbance, level of functioning in one or more major areas, such as work, interpersonal relations, or self-care, is markedly below the level achieved prior to the onset (or when the onset is in childhood or adolescence, there is failure to achieve expected levels of interpersonal, academic, or occupational functioning)" (APA, 2013, p. 99).

Simon therefore, while satisfying DSM's symptomatic criterion (Criterion A) for schizophrenia, fails to satisfy its Criterion B. This is why DSM offers scope for understanding Simon's experiences in non-pathological rather than pathological terms. But now notice this: DSM, although strongly evidence-based, requires for the determination of its criteria of clinical significance a series of *value judgments*. To satisfy Criterion B, it is not enough that there should be merely a *change* in functioning; such could indeed be defined value-free. But, to satisfy Criterion B, there must be a change in functioning *for the worse*: functioning, as the language of DSM has it, must be "markedly *below the level* achieved prior to the onset" or, in children and adolescents, there must be "*failure* to achieve expected levels."

7.2.2 Simon's story and *The Myth of Mental Illness*

Understood through the language of DSM, Simon's story is thus on the face of it consistent with Szasz's thesis in his *Myth of Mental Illness* that mental illnesses are defined by evaluative norms. The norms in question, furthermore, have been adduced here, not by way of an external critique of psychiatry, but from the language of psychiatry itself as exemplified by DSM. Simon, it is important to point out, is no "exception that proves the rule." Normal (as opposed to pathological) psychotic experiences are now recognized to be commonplace in the general population (Johns and van Os, 2001), and ordinary language studies of both DSM (Sadler, 2005) and ICD (Fulford, 1994, 2002) show values to be pervasive in psychiatric diagnosis.

Those opposed to Szasz's view would, of course, bring a range of counterarguments to bear at this point. Rather than trying to do justice to these, however, I will stick to my ordinary language approach by focusing, not on the content of the relevant arguments and counterarguments, but rather on the *form of argument* adopted. This will suggest that thesis and antithesis, in this instance, are not as far apart as they appear. This in turn will lead to the synthesis from which contemporary VBP is derived.

7.2.3 Thesis and antithesis: parallel forms of argument

One way to see the closeness of thesis and antithesis in the debate about mental illness is by comparing Szasz's argument directly with that of one of his contemporary opponents, the British psychiatrist and epidemiologist, R.E. Kendell. Szasz and Kendell were well matched. Both were psychiatrists; both achieved full professor status as relatively young men; and both were widely read and scholarly. Kendell, besides his empirical work in epidemiology, wrote a still important book on the conceptual challenges of psychiatric diagnosis (1975a). They came to directly opposite conclusions about mental illness. Whereas Szasz concluded that mental illness is a myth, Kendell (1975b) argued to the contrary that at least many mental illnesses are properly part of medicine. Yet the forms of argument they adopted are closely similar.

Table 7.1 shows just how close are the forms of argument adopted by these well-matched protagonists. Both take the concept of mental illness to be "the problem"; both assume that the concept of bodily illness is relatively unproblematic and thus provides a resource for tackling the problem; and both proceed by comparing mental illness with bodily illness. From there, of course, their paths diverge. Szasz argues that mental illness is essentially different from bodily illness in being defined by evaluative norms (his "ethical, legal, and social" norms) rather than factual (his "norms of anatomy and physiology"). Kendell argues that mental illnesses are similar to bodily illnesses in the conceptually key respect that both are biologically dysfunctional (both are associated with reduced longevity and reduced fertility).

But the point to take from their shared form of argument is this: In diverging as they do on what they take to be the meaning of bodily illness, Szasz and Kendell show their shared understanding of "the problem" to have been radically mistaken. For what

Table 7.1 Key features of the shared form of argument adopted by Szasz and Kendell

Shared form of argument	Szasz (1960)	Kendell (1975b)
Problem: concept of mental illness	"My aim . . . is to raise the question ' Is there such a thing as mental illness?' "	My aim is "to decide whether mental illnesses are legitimately so called."
Resource: concept of bodily illness	Bodily illness is defined by "deviation from . . . some clearly defined norm[s] . . . of the structural and functional integrity of the human body."	Body illness is defined by "biological disadvantage" which "must embrace both increased mortality and reduced fertility."
Method: concept of mental illness "tested" against concept of bodily illness	"The norm[s] deviation from which [are] regarded as mental illness" are "psychosocial, ethical and legal."	At least some mental illnesses "carry with them an intrinsic biological disadvantage."

their debate has turned out to be about is not primarily, as they had supposed, the concept of mental illness, but that of *bodily illness*. Further, and more remarkably still, far from bodily illness being a resource supporting an argument by comparison, it is the *differences between them in what they take bodily illness to mean* that drives their different conclusions about mental illness.

Once again, there are different directions in which the argument might run from here. The standard line has been to hang on to the argument by comparison by digging deeper into the meaning of bodily illness. The assumption behind this approach, consistent with the Szasz versus Kendell parallel forms of argument, has been that bodily illness (or its cognates) is at any rate the *lesser* problem and as such remains an appropriate reference point against which the status of mental illness stands or falls. According to this standard line of argument, therefore, if mental illness is shown to be essentially similar to (whatever analysis is offered of) bodily illness, then Kendell was right and mental illness is legitimately so-called. If it does not, then Szasz was right, and mental illness is a myth.

This standard line has been highly productive, generating, in particular, a rich literature on the reducibility or otherwise of concepts of disorder to terms that are value-free (Fulford, 2000, 2014; Thornton, 2000, 2014). Ordinary language philosophy, however, starting as it does from language use, invites a different approach. Instead of debating whether mental illness is relevantly similar to bodily illness, ordinary language philosophy seeks rather to explain even-handedly, and within a general account of illness concepts, the differences (as well as the similarities) between bodily illness and mental illness (Fulford, 1989). The operative difference in this case is just why mental illness is value-laden while bodily illness (to the same extent at least) is not. In terms of Simon's story, then, the challenge is to explain why DSM includes a (diagnostically crucial) Criterion B, while its counterpart, bodily disorder diagnostic manuals, do not. Philosophical value theory, as exemplified by the philosophy of R.M. Hare

(Austin's successor as White's Professor and one of my D.Phil. supervisors), offers one such explanation (Hare, 1952, 1963).

7.2.4 Synthesis: explicit values equal diverse values

Hare's work in philosophical value theory remains controversial, turning as it does on issues within the wider "is-ought" debate (Warnock, 1971; Fulford, 2000, 2014; Thornton, 2000, 2014). In the "small print" of his work though, as I have called it else-where (Fulford, 2014), there are to be found a number of insights helpful for clinical practice.

One such insight is Hare's observation that values tend to become *explicit where they are diverse* and hence (for this or other reasons) cause difficulties. Values, in other words, are in this respect like the air we breathe: Air is everywhere and ultimately important, but we notice it only when, for one reason or another, we have difficulty breathing. Figure 7.1 summarizes one of Hare's own examples (his comparison be-tween strawberries and pictures) and shows how it parallels the difference in visibility of values between bodily illness and mental illness.

Shared values = Implicit values	Diverse values = Explicit values
Strawberries and bodily Illness	Pictures and mental Illness
"Good" in **"good strawberry"** is a value term.	"Good" in **"good picture"** is a value term.
But people have **shared** ideas about what kinds of strawberry are good (red, sweet, tasty, etc.).	But people have **different** ideas about what kinds of picture are good.
Hene "good" in "good strawberry" **attracts the factual meaning,** "red, sweet, tasty, ect., strawberry" and its evaluative meaning becomes **implicit.**	Hence "good" in "good picture" **fails to** attract any factual meaning and its evaluative meaning remains **explicit.**
Bodily illness is in this respect like **strawberries.**	Mental illness is in this respect like **pictures.**
It involves areas of human experience and behavior (such as pain) where our values are largely **shared.**	It involces areas of human experience and behavior (such as emotion, desire, beliefs, etc.) where our values are highly **diverse.**
Hence the meaning of bodily illness **attracts correspondingly factual content** and its evaluative meaning becomes **implicit.**	Hence the meaning of mental illness **attracts no consistent factual content** and its evaluative meaning remains **explicit.**

Figure 7.1 Strawberries/pictures compared with bodily/mental illness.
(Photographs: photastic/Shutterstock and ChooChin/Shutterstock)

To follow Hare's argument through, start with the top part of Figure 7.1. Hare's point is that "good strawberry" and "good picture" are both value terms. But "good strawberry" carries the factual meaning "red, sweet, grub-free strawberry" (or some similar set of value-free descriptive terms), because the factual criteria by which we judge strawberries to be good are largely *shared*. Most people judge a strawberry that is a "red, sweet, grub-free strawberry" to be a good strawberry. Hence the meaning of "good strawberry" has come, by association, to be thought of as "red, sweet, grub-free strawberry," with the evaluative element in its meaning dropping out of sight. For "good picture," by contrast, there are no such shared factual criteria. People disagree widely over what makes a picture good. In the case of pictures then, our values, although not inchoate, are *highly diverse* and the evaluative element in the meaning of "good picture" thus remains explicit.

The lower part of Figure 7.1 shows how an essentially parallel argument explains why values are explicit in the meaning of mental illness while implicit (according to this account) in bodily illness. Like strawberries, the criteria by which we evaluate the symptoms of bodily illness are largely *shared*. Pain, for example, is widely (though of course not universally) judged to be (in itself) a bad thing—most people in pain want to be free of it. The areas of human experience and behavior with which bodily medicine is concerned are, in this sense, values-simple. But the areas of human experience and behavior with which psychiatry is concerned are, to the contrary, values-complex. Emotion, desire, belief, volition, sexuality, and so forth, are all areas in which (as with Hare's example of pictures) our values, although not inchoate, are *highly diverse*.

There is, of course, yet again more to be said about all this. The relationship between the experience of illness and underlying causal theories of disease remains to be spelled out, as does that between disease and dysfunction. I explore these and other issues in *Moral Theory and Medical Practice* (1989), applying a range of ideas from philosophical value theory to the language of values to the language of medicine. The argument, as a whole, furthermore prompts many questions in philosophical value theory about the relationship between (indeed the very distinction between) descriptive and evaluative meaning (Putnam, 2004).

Hare's observation, as it stands, however, gives us a new and completely different way of understanding the visibility of values in mental illness as compared with bodily illness. Szasz took this as showing that mental illness is a myth. To paraphrase, mental illness is "about values," while bodily illness is "about facts." Kendell, focusing instead on scientific norms of biological dysfunction, later went on to argue with others, such as Boorse (1976), that the appearance of values in mental illness reflects (what they took to be) the primitive state of psychiatric science. Hare's observation, by contrast to both of these positions, suggests that we should understand the visibility of values in mental illness, neither (with Szasz) as showing mental illness to be outside the scope of medicine, nor (with Kendell and others) as provisional on future advances in psychiatric science, but rather as a reflection of *the diversity of individual human values* in the areas of human experience and behavior with which psychiatry is characteristically concerned.

Szasz then, according to this Hare-led view, was right to point to the relatively value-laden nature of mental illness, but wrong to take this as showing that mental illness is a myth. Kendell, and successor critics of Szasz, were right to resist Szasz's exclusion of mental illness from medicine, but wrong to do this by denying the importance of values in mental health (and indeed in the rest of medicine). The synthesis to which a Hare-led understanding leads is that mental illness is indeed a part of medicine, but engages in areas of human experience and behavior where our values are particularly diverse. This synthesis is the starting point for VBP.

7.3 Applying the new values-based synthesis

VBP is a new skills-based approach to balanced health care decision-making where diverse values are in play (Fulford et al., 2012). Developed originally as a response to the values-complex challenges presented by mental health (Fulford, 2004), VBP is now extended to bodily medicine.

This section gives a brief overview of VBP, illustrates its applications in mental health (in the case of involuntary psychiatric treatment) and in bodily medicine (in the case of surgery), then indicates a key challenge—namely, that of pluralism—which VBP shares with evidence-based practice (EBP).

7.3.1 Values-based practice

VBP, as its name suggests, is a partner to EBP. Just as EBP provides a process that supports clinical decision-making where diverse evidence is in play, so VBP provides a (different though complementary) process that supports clinical decision-making where diverse values are in play.

The process of VBP is summarized in Figure 7.2. Building on a premise of mutual respect, the ten process elements of VBP support balanced decision-making within locally derived frameworks of shared values. Of the process elements of VBP, learnable clinical skills (covering awareness of values, reasoning, knowledge, and communication) are foundational. These skills, however, have to be used within a particular service environment (one that is person-centered and multi-disciplinary), in close partnership with EBP, and in a dissensual model of shared decision-making.

Premise of mutual respect for differences of values		
Ten key process elements:	Together these support: ⟶	Balanced dissensual decisions **made within** frameworks of shared values.
4 clinical skills.		
2 aspects of clinical relationships.		
3 principles linking VBP and EBP.		
Partnership in decision-making.		

Figure 7.2 A flow diagram of values-based practice.

VBP has been applied in a variety of areas of mental health and primary care. The challenges presented by involuntary psychiatric treatment illustrate the strengths, though also the limitations, of this approach.

7.3.2. **Applying values-based practice to involuntary psychiatric treatment**

Involuntary psychiatric treatment was one of Szasz's particular targets (Szasz, 1963, 1984, 2003). It has been a target too of many others within psychiatry (Szmukler and Holloway, 1998). The concern is that the mere possibility of involuntary treatment renders psychiatry vulnerable to abusive misuses as a means of social control. Such abuses are all too common in the modern history of psychiatry (Bloch and Reddaway, 1977). Yet the balancing concern is that absent the possibility of involuntary treatment and, in Appelbaum's and Gutheil's (1979) critique of Szasz, patients are at risk of "rotting with their rights on."

The issues raised by involuntary psychiatric treatment came to a head in the U.K. recently with the launch of a public consultation in the run-up to a revision of the relevant mental health law. As it was launched on a "public safety" ticket, mental health stakeholders were naturally concerned that any revisions would shift mental health law away from its proper purpose of facilitating medical treatment toward social risk management. The result was that a planned five-month consultation stretched out to five years of deeply divisive debate. From this process, though, emerged a number of principles shared by proponents and opponents of the new law. It was these principles—the "Guiding Principles" as they came to be called— that provided the basis for a range of values-based training materials produced by the U.K. Department of Health to support implementation of the new law (CSIP/ NIMHE, 2008b).

The approach adopted in the training materials is shown diagrammatically in Figure 7.3. The five Guiding Principles are shown here as a round table of shared values that have equal weight in practice. The idea (which was formalized in the legislation) was that these principles should guide the way that the new law would be applied in individual cases. This was easy to state, but difficult to do. For the Guiding Principles, reflecting the diversity of human values in play in mental health, are (individually) complex and (together) conflicting. The Respect Principle, for example, is complex in the sense that it means different things to different people in different circumstances. Respect, moreover, important as it is, is, from the perspective at least of the person resisting treatment, in conflict with the Purpose Principle (which includes treating patients in certain circumstances against their express wishes). This is why VBP is shown at the center of the round table. The skills and other elements of VBP are required if the Guiding Principles are to be used in a balanced way according to the particular circumstances presented by individual cases.

Examples of how this values-based approach works are given in the training materials, a full-text version of which is downloadable from the Collaborating Centre for Values-Based Practice, St. Catherine's College, Oxford (2018). The website for this

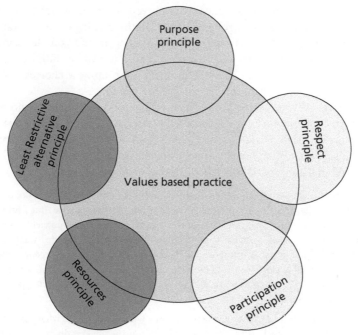

Figure 7.3 The "Guiding Principles" as a framework of shared values.

center also gives details of many other applications of VBP in mental health and primary care. These include a Department of Health program on values-based assessment in mental health (the "three keys" program), which is directly relevant to Simon's story (CSIP/NIMHE, 2008a). The hot news though is that, supported by the Collaborating Centre, VBP is now being extended from mental health into areas of frontline bodily medicine, such as vascular surgery.

7.3.3 Applying values-based practice in vascular surgery

That VBP is finding application in an area of bodily medicine like vascular surgery contradicts the expectations of those (like Kendell and his successors) who regarded the value-laden nature of mental illness to be a reflection of (what they took to be) the relatively primitive stage of the development of psychiatric science. Accordingly, more science should mean less values. Contemporary developments in VBP show, to the contrary, that more science means *more* values.

That more science means more values is readily explained from the perspective of philosophical value theory. When Szasz and Kendell were engaged in their original debate in the 1960s and 1970s, bodily medicine was still preoccupied mainly with acute life-threatening illnesses. These are, in the terms of philosophical value theory, values-simple; for example, when someone has a heart attack, the values engaged (of saving life) are (very largely) *shared values*. Today's medicine, though, driven by scientific advances, has moved on to the point that its principle preoccupations are no longer with acute life-threatening situations (although these, of course, remain important), but with long-term and complex conditions where the values involved are *highly diverse*. There is a direct link here. For the impact of scientific advances in medicine is to open up new choices—and with choices goes diversity of values.

It is this link—between scientific advances and values diversity in medicine—that is behind the contemporary expansion of VBP from its origins in mental health into bodily medicine. Ashok Handa, a vascular surgeon in Oxford and Co-Director of the Collaborating Centre, described (in a personal communication to me in 2015) how VBP has shifted his approach to decision-making with his patients:

> For me the crunch comes clinically when a patient asks 'What would you do, doctor?' Sometimes we have the luxury of unambiguous evidence-based advice. But I find most clinical decision-making is in grey areas where discussion often comes down to the patient not unreasonably asking: So what would you do, doctor? And I wouldn't want to duck that. It's not helpful to patients to push the decision back to them. As surgeons, after all, we have considerable experience of how different options work out in practice; this can help a patient who is trying to make difficult choices in the context of facing potentially life-limiting diagnoses.
>
> But it's also not helpful to push our own decisions willy-nilly. This is what patient feedback from the workshops suggests we have been too inclined to do. It is what I now realize I have been in effect doing. What these workshops have brought home to me is that my answer to 'What would you do?' has reflected my own values, not those of the patient. So we may think we are being patient-centered but we end up being clinician-centered. Of course, it's not easy. But instead of just replying with this or that option (however obvious it seems to me) I now start by finding out more about what matters to this patient. Then I'm better able to look at what 'I' would do in terms of what matters from their point of view rather than from mine. So now when asked 'What would you do, doctor?' my answer starts with 'Well, that depends on what is important to you? If you tell me that I can help you make a better decision.' The dialogue then develops from there.

The shift that Handa describes here may seem a small change in practice—but it is vital. Previously he had (inadvertently) been advising patients according to his own values. Now he finds out first what matters to each particular patient in question so that he can advise patients according to their own values. Notice here that in both cases the evidence base remains crucial. This is not a "customer knows best" approach. The advice offered from either value perspective is guided by the evidence-based options available.

Values-based decision-making of the kind described by Handa has been given a strong boost by a 2015 decision in the U.K.'s Supreme Court (Montgomery v Lanarkshire, 2015). The Montgomery case, as it is called, consolidated recent legal and ethical thinking away from the traditional "prudent clinician" principle of consent to that of an "informed patient." The detail, though, makes clear that "informed" means (as in Handa's example) informed by what matters to the particular patient concerned (i.e., that particular patient's individual values). Consent, the Montgomery judgment establishes, does not mean "bombarding the patient with technical information . . . let alone . . . demanding her signature on a consent form" (Montgomery v Lanarkshire, 2015, paragraph 90). Rather, "the doctor's advisory role involves dialogue, the aim of which is to ensure that the patient understands . . . her condition" (paragraph 90) sufficiently to make a choice taking "into account *her own values*" (paragraph 115, italics added).

7.3.4 The challenge of pluralism

In spelling out the basis of consent in this way, the Montgomery judges were clearly minded of the danger of rights being used as an excuse for neglect. They did not actually cite Appelbaum and Gutheil (1979) on patients "rotting with their rights on," but they might well have done. What is needed in bodily medicine, as in psychiatry, is balanced decision-making. It is this that VBP, working in partnership with EBP, seeks to achieve.

The importance of partnership in decision-making between values-based and evidence-based approaches was well recognized by the founders of evidence-based medicine. EBP today is largely focused on best research evidence. VBP is commonly misread as a counter to evidence-based approaches. But in his pathfinder book, David Sackett, writing as the founding Director of Oxford's Centre for Evidence-Based Medicine (CEBM), actually defines evidence-based medicine as combining best research evidence with clinical experience *and values* (Sackett et al., 2000, p. 1). The values of patients, Sackett continues, again consistent with contemporary VBP, are "the unique preferences, concerns, and expectations each patient brings to a clinical encounter" (2000, p. 1), and "when these three elements [best evidence, clinical experience, and patient values] are integrated, clinicians and patients form a diagnostic and therapeutic alliance which optimizes clinical outcomes and quality of life" (2000, p. 1).

The collapse of EBP from David Sackett's original three-factor (evidence plus experience plus values) to a one-factor (evidence-only) model, and the misreading of VBP as an opponent rather than partner of EBP, are examples of what the Oxford political philosopher Isaiah Berlin (1958) called the challenge of pluralism. Writing in the 1950s, in the shadow of National Socialism, Berlin pointed out that, as a species, we consistently default from pluralism to monism. Faced with Sackett's pluralistic demand to "integrate" evidence with experience and values in clinical decision-making, people default to the monism of an evidence-only model. The corresponding danger for VBP is a collapse to a values-only, one-factor monism.

The challenge then for the values-based synthesis is Berlin's challenge of pluralism. The debate between Szasz's thesis and his critics' antithesis is a debate between competing monisms. VBP, derived as it is from philosophical value theory, is by contrast irreducibly pluralistic. As such, and for all its progress to date, it is at risk of collapsing into some new form of monism. There is evidence already of a collapse within VBP from a values-only to a one-value-only monism (Fulford et al., 2015). But if the pluralistic model of balanced decision-making offered by VBP can be sustained in practice, then patients may, as Szasz wished, have their rights upheld without, as his critics feared, being left to rot "with their rights on."

7.4 **Conclusions**

In this chapter, I have shown how ideas derived from a branch of Oxford analytic philosophy called philosophical value theory provide the basis for a synthesis between Szasz's thesis that mental illness is a myth and the antithetical biomedical models of his critics. According to this synthetic third way, Szasz is right to emphasize the importance of values in concepts of mental illness, but wrong to conclude thereby that mental illness is a myth. His critics, on the other hand, are right to insist that mental illness is properly a part of medicine, but wrong to base their insistence on the denial of the values to which Szasz had drawn attention.

According to the synthetic third way, the visibility of values at the heart of psychiatric diagnostic concepts (as illustrated by Simon's story) reflects the diversity of values in the areas of human experience and behavior (emotion, desire, volition, belief, sexuality, and so forth) with which psychiatry is characteristically concerned. Recognizing this opens psychiatry to the resources of VBP for balanced decision-making where diverse values are in play in clinical care. I have illustrated these resources with training materials produced in the U.K. to support implementation of a recently revised mental health law on involuntary psychiatric treatment, and with a recently launched program on values-based surgical care in Oxford.

I promised a personal anecdote by way of conclusion. I have in fact two anecdotes, one from what was sadly to be my last meeting with Tom, and one from my first meeting with him some thirty years earlier. My last meeting with him was in my role as chair of a plenary lecture he gave at the Royal College of Psychiatrists as a guest of the U.K.'s Critical Psychiatry Network. Programmed as a parallel session, the lecture was allocated a small auditorium in anticipation of a small turnout. We were packed! Now well into his eighties, the public Tom Szasz never lost his rhetorical "Wow!" factor. My earlier recollection was of a very different private Tom Szasz who, with his wife, joined us for lunch at our home in London. The occasion, as I recall, was a sunny Saturday and our three teenage children were also there. Having drawn so deeply on his *Myth of Mental Illness* in my early work in philosophical value theory, I was keen to engage our distinguished visitor in debate. But Tom was interested instead in my wife, Jane's, work as a teacher, and in our children's ambitions for the future.

There was no contradiction here. It was the private humanist Tom by whom the public rhetorical Tom was motivated. His thesis in *The Myth of Mental Illness* and subsequent publications was driven by a humanitarian concern for the adverse consequences for patients of a naively simplistic biomedical model of psychiatry. We should take that concern seriously. We should, though, by the same token, take no less seriously the antithetical humanitarian concerns of Szasz's critics. Appelbaum's and Gutheil's (1979) evocative image of patients "rotting with their rights on" precisely captures the adverse consequences for patients of a naively *anti*biomedical model. Thesis and antithesis are thus nicely reconciled in these equal and opposite humanitarian concerns. VBP is the synthesis that comes from taking Szasz seriously—and his critics, too.

Acknowledgment

Simon's story is based on one of a number of cases collected by Mike Jackson as part of his doctoral work and published with philosophical implications and a series of commentaries in Jackson and Fulford (1997).

References

American Psychiatric Association (APA). 2013. *Diagnostic and Statistical Manual of Mental Disorders [DSM-V]*, 5th edn. Arlington, Virginia: American Psychiatric Association.

Appelbaum, Paul S., and Thomas G. Gutheil. 1979. "'Rotting With Their Rights On': Constitutional Theory and Clinical Reality in Drug Refusal by Psychiatric Patients." *Bulletin of the American Academy of Psychiatry Law* **7** (3): 306–15.

Austin, John Langshaw. 1956–1957. "A Plea for Excuses." *Proceedings of the Aristotelian Society* **57**: 1–30.

Berlin, Isaiah. 1958. *Two Concepts of Liberty*. Oxford: Clarendon Press.

Bloch, Sidney, and Peter Reddaway. 1977. *Russia's Political Hospitals: The Abuse of Psychiatry in the Soviet Union*. London: Gollancz.

Boorse, Christopher. 1976. "What a Theory of Mental Health Should Be." *Journal for the Theory of Social Behavior* **6** (1) (April): 61–84.

Care Services Improvement Partnership (CSIP); National Institute for Mental Health in England (NIMHE). 2008a. *Three Keys to a Shared Approach in Mental Health Assessment*. London: Department of Health.

Care Services Improvement Partnership (CSIP); National Institute for Mental Health in England (NIMHE). 2008b. *Workbook to Support Implementation of the Mental Health Act 1983 as Amended by the Mental Health Act 2007*. London: Department of Health.

Collaborating Centre for Values-Based Practice in Health and Social Care, St. Catherine's College, Oxford. 2018. "Full Text Downloads." Accessed April 20, 2018. <valuesbasedpractice.org/more-about-vbp/full-text-downloads/>

Fulford, K.W.M. 1989. *Moral Theory and Medical Practice*. Cambridge: Cambridge University Press.

Fulford, K.W.M. 1994. "Closet Logics: Hidden Conceptual Elements in the DSM and ICD Classifications of Mental Disorders." In *Philosophical Perspectives on Psychiatric Diagnostic Classification*, edited by John Z. Sadler, Osborne P. Wiggins, and Michael A. Schwartz, pp. 211–32.

Fulford, K.W.M. 2000. "Teleology Without Tears: Naturalism, Neo-Naturalism and Evaluationism in the Analysis of Function Statements in Biology (and a Bet on the Twenty-First Century)." *Philosophy, Psychiatry, and Psychology* **7** (1) (March): 77–94.

Fulford, K.W.M. 2002. "Values in Psychiatric Diagnosis: Executive Summary of a Report to the Chair of the ICD-12/DSM-VI Coordination Task Force (Dateline 2010)." *Psychopathology* **35** (2–3) (March–June): 132–8.

Fulford, K.W.M. 2004. "Facts/Values: Ten Principles of Values-Based Medicine." In *The Philosophy of Psychiatry: A Companion*, edited by Jennifer Radden, pp. 205–34. Oxford: Oxford University Press.

Fulford, K.W.M. 2014. "Living with Uncertainty: A First-Person-Plural Response to Eleven Commentaries on Values-Based Practice." In *Debates in Values-Based Practice: Arguments*

For and Against, edited by Michael Loughlin, pp. 150–70. Cambridge: Cambridge University Press.

Fulford, K.W.M., Ed Peile, and Heidi Carroll. 2012. *Essential Values-Based Practice: Clinical Stories Linking Science with People*. Cambridge: Cambridge University Press.

Fulford, K.W.M., Sarah Dewey, and Malcolm King. 2015. "Values-Based Involuntary Seclusion and Treatment: Value Pluralism and the UK's Mental Health Act 2007." In *The Oxford Handbook of Psychiatric Ethics*, edited by John Z. Sadler, C.W. van Staden, and K.W.M. Fulford, Chapter 60. Oxford: Oxford University Press.

Hare, Richard Mervyn. 1952. *The Language of Morals*. Oxford: Oxford University Press.

Hare, Richard Mervyn. 1963. "Descriptivism." *Proceedings of the British Academy* 49: 115–34.

Jackson, Mike, and K.W.M. Fulford. 1997. "Spiritual Experience and Psychopathology." *Philosophy, Psychiatry and Psychology* 4 (1) (March): 41–66.

Johns, Louise C., and Jim van Os. 2001. "The Continuity of Psychotic Experiences in the General Population." *Clinical Psychology Review* 21 (8) (November): 1125–41.

Kendell, Robert Evan. 1975a. *The Role of Diagnosis in Psychiatry*. Oxford: Blackwell Scientific.

Kendell, Robert Evan. 1975b. "The Concept of Disease and Its Implications for Psychiatry." *British Journal of Psychiatry* 127 (October): 305–15.

Montgomery (Appellant) v Lanarkshire Health Board (Respondent) (Scotland). 2015. (March 11). Accessed April 16, 2018. <www.supremecourt.uk/cases/uksc-2013-0136.html>

Putnam, Hilary. 2004. *The Collapse of the Fact/Value Dichotomy and Other Essays*, revised edn. Cambridge, Mass.: Harvard University Press.

Sackett, David L., Sharon E. Straus, W. Scott Richardson, W., et al. 2000. *Evidence-Based Medicine: How to Practice and Teach EBM*, 2nd edn. Edinburgh: Churchill Livingstone.

Sadler, John Z. 2005. *Values and Psychiatric Diagnosis*. Oxford: Oxford University Press.

Szasz, Thomas S. 1960. "The Myth of Mental Illness." *American Psychologist*, 15 (2): 113–18.

Szasz, Thomas S. 1961. *The Myth of Mental Illness. Foundations of a Theory of Personal Conduct*. New York: Hoeber-Harper.

Szasz, Thomas S. 1963. *Law, Liberty, and Psychiatry: An Inquiry into the Social Uses of Mental Health Practices*. New York: Macmillan.

Szasz, Thomas S. 1984. *The Therapeutic State: Psychiatry in the Mirror of Current Events*. Buffalo: Prometheus.

Szasz, Thomas S. 2003. "Psychiatry and the Control of Dangerousness: On the Apotropaic Function of the Term 'Mental Illness'." *Journal of Medical Ethics* 29 (4) (August): 227–30.

Szmukler, George, and Frank Holloway. 1998. "Mental Health Legislation Is Now a Harmful Anachronism." *Psychiatric Bulletin* 22 (11) (November): 662–5.

Thornton, Tim. 2000. "Mental Illness and Reductionism: Can Functions Be Naturalized?" *Philosophy, Psychiatry, and Psychology* 7 (1) (March): 67–76.

Thornton, Tim. 2014. "Values-Based Practice and Authoritarianism." In *Debates in Values-Based Practice: Arguments For and Against*, edited by Michael Loughlin, pp. 50–61. Cambridge: Cambridge University Press.

Warnock, Geoffrey James. 1971. *The Object of Morality*. London: Methuen.

Williams, Arthur R., and Arthur L. Caplan. 2012. "Thomas Szasz: Rebel with a Questionable Cause." *Lancet* 380 (9851) (October 20): 1378–9.

Wing, John Kenneth, John Edward Cooper, and Norman Sartorius. 1974. *Measurement and Classification of Psychiatric Symptoms*. Cambridge: Cambridge University Press.

World Health Organization (WHO). 1992. *The ICD-10 Classification of Mental and Behavioural Disorders: Clinical Descriptions and Diagnostic Guidelines*. Geneva: World Health Organization.

Chapter 8

Schizophrenia: Sacred symbol or Achilles heel?

E. Fuller Torrey

8.1 Introduction

I first met Tom Szasz in 1966, when I was working in the state psychiatric hospital in Syracuse. I invited him to contribute a chapter to a book on medical ethics which I was editing, and he did so (Szasz, 1968a). I stayed in touch with him intermittently over the years and met him for lunch one year prior to his death. He was unfailingly good company—bright, witty, an excellent historian, certain that he was right, but sometimes wrong.

Szasz's early books—*The Myth of Mental Illness* and *Law, Liberty and Psychiatry*—influenced my thinking about what we call mental illness and what psychiatrists do. This was the 1960s, the zenith of psychoanalytic theory and practice in the United States, and an era of unlimited expectations regarding the role of psychiatrists. G. Brock Chisholm, the former Director-General of the World Health Organization and President of the World Federation of Mental Health, captured this hubris: "If the [human] race is to be freed from its crippling burden of good and evil, it must be psychiatrists who take the original responsibility . . . With the other human sciences, psychiatry must now decide what is to be the immediate future of the human race. No one else can. And this is the prime responsibility of psychiatry" (Chisholm, 1946).

Szasz argued logically that to be a mental illness, a condition must also be a brain disease, like syphilis of the brain. He disagreed passionately with the increasing psychiatrization of human behavior which was underway at that time and has continued ever since: "Psychiatric activity is medical in name only. For the most part, psychiatrists are engaged in attempts to change the behavior and values of individuals, groups, institutions and sometimes even of nations. Hence, psychiatry is a form of social engineering. It should be recognized as such." (Szasz, 1968b, p. vii).

The practice of outpatient psychiatry at that time focused predominantly on such problems as finding meaning in life, unfulfilled relationships, and exploration of unconscious thoughts—problems which Szasz called "problems in living" (Szasz, 1968b, p. 12). He also argued strongly against the use of psychiatric hospitalization for individuals who did not really have a mental illness. The American poet Ezra Pound, who was charged with nineteen counts of treason for his collaboration with the Italian government during World War II, was not brought to trial after the War but instead was confined for thirteen years in a government psychiatric hospital. Szasz used the

Pound case to illustrate his point. Szasz had most of his facts correct, except that he portrayed Pound as a political prisoner. In reality, Pound voluntarily conspired with the government's psychiatrists to be hospitalized in order to avoid going to trial, as I later demonstrated in my book about this case, *The Roots of Treason* (Torrey, 1984).

In 1974, I published *The Death of Psychiatry*, expanding on Szasz's ideas and recommending that problems in living be dealt with by psychologists, social workers, and other psychotherapists—not by psychiatrists. Individuals with true brain diseases would become the province of neurology, thereby leaving nothing for psychiatrists to do. Szasz contributed a cover comment, warmly praising the book as "a reasoned review of the mythology of mental illness . . . I commend his courage and recommend his book" (Torrey, 1974). I have always suspected that Szasz did not read the entire book, since I clearly stated that schizophrenia is a brain disease: "The evidence that these people have a true brain disease has become increasingly strong in recent years" (Torrey, 1974, pp. 158–9). I then went on to cite neurological studies as well as studies of the blood and spinal fluid pointing in this direction, and speculated that infectious agents might be the cause. Publicly and privately, Szasz and I would argue about this issue for the next thirty-eight years until his death.

8.2 **The reality of schizophrenia**

It is interesting to speculate why Szasz got caught off-base so badly regarding the nature of schizophrenia. He trained in psychiatry at the Chicago Institute for Psychoanalysis from 1951 to 1956. Like the majority of psychoanalytic institutes, most of the patients treated there had neuroses of various kinds, not schizophrenia or other psychoses. The director of the Institute at that time was Franz Alexander, whose main interest was in psychosomatic conditions. The associate director was Karen Horney, who specialized in theories of neuroses, especially revising Freud's ideas about penis envy and the Oedipal complex. There was apparently no psychoanalyst on the staff of the Institute with any interest in schizophrenia, such as Frieda Fromm-Reichmann or Silvano Arieti had at the William Alanson White Institute in New York.

It is thus quite possible that Szasz never diagnosed or treated any patient with schizophrenia. Szasz said in 1992: "I have never, ever given drugs to a mental patient" (Maugh, 2012), which would be consistent with his lack of patient experience. It would also explain some of his statements regarding the nature of schizophrenia, statements that appear fatuous in retrospect. For example: "The typical madman behaves the way he does because of his particular adaptation to the events that make up his life" (Szasz, 1994, p. 109). "Most people believe that psychotic persons have delusions and hallucinations, engage in senseless or unmotivated acts, and deny their illness. The truth is simpler and more painful. What psychotic persons do and say makes perfectly good sense, but it is so disturbing that we prefer not to hear or understand it" (Szasz, 1994, p. 182). "The facts are that, in the main, so-called madmen—the persons whom we now call schizophrenic and psychotic—are not so much disturbed as they are disturbing; it is not so much that they themselves suffer (although they may), but that they make others (especially members of their family) suffer" (Szasz, 1976, p. 36).

It is perhaps easiest to understand Szasz's views on schizophrenia as a product of his time, without the correcting factors of patient experiences or later learning which should have led him to revise his views. The theories about schizophrenia that were being taught when Szasz was receiving his psychiatric training were predominantly psychoanalytic. For example, the section on schizophrenia in the 1959 *American Handbook of Psychiatry* is almost completely psychodynamic in formulation. The "road leading to schizophrenia" is said to have "its beginning in the remote past of the patient, perhaps shortly after his birth" (Arieti, 1959, p. 468). This road was said to lead to a "schizophrenic mother," "marital skew," and other family problems which then produced the symptoms of schizophrenia in the unfortunate child. Although psychiatry had almost completely discarded such formulations by the 1990s, they apparently continued to shape Szasz's thinking.

Szasz, however, did acknowledge that diseases of the brain existed, and often used syphilis of the brain and epilepsy as examples. In *Schizophrenia: The Second Symbol of Psychiatry* (1976), he said that "a suspected brain disease does not become an actual brain disease until it is so proved by appropriate and consistently repeatable histopathological or pathophysiological findings" (Szasz, 1976, p. 110). Similarly, he said that a disease should be regarded as a disease only when the disease processes can be identified, reasoned, and demonstrated "in an objective, physicochemical manner" (Szasz, 1976, p. 4). In a letter to me (August 15, 1994), he acknowledged that "my view does not exclude the possibility that there [are] as yet undiscovered brain diseases (or perhaps discovered but not fully accepted or validated), and that some persons diagnosed as suffering from schizophrenia or manic-depression are the victims of a brain disease."

Since that time, the evidence has become overwhelming that schizophrenia is indeed a disease of the brain, involving multiple brain regions and the connections between them. Well over a hundred neuroimaging studies have reported the cerebral ventricles as being on average 15 percent larger in individuals with schizophrenia, compared to controls, suggesting the loss of brain tissue. Subtle neuroimaging and neuropathological abnormalities have been reported for several brain regions, especially the anterior insula. More than sixty neurological studies have reported that neurological abnormalities, especially what are referred to as "soft signs," occur much more frequently in individuals with schizophrenia than in matched controls. There have also been literally hundreds of studies of cognition in schizophrenia; the cognitive functions that are most often impaired in this disease are attention, certain types of memory, executive function (planning, problem solving, abstracting, etc.), and awareness of illness.

Brain abnormalities such as these have been reported in individuals with schizophrenia who have been treated with antipsychotic drugs, as well as in those who have never been treated. There is no single abnormality which is specific to schizophrenia as a diagnostic signature, but this is not unusual for brain diseases. For example, amyloid plaques in the brain are regarded as the hallmark of Alzheimer's disease, but such plaques can be found in some individuals with other brain diseases and even in some normal controls with no brain disease. Periodically, I would send Szasz published studies to try and convince him that schizophrenia met his criteria for being a brain disease. He would usually politely acknowledge receipt, but as he replied in one personal communication (August 15, 1994): "You probably cannot 'change' my mind, [but] you can certainly influence it."

8.3 The necessity of involuntary treatment

In addition to the reality of schizophrenia, the other issue which I discussed with Szasz was the occasional necessity for involuntary treatment. On this issue he felt very strongly, and I never really harbored any hopes of changing his mind. His strong feelings probably came in part from having grown up in Hungary under both Nazi and Communist regimes, which had influenced his libertarian views. However, his views had also been shaped by having never taken care of any patients who needed to be involuntarily hospitalized or treated. Allen Frances, in Chapter 13 of this volume, said that during his psychiatric training, Szasz "refused on principle to see involuntary, severely ill inpatients and focussed instead on his psychoanalytic training with relatively healthy outpatients." When Szasz was "faced with an ultimatum" that he must work with inpatients, according to Frances, Szasz left Chicago and went to Syracuse. Thus, in 1992 Szasz could boast: "I have never committed anyone" (Maugh, 2012).

Because Szasz had had no personal experience with psychiatric patients who had been involuntarily committed, he had no understanding of its necessity. In *Schizophrenia* he simply states that "the functions of the involuntarily hospitalization of the 'schizophrenic' is to relieve his relatives of the burden which he is to them" (Szasz, 1976, p. 23). His categorical opposition to all psychiatric involuntary hospitalizations led Szasz and two colleagues, in 1970, to establish the American Association for the Abolition of Involuntary Mental Hospitalization (AAAIMH), whose main activity was "securing help for individuals in need of legal assistance" to get out of the hospital (Szasz, 1998). It also led Szasz, in 1969, to join with Scientologists to form the Citizens Commission on Human Rights (CCHR). In retrospect, Szasz tried to justify this action by saying that Scientology was "the only organisation who had money and had some access to lawyers and were active in trying to free mental patients who were incarcerated in mental hospitals with whom there was nothing wrong, who had committed no crimes, who wanted to get out of the hospital. And that to me was a very worthwhile cause" (Szasz and Mitchell, 2009, p. 2). Szasz's association with Scientology has probably done more to undermine his reputation, and thus lose the benefit of his many useful ideas, than any other factor.

Finally, Szasz's categorical opposition to any involuntary psychiatric hospitalization has been used by others, especially civil liberties lawyers, to justify their actions. For example, Bruce Ennis, one of the original lawyers who formed the Mental Health Law Project (which later became the Bazelon Center), cited Szasz's writings as his original guide. In *Prisoners of Psychiatry* (1972), for which Szasz wrote the introduction, Ennis says that "the goal should be nothing less than the abolition of involuntary hospitalization" (Ennis, 1972, p. 232). Similarly, the seminal 1976 Lessard decision in Wisconsin (Lessard v. Schmidt), which made the involuntary hospitalization of psychiatric patients almost impossible, was brought by two young lawyers. One of them, Robert H. Blondis, explained to me that when he took on the case he "knew nothing about mental health law . . . I had read a few things, including Thomas Szasz's *The Myth of Mental Illness*, and that is where I was coming from" (Torrey, 2008, p. 77).

Szasz acknowledged that involuntary hospitalization was sometimes necessary for individuals with other diagnoses, such as "adults who are severely mentally retarded or who have been rendered temporarily or permanently unconscious, delirious, or demented by injury or illness" (Szasz, 1994, p. xiii). But he did not believe that any psychiatric patients fell into these categories. On occasion, I would send him information on how it is now known that half of all individuals with schizophrenia have lost the ability to recognize their own illness and are like individuals with Alzheimer's disease in this regard. In neurological terms, they have some degree of anosognosia. When I met with him one year prior to his death, I explained that we now had nineteen imaging studies showing that the brains of individuals with schizophrenia who have anosognosia are different than the brains of individuals with schizophrenia who are fully aware of their illness. Szasz just smiled politely. In retrospect, I realize that he was devoid of any framework to understand the problem, since he had had no firsthand experience with such patients.

8.4 **Dr. Szasz or Dr. Seuss**

In 1996, at Towson State University in Baltimore, I debated Szasz on "Serious Mental Illness: What Is It and What Should We Do About It?" As usual, I strongly urged him to recant his errors and publicly agree that schizophrenia is a legitimate brain disease. I said that his doing so would allow the next generation of mental health professionals to pay attention to his writings on the inappropriate psychiatrization of normal human behavior. I said that if he did so, he would be remembered as "a critic of American psychiatry, initially in error about schizophrenia, but he admitted his error, and was right about a lot of other issues." If he did not do so, I predicted that his legacy would be as the possible author of *The Cat in the Hat* (Seuss/Geisel, 1957), *Hop on Pop* (Seuss/Geisel, 1963), and *Horton Hatches the Egg* (Seuss/Geisel, 1940).

References

Arieti, Silvano. 1959. "Schizophrenia." In *American Handbook of Psychiatry*, edited by Silvano Arieti. New York: Basic Books.

Chisholm, G. Brock. 1946. "The Reestablishment of Peacetime Society: The Responsibility of Psychiatry." *Psychiatry* **9** (1) (February): 3–20.

Ennis, Bruce J. 1972. *Prisoners of Psychiatry: Mental Patients, Psychiatrists, and the Law.* New York: Harcourt Brace Jovanovich.

Lessard v. Schmidt. 1976. 413 F. Supp. 1318 (E.D. Wis.).

Maugh, Thomas H. 2012. "Dr. Thomas Szasz dies at 92: Psychiatrist Who Attacked Profession." *Los Angeles Times* (September 17). Accessed April 9, 2018. <articles.latimes.com/2012/sep/17/local/la-me-thomas-szasz-20120916>

Seuss, Dr. (pseudonym of Theodor Seuss Geisel). 1940. *Horton Hatches the Egg.* New York: Random House.

Seuss, Dr. (pseudonym of Theodor Seuss Geisel). 1957. *The Cat in the Hat.* New York: Random House.

Seuss, Dr. (pseudonym of Theodor Seuss Geisel). 1963. *Hop on Pop.*
New York: Random House.

Szasz, Thomas S. 1968a. "Problems Facing Psychiatry: The Psychiatrist as Party to Conflicts."
In *Ethical Issues in Medicine: The Role of the Physician in Today's Society*, edited by E. Fuller
Torrey, pp. 249–64. Boston: Little, Brown.

Szasz, Thomas S. 1968b. *Law, Liberty, and Psychiatry: An Inquiry into the Social Uses of Mental
Health Practices.* New York: Collier Books.

Szasz, Thomas S. 1976. *Schizophrenia: The Sacred Symbol of Psychiatry.* New York: Basic Books.

Szasz, Thomas S. 1994. *Cruel Compassion: Psychiatric Control of Society's Unwanted.*
New York: John Wiley & Sons.

Szasz, Thomas S. 1998. "The Abolitionist Archive" (July 21). Thomas S. Szasz Cybercenter for
Liberty and Responsibility. Accessed April 9, 2018. <www.szasz.com/abolitionist.html>

Szasz, Thomas S., and Natasha Mitchell. 2009. "All in the Mind: Thomas Szasz Speaks (Part 2
of 2)." (April 11). Accessed April 9, 2018. <www.abc.net.au/radionational/programs/
allinthemind/thomas-szasz-speaks-part-2-of-2/3138880#transcript>

Torrey, E. Fuller. 1974. *The Death of Psychiatry.* Radnor, Penn.: Chilton.

Torrey, E. Fuller. 1984. *The Roots of Treason: Ezra Pound and the Secret of St. Elizabeths.*
New York: McGraw-Hill.

Torrey, E. Fuller. 2008. *The Insanity Offense: How America's Failure to Treat the Seriously
Mentally Ill Endangers Its Citizens.* New York: Norton.

Chapter 9

Suicide prohibition: Shame, blame, or social aim?

James L. Knoll IV

9.1 Introduction and disclosures

Before beginning to comment on the substance of Szasz's final book, *Suicide Prohibition: The Shame of Medicine* (2011), especially its Chapter 4, I feel obliged to disclose fully my relationship to Szasz, who was a friend and colleague for many years. I readily acknowledge that I admired his intellect, passion for liberty, and fierce independence. At the same time, one could only argue with him on his own terms. This limited my ability to have a mutually exploratory dialogue with him, so I remained at the level of appreciating him in the abstract. That is to say, I saw him as an icon of independence and intellectual freedom.

Readers should not be surprised that Szasz was a beloved emeritus professor in the psychiatry department at SUNY Upstate. This owed largely to his passionate, yet collegial, cultivation of intellectual freedom. He devoted his life to independence of thought, and this was respected by his colleagues. Dating back to when he wrote *The Myth of Mental Illness*, he was instrumental in cultivating a departmental culture that embraced a variety of views and scholarly explorations. Ultimately, I chose to view Szasz as the torchbearer for the vital importance of protecting the diversity of thought in psychiatry.

Intellectual freedom seems all the more important upon cataloging the progress, or lack thereof, in psychiatry over the past fifty years. What will be discovered is a hegemonic exertion of psychiatric power or knowledge by so-called evidence-based medicine that caters primarily to biological psychiatry and the pharmaceutical industry (Robertson, 2005). As a hybrid profession of clinical science and humanities, however, psychiatry cannot flourish without the creativity fostered by intellectual freedom. Otherwise, it becomes merely what those in positions of power define it to be. Technical, empirical knowledge requires balance with what Jürgen Habermas calls "emancipatory cognition" or "emancipatory knowledge" (1971)—a process of critical reflection. To emancipate one's thinking is to think about what we think, why we think it, and what has influenced us to think this way.

Too few psychiatric "thought leaders" are now afforded the opportunity to engage in this type of speculative work. It neither pays well nor typically secures the research grant funding that academic psychiatry departments require to sustain themselves. Nevertheless, as "heroes of uncertainty" (Brooks, 2013), psychiatrists must rely on self-reflection, improvisation, and creativity—in addition to clinical research. I would like to believe that Szasz, the libertarian, valued emancipatory knowledge. He clearly understood that, without the balance of self-reflection provided by emancipatory knowledge, there is enslavement to scientism along with the potential for governmental misuse (Furedi et al., 2009).

In the last few years of his life, Szasz graciously gave some teaching sessions to my forensic psychiatry trainees. His Socratic discourse remained impressive even when he was ninety-two, just before his death. He spoke with a vast perspective and knowledge of history and literature. The exchanges between Szasz and my forensic fellows were, to me, endearing and illuminating. He put forth compelling arguments about power, control, and liberty. I always made sure to write down the potent statements he made during these sessions, that very day, before my memory faded. A number of his points still linger in my mind for a variety of reasons. One was: "Being alive is a great existential responsibility. We free or enslave ourselves with language." Another came when we began discussing *Suicide Prohibition*. He offered a premise that was hard to dispute: "Psychiatry has been yoked with the burden of controlling other people's suicidal and dangerous behavior." His second premise amounted to a complex, provocative assertion that could never be resolved in a single session: "This is a fraud, limits one's ability to help others, and is intellectually stifling." He capped all this off with a third premise, which seemed to be the motivating principle and distillation of his final book: "Suicide is a decision. It is an act of expression. We communicate all the time. Everything we do is an expression with meaning—and we should be free to do this."

A few preliminary comments about the title of this chapter seem warranted: By "shame," I refer not only to Szasz's book but also to the guilt induced by the internalized parent, otherwise known as the superego in psychoanalytic theory. "Blame" signifies the magical thinking seen in child development, wherein all tragic or unacceptable acts must, without fail, have a blameworthy scapegoat. This is particularly salient in the areas of community harm and psychiatric malpractice. Finally, by "social aim," I refer to the extant observing ego of a given society. Considering our undeniable interconnectedness as a species, there are certain human tragedies that are, arguably, shameful to ignore.

9.2 Suicide prohibition: Szasz's position

Szasz had previously explored the topic of suicide in his book *Fatal Freedom* (2002), but in *Suicide Prohibition* he placed the issue fully center stage, covering a broad range of suicide-related topics. His argument in support of the freedom to choose to die by suicide remained identical between the two books; specifically, that choosing to die by suicide is an intrinsic human experience and is simply *not* a medical problem. For the purposes of this discussion, I have chosen to focus primarily on Chapter 4 of *Suicide Prohibition*, "Separation: Emigration, Secession, Suicide" (Szasz, 2011, pp. 75–94). This chapter seems particularly meaningful, in terms of both suicide and Szasz's own personal history as an emigrant. As with virtually all of Szasz's work, the subject matter serves as a forum for emphasizing the significance of autonomy and freedom. In Chapter 4, though, Szasz analogizes suicide to emigration and secession. He reasons that the commonality between the two is an escape from "it"—meaning whatever it is that makes life seem intolerable. For Szasz, the act of suicide is to escape a life that is seen as worse than death, due to unendurable pain or perhaps the loss of autonomy that may come with advancing age, illness, or disability. Szasz would have this form of "emigration" also available to anyone who saw life as intolerable, whether due to physical illness or psychological turmoil.

In cases of psychological distress, Szasz's emigration analogy comes close to invoking the psychological "escape theory" of suicide (Baumeister, 1990), which has existed in some form since antiquity, mainly through Stoics such as Epictetus (Oates, 1957, pp. 264–8). This theory of suicide has been used to explain the suicidal individual's motivation to escape from aversive (excessively painful) self-awareness. When the drive to avoid painful emotions becomes strong enough, the individual experiences distorted judgment (cognitive deconstruction) that may lead to suicide or other self-destructive behaviors. In escape theory, the process of cognitive deconstruction involves rejection of meaning, increased irrationality, and disinhibition. Suicide then becomes the ultimate step in the effort to escape from meaningful awareness and its implications about the self. The thorny issue here is that escape via suicide comes about only if the individual's coping options or problem-solving abilities become overwhelmed, so that no viable solution can be perceived. This is a serious problem if we are concerned about whether the individual possesses the mental autonomy and freedom to make an irrevocable, life-ending decision. When Szasz uses the analogy of emigration, clearly a personal subject for him, he seems to express himself with a certain intellectual sincerity missing from the rest of the book. For example: "Interpreted as a kind of emigration, the suicide decides to move from the land of the living to the land of the dead. Viewed as a kind of secession, the suicide chooses to firmly separate himself from his family and society. Every emigrant knows from personal experience that it is painful to leave one's home and exchange one's mother tongue for a 'foreign' language" (Szasz, 2011, p. 77). These powerful passages use a persuasive analogy. Nevertheless, the analogy contains a decisive flaw.

In my view, the emigration analogy is handy but imprecise. It is not a good fit for the simple reason that emigration and separation are not the equivalent of death, which is irreversible. Szasz does not adequately analogize the irrevocable, life-negating reality of suicide. Indeed, the motive of emigration is typically altogether different and *life-affirming*. In the case of emigration, the leaver (or emigrant) is motivated by hopes for a better set of *life* circumstances, and this is the critical difference. In some cases, the emigrant may simply be seeking to broaden his or her experience of the world, to obtain better education, or to achieve more favorable financial circumstances. But in other cases, the emigrant may be literally fleeing his or her country due to intolerable circumstances, oppressive dictatorship, or threatened death. In all these cases, the common theme follows the pleasure principle—either avoid pain in some way or seek the pleasure of better circumstances. Not only does the emigrant hope to achieve a better set of circumstances *while living*, but he or she sometimes also has the option of returning to the country of origin at some future point. But death by suicide is infinitely final and precludes any return.

Alongside unilateral arguments in the name of autonomy are profound philosophical and existential issues. Szasz relies on his knowledge of psychoanalytic theory and social anthropology when he asks: "Why else would man create God, if not to love him and be loved by him in return? I suspect this point is why the gods of the monotheistic religions condemn suicide" (Szasz, 2011, p. 78). He explains his view that suicide prohibition is "God's command" to never abandon him, finally concluding that the divine prohibition of suicide represents our own fear of abandonment and loss of love from the internalized parent. Szasz's intellectual acumen is on display in his apparent concession that pure autonomy is an illusion: "Our sense of existence is intrinsically dialogic. We are social creatures through and through. Strictly speaking, there is no such thing as an independent, self-sufficient, autonomous individual. That fact does not render the term autonomous less useful. It requires only that we keep in mind that our need for autonomy is permanently at odds with our need for relationships with other human beings" (Szasz, 2011, p. 78, some italics added). We can view this statement in reference to the ubiquitous compromise formation—we all relinquish some portion of independence in exchange for something. But Szasz concedes some measure of interdependence with others. Further, he states that our freedom may run contrary to our relationships with others. Here, we reflect upon the impact on others of a decision to die by suicide and how well this squares with Szasz's admission of our interdependence. I argue this point more forcefully later, when I discuss communal harm.

Szasz reasons that suicide is exclusively a philosophical and moral problem, and as such it is not to be managed as a medical problem. The wealth of data from psychological autopsies over recent decades, finding that the vast majority of suicides are associated with serious mental health symptoms, impaired judgment, or substance dependence, would seem to militate against confining suicide purely to the realm of the philosophical (Simon, 2002; Maris et al., 2000, pp. 268–70, 319–20; Knoll, 2008, 2009). At best, we are left on shaky ground with the proposal of suicide as the autonomous, freely chosen act of an individual who is mentally competent to make such a decision.

9.3 My views on suicide and suicide prohibition

I partially agree with Szasz's analytic formulation suggesting that suicide prohibition has at least some of its origins in the fear of abandonment and loss of love from the internalized parental figure. I also partially agree with his suggestion about religious contributions to suicide prohibition; however, I argue that undergirding religious prohibitions were clear concerns about communal harm reduction (i.e., religious prohibitions cannot all be ascribed to unconscious fears).

As far back as ancient Greece and Rome, we find social, legal, and religious viewpoints on suicide that oscillated according to the zeitgeist (Lykouras et al., 2013). Suicide appears as a theme in Greek literature, mostly in connection with tragedies that invoked mortals' relationship to the gods (Laios et al., 2014). The Stoic philosopher Epictetus believed that suicide could be a reasonable choice if suffering were to become unbearable or if life became otherwise pointless (Oates, 1957, pp. 267–8). Yet ancient Greek philosophy addressed concerns about the impact of suicide on society. For example, Plato expressed a societal obligation in which suicide was inconsistent with the greater good (Plato, 1973, pp. 44–52, 1432; *Phaedo* 61e–69e, *Laws* 873c–e). Physicians in ancient Greece did not approve of suicide on principle and viewed the behavior as likely a manifestation of mental diseases, such as melancholia or mania. Indeed, they tried to use the medications of their time to assuage the mental suffering of suicidal persons. These treatments were primarily aimed at inducing calm mental states and involved plant-based drugs such as mandragora (Laios et al., 2014). Of course, the ancients recognized the motivations of those who chose to die by suicide to avoid capture, torture, or slavery. Yet these types of suicide were understood as fundamentally different from those induced by mental afflictions.

It was not until approximately the time of the ascendancy of Christianity that suicide came to be seen in the Western world as an act of betrayal (Luft, 2013). In the more widely accepted versions of the New Testament, Judas betrayed Christ and then took his own life by hanging himself. The origins of the word "betrayal" are of interest here—the root word *tradere* meaning to hand over, surrender, or break a trust or a contract. The underlying theme of the Judas story is disloyalty to a loving, blameless, parental figure. Yet early Christian objections to suicide were also concerned with communal harm as well as with betrayal, guilt, and personal fears. For example, Augustine's argument against suicide in Book I of *City of God* was partially an effort to stop the wholesale martyrdoms that were occurring at that time (Augustine, 1958, pp. 50–9; Mayo, 1986). The First Council of Braga (561) transformed suicide prohibition into canon law, mandating that the individual who committed suicide would be refused formal funeral rights.

History documents our apparent struggle to comprehend fully the reality of suicide, perhaps as evidenced by the fact that a generally accepted term for suicide (*suicidium*) did not emerge until the seventeenth century (Lykouras et al., 2013). Perhaps our struggle to comprehend continues to this day, as there remains a curious lack of standard nomenclature in the field of suicidology (Silverman, 2006). It may be too difficult to organize clearly and classify any human behavior with multiple, complex underpinnings. In psychiatry, we frequently rely upon the biopsychosocial model to conceptualize the many complex phenomena we encounter. This model was never meant to diagnose—rather, its place is to keep our awareness on the multidetermined nature of mental experiences. This necessarily results in a very broad consideration of an individual's life circumstances. When a profession, particularly a medical specialty, claims special expertise in an area, then that profession incurs duties (legal, clinical, or ethical) when practicing in that area. This presents complex problems for psychiatry, which has proclaimed its province of expertise to be the hydra-headed challenge of biopsychosocial *dis*-ease. In contrast, other fields of medicine are not typically held responsible for monitoring and changing psychological or social aspects of patients' life choices—in addition to treating any underlying biological processes.

9.4 **Social factors**

To speak about suicide without addressing social causes is akin to speaking about skin cancer without mentioning the sun. Social causes of suicide have been noted since the earliest recorded history and became a subject of social science theory with Émile

Durkheim (1966). Social factors associated with increased risk of suicide continue to be studied and catalogued. For example, Thomas Joiner's interpersonal theory of suicide proposes "thwarted belongingness" (2005, p. 23) as one of three key components leading to suicide. Social factors associated with an increased risk of suicide include various life crises such as loss of job, divorce, or legal or financial troubles (APA, 2003). Social factors may also act as so-called protective factors (decreasing the risk of suicide), such as having a stable, supportive spouse, having a good social support network, or being invested in a religious faith that dissuades suicide. Indeed, social factors have been gaining increased attention lately due to rising suicide rates in the United States.

Suicide appears to have increased relatively recently, even while overall mortality rates have been declining (Heron, 2016). According to the Centers for Disease Control and Prevention (CDC), suicide rates in the United States have been on the rise over the past decade, particularly among middle-aged adults (CDC, 2013; Curtin et al., 2016). The CDC does not offer any concrete explanations for this, but suggests the economy as a strong possibility. This would be consistent with historical observations of higher suicide rates during times of economic hardship. None of this would surprise Szasz, as he would view it as more self-evident data supporting the common-sense notion that suicide is an escape from an intolerable situation. Clearly, social science data support him in this view—to a point. We have only hypotheses about why so many who experience adverse social circumstances *do not* choose to die by suicide.

Edwin Arlington Robinson's famous poem "Richard Cory" (1897) reminds us of the conundrum of those who die by suicide despite their enviable social circumstances. This poem is believed to have been inspired by the Panic of 1893. The notion that a rich person in a highly desirable socioeconomic position would choose to kill himself is part of what gives the poem its shockingly dark appeal. We imagine that anyone would be happy in Cory's situation. We who envy him are left dumbfounded and alarmed when he kills himself. Yet this situation can and does occur in real life. It demands an explanation, which may be supplied on the prongs of the biopsychosocial model. Did Cory hide some unacceptable secret from the townspeople? Or did he labor under a crushing biological depression inherited from his family? Or was there an exogenous depression due to opium or cocaine abuse? Some combination of all three? We want, even need, an understanding. Make no mistake, *there is always an explanation*—whether we are able to find it or not. Every single family, every friend of a person who has lost someone to suicide, wants to understand why. I have never met anyone who was affected by someone's suicide who did not want to know why it happened. This brings us to another social aspect of suicide—the effects on the community.

Szasz makes clear that he believes the act of suicide should be undertaken only in private. Why? If done in public, he reasons, the behavior is "an interference with the everyday activities of others and a violation of their rights" (Szasz, 2011, p. 3). This key point leads us unswervingly toward concern about societal harm. Suicide prohibition is, and always has been, rooted in communal harm reduction. Too little research to date has focused on the impact of suicide on the decedent's social network (Cerel et al., 2008). What research exists tells us that the harm caused to others by an individual's suicide is substantial and includes complicated bereavement, depression, survivor guilt, and feelings of betrayal. This psychological trauma is in addition to social and often financial upheaval (McMenamy, Jordan, and Mitchell, 2008). While data is still accumulating on the effects of suicide on the decedent's extended social network, the data on close relatives is already impressive. Losing any first-degree relative to suicide increases a mourner's chance of suicide by about threefold (Agerbo, 2005). Losing a spouse to suicide increases one's risk of suicide some ten to sixteenfold (NAASP, 2015, p. 18). A number of studies have found elevated rates of suicide attempts and completions in children and adolescents who lost a parent to suicide (Burke et al., 2010; Kuramoto et al., 2013; Spiwak et al., 2011).

As my colleague Ron Pies has argued, there is a genuine and profound ethical obligation to consider the community at large involving suicide and *communal harm* (Pies, 2014). One's family, friends, and community bear the emotional and psychological burden of the aftermath of a death by suicide. This is one of the strongest arguments in favor of efforts to prevent suicide. Pies describes the clinical reality of depressed individuals, whose distorted judgment leads them to conclude irrationally that their loved ones would be better off without them—a view that is "virtually never shared by the patient's friends and family, who believe that their lives would be immeasurably diminished by the patient's death" (Pies, 2014). This real-world clinical example is familiar to mental health professionals, and it is difficult to argue that such distorted perception is the product of an autonomous mind that accurately knows reality. With Szasz's concession of our interdependence and his stance against public suicide in mind, I would extend the principle of communal harm reduction to include Robert Jay Lifton's concept of "species consciousness" (2011), which describes our sense of shared fate and our undeniable interconnectedness as evolved sentient beings on this planet. I imagine that Szasz understood this concept clearly, even acknowledging it by admitting that the truly independent, self-sufficient, autonomous individual is a myth. Tragedies such as war, natural disasters—and suicides—press us toward developing species consciousness and extending communal harm reduction beyond immediate social circles.

In light of this brief historical review of the Western view of suicide, it may be instructive to examine the views of our current supreme judicial power as they relate to suicide and societal interests. The closest the U.S. Supreme Court has come to an analysis of suicide prohibition can be found in the cases of Washington v. Glucksberg (1997) and Vacco v. Quill (1997). The Court ruled on these cases together. Both dealt with whether a state's ban on assisted suicide violated the Constitution. Specifically, in Washington v. Glucksberg, the issue was whether Washington's ban violated due process. In Vacco v. Quill, the issue was whether New York's ban violated equal protection. Thus, the cases together amounted to a two-pronged claim that the states' ban on assisted suicide violated the Fourteenth Amendment. The Court found that, in both cases, the states' banning of assisted suicide did not violate Fourteenth Amendment rights, but it made a critical distinction between *allowing* death versus *hastening* death. Whereas everyone has a constitutional right to allow death by refusing life-saving treatment in certain circumstances, as in Cruzan v. Missouri (1990), no one was permitted to hasten death by assisted suicide. The Court's reasoning about its general stance on suicide made clear that there are compelling government interests in preventing suicide. The term "compelling government interests" is legal code for something that the government considers so important that it outweighs individual rights. In the Court's consideration of assisted suicide, these interests include the preservation of life, the prevention of harm to society, and the protection of vulnerable populations (e.g., the elderly or the disabled). Thus, from at least the time of ancient Greece until now, suicide prohibition has been rooted in concerns about societal harm and protecting the vulnerable.

9.5 **In search of the rational suicide**

Schur, you remember our 'contract' not to leave me in the lurch when the time had come. Now it is nothing but torture and makes no sense.

Sigmund Freud to Max Schur (Gay, 2006, pp. 650–1)

Having discussed the biopsychosocial underpinnings of suicide, the communal harm caused by suicide, the Supreme Court's assertion of compelling government interest in preserving life, and an important distinction between allowing versus hastening death, the next question is whether suicide can be a rational act. Several key aspects of this important issue must be clarified: capacity, the current state of suicidology research, and legal competence to die by suicide. The law and courts must see the person as capable of practical reason and able to form and act on intentions (Morse, 2007). As law professor Stephen Morse notes, it could not be otherwise—or the law would be powerless to affect human action. This is precisely why "free will," or its lack, is not a criterion for any legal doctrine. Even in the case of "excusing" mental health laws, they are virtually all tests of rationality, not free will. The law does not deal with free will, but Szasz's libertarian arguments not only presuppose free will but also are substantiated upon it. It is surely to Szasz's advantage that the libertarian view of free will as "true" is the default view among lay people, in contrast to hard determinism or compatibilism (Schooler, 2010). The question of free will is a metaphysical problem, plagued by dualism, and remains elusive. While we can be certain that consciousness exists, when it comes to free will (or at least contracausal free will), philosophers are uncertain and neuroscientists express doubt (Searle, 2010; Harris, 2012).

It has been argued that language and culture are responsible for our awareness of the concept of free will (Baumeister et al., 2010). Culture requires individuals to conform their behavior to rules, which are created by the language of law. Making matters even more complex, social psychology research has shown that our beliefs about free will can be influenced by exposure to claims that science has disproven the existence of free will (Baumeister et al., 2010). Further, discouraging belief in free will can lead to increased amoral behavior. This has prompted researchers to speculate that "free will might be the *capacity* of consciousness to control, perhaps through effort or interpretation, which direction in time the next moment realizes" (Schooler, 2010, p. 211, italics added). But free will still hinges on the individual's "capacity," which will always be unique to each individual and may be subject to diminishment from a variety of factors.

It is no coincidence that the dualism seen in the free will problem can also be found in public attitudes toward suicide (Hewitt, 2013). While society accepts the rationale of suicide in response to intractable physical suffering, it rejects the behavior in response to psychological pain. Why might this be? Suicide has proven to be a traumatic phenomenon throughout history—one that engenders a range of emotional responses from curious ambivalence to abject horror and strident condemnation. On the one hand, seeing suicide as a rationally chosen act of free will allows us to conquer our fears in a seemingly logical manner that keeps inconvenient fears at bay. On the other hand, seeing suicide as the product of mental *dis-ease* that may be (to some unknown extent) beyond our control does no work toward assuaging our lingering doubts. This latter view either leaves us frightened and hopeless, or demands that we give the mind more attention and study. Clearly, the latter view is the path of greater difficulty, yet also one that promises greater reward in terms of discovery and growth. While the free will problem may not yet be solved, the compatibilist view of having some individualized "degrees of freedom" appears sound. Operating within this framework to understand the mind, suicidal or otherwise, provides less comforting exactitude but holds the potential for greater breadth and depth of understanding. This is how, paradoxically, eschewing the notion of hard libertarianism (or any other dogma for that matter) leads to greater intellectual freedom.

Given Szasz's views on suicide (and mental illness generally), one must conclude that he views suicide as a largely rational and autonomous act. Thus, we discuss so-called "rational suicide," starting with the classic Golden Gate Bridge study (Seiden, 1978), which traced 515 individuals who were restrained from jumping off the bridge to their deaths. Follow-up on these individuals many years later revealed that the vast majority (94 percent) were either still alive or had died of natural causes. This data emphasizes the impulsive nature of suicide. Another lesson from the Golden Gate Bridge study, as well as from clinical case studies, is that individuals may form plans to commit suicide, and even act on those plans, yet remain so ambivalent that impulsiveness in the final moment determines the outcome. The large body of suicidology research shows that the act of suicide is often undertaken in a transitory state of acute distress and impulsivity. Psychological autopsy research supports this, along with the fact that the vast majority of deaths by suicide are associated with such significant psychological turmoil that the individuals' judgment and perception of reality were markedly distorted at the time that they decided to take their own lives.

Rather than detail the results of over three decades of neurobiological research on suicide, let it suffice here to say that this research has focused on postmortem human brain tissue, peripheral tissues, and cerebrospinal fluid obtained from suicide victims. Although no single "lesion" has been found, as Szasz would likely demand, the research findings clearly show neurobiological as well as genetic differences in the brains of those who died by suicide, when compared to controls. Interested readers are encouraged to explore this rapidly advancing area of study (Pandey, 2013; Preti, 2011). Findings from a broad range of studies "using diverse designs and postmortem and *in-vivo* techniques show impairments of the serotonin neurotransmitter system and the hypothalamic-pituitary-adrenal axis stress-response system in the diathesis for suicidal behavior" (van Heeringen and Mann, 2014, p. 63; Almeida and Turecki, 2016; Oquendo et al., 2014). Further, the overwhelming evidence from medical and mental health research makes it virtually impossible to argue that rational suicide occurs with any significant frequency relative to all deaths by suicide. This argument alone calls into question the notion of lifting a prohibition against a behavior that (1) is almost never carried out in a rational state of mind, (2) is irreversible, and (3) carries significant communal harm.

While there is an abundance of research suggesting that mental and emotional impairment is associated with suicide (Hankoff, 1982; Robins, 1981), most of the literature on rational suicide deals with the subject in the hypothetical. The first generation of research to use the psychological autopsy technique found that more than 90 percent of individuals who completed suicide suffered from mental disorders, mostly mood disorders and substance use disorders (Simon, 2002; Maris et al., 2000). When suicides are carefully investigated by reviewing medical records, interviewing family, etc., finding a "rational" suicide will be a rare event, at best. Yet arguments persist that "contemporary opinion and public policy may have gone too far in seeing suicide as the product of mental illness" (Miller, 2016, p. 736). These arguments, typically raised in the context of concerns about psychiatric "coercion" and overreaching, generally tend toward the specious and assume that psychiatry somehow benefits from involuntarily detaining patients. It does not. In fact, psychiatric care is now a losing financial proposition for the vast majority of hospital systems. I have yet to meet a psychiatrist who does not loathe the proposition of having to commit a patient involuntarily. It often damages the treatment alliance and obligates the psychiatrist to defend the decision under cross-examination in court. It is viewed as an option of last resort—to prevent a patient from injuring self or others, to obtain emergently needed care for a patient, or, of course, to prevent legal liability that would be incurred by a tragic loss of life.

9.6 Competence to die by suicide?

I would like to clarify better the concept of competence and rational decision-making, and how it might relate to suicide. The word "competence" is a legal term of art defined as that degree of mental capacity required to carry out a specific decision-making task. In the law's view, there are many different types of competence, each with its own specific demands (e.g., competence to stand trial, to be executed, to make a will). In most cases, the law operates according to a presumption of competence—that is, competence is considered to be a rebuttable presumption. A common example in medicine is competence to make treatment decisions, which is sometimes called "treatment capacity." In New York, this capacity is "the patient's ability to factually and rationally understand and appreciate the nature and consequences of proposed treatment, including the benefits, risks, and alternatives to the proposed treatment, and to thereby make a reasoned decision about undergoing the proposed treatment" (New York Mental Hygiene Law, 2018, § 527.8). Many, if not most, substantive medical treatment decisions are simultaneously moral and ethical decisions. It is impossible to disentangle the rational, medical decision and its consequences from the associated ethical and moral decision. So, the notion of a medical decision as a pure logic, key-in-lock determination is an illusion. If one accepts that medical decisions are also moral and ethical decisions, one must also conclude that any life-sustaining-versus-negating decision must be made by a mind that is competent for that particular decision.

In organized medicine, physicians have always had to act in the best interests of patients. Part of doing so involves obtaining informed consent from patients, so that each patient is able to make better treatment decisions and to understand risks, benefits, and alternatives. The right to consent, an attribute of personal autonomy, is a fundamental ethical principle in medicine and was greatly strengthened by the Nuremberg Code. The doctrine of informed consent has three main elements: (1) provision of reasonable information needed to make the decision in question; (2) voluntariness on the part of the patient; and (3) mental competence on the part of the patient. I focus on the third element, because it stresses the fundamental concept that a person must have intact mental faculties and be free of any emotional or cognitive deficits that may have an adverse impact on the decision-making task at hand.

Indeed, the physician can go no further if it is suspected that the patient is not mentally competent to absorb and then act upon relevant information for making the decision. The test is not whether the patient decides as the physician believes that the patient should. Rather, to be competent to perform a given decision-making task, one must be capable of making a reasoned choice among alternatives (Appelbaum, 2007). An objective determination of whether an individual can make such a choice requires an assessment of the individual's ability to:

(1) *appreciate* his or her situation and its consequences (which requires awareness of illness, consequences of treatment refusal or acceptance, treatment risks and benefits, etc.);

(2) *understand* the relevant information needed to make the decision (which requires the ability to learn new information, keep attention intact, and concentrate);

(3) *communicate* a choice (which requires lack of ambivalence and the ability to communicate stable choices and maintain them long enough for them to be implemented); and

(4) *reason* by manipulating the relevant information in a rational, logical, and meaningful manner (Grisso and Appelbaum, 1998).

The underlying principles of competence to make treatment decisions and genuinely autonomous decision-making are of key importance in relation to any decision to end one's life. Surely one can apply each of the aforementioned four elements to suicidal individuals and see how many, if not most, of them will not possess the requisite capacity to make "rational" decisions to end their lives. If we require individuals to be competent to make decisions about financial matters, medical treatment, and legal issues, why do we falter when it comes to a life-or-death decision that is well-known to be often made in the context of distorted cognition and irrational judgment? We encounter the familiar problem of doubt about the individual's decision-making capacity, whether justified or not, whenever the specter of mental illness can be raised. A teaching anecdote may provide further clarification of this real-world issue. As a forensic psychiatry trainee, I was fascinated by an opening "teaser" question posed by my mentor, Phillip J. Resnick, whenever he gave his lecture on the right to refuse treatment. I will paraphrase the two scenarios he posed:

Scenario 1: A man with a history of heart disease is brought to the emergency room for chest pain. After a quick exam and blood work, it is determined that he has likely suffered another heart attack. The physician strongly recommends that the patient stay overnight in the hospital to be further evaluated and treated. The patient states he now feels fine and demands to leave. The man has no psychiatric history and his mental status is assessed as "within normal limits." The physician allows him to leave, but only after he signs himself out "against medical advice," which he promptly does.

Scenario 2: A woman is brought to the emergency room by ambulance after taking an overdose of Tylenol in a suicide attempt. She is treated for the overdose and is now medically stable. She acknowledges feeling sad due to a recent breakup with a boy-friend. She has a history of being treated for depression, three past suicide attempts, and borderline personality disorder. She begins demanding to leave the hospital and refuses to be admitted voluntarily to the psychiatric inpatient unit. Despite her angry demands to leave the hospital immediately, the emergency room psychiatrist signs a seventy-two-hour emergency hold and has her involuntarily admitted to the inpatient unit.

After presenting these cases to a variety of mental health audiences, Resnick would poll each audience for whether they agreed with the physician's decisions in each case. Typically, the vast majority would agree with the decisions. Next, Resnick would ask: "What is the difference between these two cases?" After fielding a barrage of nit-picky, off-topic questions demanding more information, Resnick would precisely clarify the crux of the lesson. In Case 2, the organ experiencing the disturbance was the same organ required to make an informed decision about accepting or refusing treatment. For virtually any mental health-related decision required of a patient, this is a common theme. The stumbling block frequently encountered in such situations involves a patient's denial of illness—also called a lack of insight into the illness. This may also affect a mentally ill patient's ability to make decisions about physical health. Insight into one's illness requires an *appreciation* of one's *situation* (i.e., realizing that one does, in fact, have an illness) and of the *consequences* of accepting or refusing treat-ment. Consider the individual who suffers from psychosis and refuses blood pressure medication despite having a blood pressure so high that he may have a stroke at any minute. He refuses treatment based on his belief that his blood pressure is fine and that all the high readings are part of a conspiracy to get him to take blood pressure medi-cation, which he believes will control his mind. This individual cannot be said to have made a competent and rational decision.

Next, consider the same psychotic patient who still does not believe that he suffers from high blood pressure, yet who agrees (for now) to take the blood pressure med-icine because the spirit of Daniel Webster has commanded him to do so. Again, this individual cannot be said to have competently made a treatment decision. Why does it matter? He has agreed to the treatment that his physician thinks is beneficial for him. The reason, in the eyes of the law, is that mere compliance does not vitiate the need for competence. Here it is important to distinguish between *assenting* to treatment and giving informed *consent*. *Assent* means mere willingness to accept the treatment. The patient may or may not have capacity to make such a decision about treatment. In other words, the patient acquiesces to treatment without having true legal capacity to do so. In contrast, *consent* implies that the patient is capable of informed consent and has legal capacity to make a decision about treatment. If mere assent is used to determine capacity, then evaluations of mental capacity become irrelevant, leading to an increased risk of improperly finding a patient to be capable of informed consent. The Supreme Court addressed this issue in Zinermon v. Burch (1990), holding that a psychiatric patient's constitutional (due process) rights were violated when he was allowed to sign into the hospital voluntarily, yet was incompetent to give informed consent to do so.

Some further details about Zinermon v. Burch may be enlightening. Darrell Burch was found by police wandering along a Florida highway in bad shape. He was taken to a mental health facility where he was found to be bloodied, bruised, hallucinating, confused, and believing he was "in heaven." He was asked to sign forms giving his consent to admission and treatment, which he did. He remained at the facility three days, was diagnosed with paranoid schizophrenia, and given antipsychotic medication. A bit later, it was determined that Burch needed continued hospitalization, and he was referred to Florida State Hospital (FSH). Upon referral, he again signed forms requesting voluntary admission. Once at FSH, Burch signed other forms for voluntary admission and treatment. The forms contained the proviso that his voluntary admission would be "in accordance with the provisions of expressed and informed consent" (Zinermon v. Burch, 1990, at 119). Dr. Zinermon's FSH notes stated that Burch refused to cooperate, would not answer questions, and appeared "distressed" and "confused." A nursing assessment indicated Burch was confused, unable to state the reason for his hospitalization, and still believed that he was "in heaven." Subsequent records described Burch as extremely psychotic, paranoid, and hallucinating. Burch remained at FSH for five months, receiving treatment that resulted in improvement. However, no hearing was ever held regarding his hospitalization or treatment. After his release, he complained that he had been admitted inappropriately and did not remember signing voluntary admission forms. His complaint reached the Florida Human Rights Advocacy Committee, which investigated his complaint. Burch filed a federal civil rights (42 U.S. Code § 1983) complaint alleging that the defendants knew, or should have known, that he was incompetent to give informed consent, and that their failure to initiate Florida's involuntary commitment procedure denied him constitutionally guaranteed procedural safeguards. Ultimately, the Supreme Court held that it was foreseeable that persons requesting treatment might be incapable of informed consent, and only hospital staff are in a position to ensure that proper procedures and safeguards are afforded to those unable to give consent. The requirement that a patient be competent to consent and to make treatment decisions is well established.

Szasz seems not to acknowledge adequately the foregoing issues of decision-making competence in the setting of mental illness. This is because he did not accept mental illness as real in the sense that cancer is real. In his view, the individual should be free to make poor, ill-informed, or impulsive decisions. In a video of Szasz lecturing that I use for teaching purposes, he states: "I am entirely in favor of psychiatric acts between consenting adults . . . You want a lobotomy? Have one. Electric shock? Have one. I believe in freedom—and responsibility. But it should be your decision. And preferably, you should know what you are doing. But if not, that's your problem." This is, in a sense, almost a social Darwinian view, or at the very least, an evolutionary psychology perspective. It is as if Szasz implies that if one's genetic burden cannot be overcome by efforts to inform oneself better, then dying by suicide may serve the purpose of reducing the likelihood of passing on one's "problem" decision-making to future generations (Shackelford and Liddle, 2014).

But perhaps, with this last hypothesis, I have gone too far and speculate too recklessly. Szasz makes clear in *Suicide Prohibition* that suicide is only "a moral and political problem" (2011, p. x). Let us assume that Szasz is correct about this. Even within this one-dimensional (perhaps inaccurate) viewpoint, intervening to prevent a suicide that flows from impulsive or flawed reasoning "where the person has temporarily lost capacity for autonomy . . . is likely to be *morally* justified" (Hewitt, 2013, p. 362, italics added). It is well known that a suicidal individual's capacity for autonomous thought and action is likely to fluctuate and sometimes become erratic. Cases involving death by suicide where the decedent lost contact with reality or otherwise had an unrealistic appreciation of present or future circumstances would be considered prima facie irrational, and thus not autonomous acts. Mental health professionals are quite familiar with cases "of persons who, in acute psychological distress caused by crisis . . . impulsively wished to die, but whose desires were rescinded once the acute nature of the crisis had passed" (Hewitt, 2013, p. 362). Consider the following real-world case from my personal forensic files. The details are modified to preserve privacy, although the case was made public due to litigation:

Case study: A bright and accomplished young public servant in his late twenties suddenly begins to act and speak oddly. Friends and family describe him as acutely different, fearful, and obsessed. He is obsessed with his newfound conviction that humanity teeters on the brink of annihilation due to religious and spiritual forces. He proclaims to his family and colleagues: "It is the eleventh hour! I must die to save humanity. I have been told by God that I must sacrifice myself. Humanity dies unless I am dead by sunrise!" After first attempting to kill himself by violently smashing his head into a metal structure, he is rushed to a hospital for treatment of his skull fracture. He remains agitated, paranoid, and expresses an urgency that he must die as soon as possible because the fate of humanity is at stake. Not long after he is placed on the hospital floor awaiting further treatment, he asphyxiates himself by tying bed linens around his neck.

Staying inside the bounds of our artificial thought experiment on suicide as a purely moral problem, we could persuasively argue that to abandon such individuals would be morally impermissible. In essence, even if one argues that suicide is a purely moral problem, there remain strong and persuasive reasons for its prohibition. But, in the final analysis, what is *rational* often ends up being what is *normative*. While many would argue that suicidal thinking flowing from an acute emotional or mental crisis is "rightly not considered relevant to any discussion of rational suicide" (Hewitt, 2013, pp. 362–3), others might argue that this is irrelevant if freedom and autonomy have primacy. Many decisions have been made that were not normative or reasonable for their time, yet could be said to have resulted in a justifiable outcome. So the question becomes: must we require all decisions to be rational, and therefore normative? We can sidestep this slippery slope with a simple disclaimer—we require any irrevocable, life-or-death decision to be made by a mind that can comprehend reality-based consequences. A decision outside the norm may be made, but it must first be held up to the yardstick of the normative, and the decision-maker must demonstrate mental competence and intelligible reasoning. Such is presently the case with physician-assisted suicide in the United States, as well as the (troubling) cases of assisted suicide for individuals "suffering from 'incurable, permanent, severe psychological disorders'" in places such as Switzerland (Appel, 2007, p. 21).

9.7 Lethal drug prescription for psychiatric patients

A currently evolving subject, internationally, is so-called physician-assisted suicide (PAS), also referred to as physician-assisted death (PAD). In *Fatal Freedom* (2002), Szasz considers the term PAS as a euphemism. Some medical ethicists also consider the nearly synonymous term PAD a euphemism (Pies, 2016). Again, I agree with Szasz. The euphemistic quality of these terms deserves comment. Both PAS and PAD, from a linguistic standpoint, misstate and obfuscate the concrete reality of what is actually being done. The physician is not giving support, help, or aid to the patient. Rather, the physician uses prescribing power to give a patient a lethal drug. Thus, the term lethal drug prescription (LDP) seems to capture the reality of the situation more accurately.

What makes the recent LDP movement unique is that LDP is offered (outside the United States) to those suffering only from chronic psychiatric illnesses (Varelius, 2016). Proponents argue that hopelessness and the desire to end one's life are not necessarily a result of mental illness (Duffy, 2015). Further, they argue that, even when an individual suffers from mental illness, a decision to die by suicide can still be "rational." In the United States, mental illness is prohibitive of LDP, whereas it may be a valid reason for LDP in other countries. The central problem is how to ensure that the suffering organism possesses the capacity to decide to extinguish itself. A secondary, yet equally serious problem, lies in ensuring that the mental illness in question is permanently unresponsive to treatment that might alleviate suffering.

The Royal Australian and New Zealand College of Psychiatrists recommends mandatory psychiatric assessment and would preclude LDP for patients suffering exclusively from a mental disorder. They cite the problem of ensuring capacity, as well as the rarity of genuinely unassuageable psychiatric suffering. Other problems not likely to be resolved soon include (1) the lack of a widely accepted capacity assessment for LDP, (2) absence of any legally defined test for capacity to consent to LDP which would clearly distinguish depressive symptoms from a "rational" wish to die, and (3) the fallibility of evaluators. Regarding this last problem, it seems worthwhile to consider carefully how many psychiatric evaluators have the confidence to distinguish a mental disorder impairing judgment from an existential motivation. Further—for those who claim to possess the confidence—how will they arrive at their opinions and how can we be assured that their determinations are not value-driven or morality-based? The possibility of psychiatrists reliably distinguishing mental from existential suffering suggests the possibility of wandering into a morass of fundamentally subjective determinations.

9.8 **Conclusions**

The struggle itself toward the heights is enough to fill a man's heart. One must imagine Sisyphus happy.–

Camus (1955, p. 91)

Already far outside the bounds of the complex, highly nuanced reality of suicide, I will continue along the winding trail of this imaginary exercise to see if it might lead to a clearing in the woods. I hope that I have left enough bread crumbs along the way to allow for an eventual return to the real world. But for now, assume, as a final thought experiment, the existence of a truly free, rational, and purely autonomous suicide. We find ourselves in a clichéd and rarified condition: sitting in a café—perplexed, not by any significant psychological turmoil, but by the *ennui* of a privileged, intellectual life. We turn the dilemmas of the absurd nature of human existence over and over in our minds, as though examining two sides of a coin. A question arises, not from sudden enlightenment, but from annoyance: Should I kill myself, or have a cup of coffee?

Camus answers this question in *The Myth of Sisyphus*. I would argue that he answers it in a way that has yet to be surpassed. He reasons that this question can only be addressed from a starting point of absolute intellectual honesty. If this is not possible, then go no further. However, if we are willing to be intellectually honest about the human condition, then we cannot avoid confronting the realization that it is absurd, futile, and ends in death without escape. For Camus, to continue living while pretending that life is not absurd amounts to evasion and denial. In fact, he would judge a decision to die by suicide instead of having a cup of coffee as just another form of evasion. How so? Because, by choosing suicide, not only do we proceed to an unknowable situation, but more importantly, we *have done no work toward changing the absurd nature of life*. Therefore, Camus posits that the only viable solution is to live fully conscious of this entire predicament. We strive to live fully conscious of the absurd nature of life, even rebelling in a sense against nihilistic fatalism. In doing so, we thereby achieve personal satisfaction by having transcended the entire struggle.

In sum, I am in partial agreement with Szasz's psychoanalytic formulation of suicide prohibition, insofar as it relates to some of the moral restrictions imposed by religion. Here, I specifically refer to Szasz's assertion that there may be a psychodynamic element in suicide prohibition where the need for love and protection from a powerful parental figure is concerned (Freud, 1950). A psychodynamic view may encompass our need to restrain violent impulses to achieve a functional civilization (Freud, 1961), despite the origins of religious anti-suicide efforts in communal harm reduction. Although *Suicide Prohibition* raises many fine philosophical and linguistic issues, Szasz's position contains too many flaws. Even viewing the issue on his terms and setting aside the growing body of suicidology research, I find that the book charges forcefully ahead with libertarian idealism, while ignoring critical moral and ethical issues. This could be the fatal flaw of hard libertarianism in general: Where does one draw the line between the ideal of liberty and the communal harm resulting from a failure to intervene in others' lives? Psychiatrists are all too familiar with this dilemma. We struggle with it daily. We are maligned for our role in it, and any praise we receive seems quite infrequent and muted by societal stigma.

We all want freedom. We psychiatrists also want psychological freedom for those whom we treat. But as the Supreme Court has put it: "One who is suffering from a debilitating mental illness and in need of treatment is neither wholly at liberty nor free of stigma" (Addington v. Texas, 1979, at 429). A person in the throes of acute psychological crisis, unable to think rationally, or laboring under a distorted perception of reality, cannot be said to be free, but is a prisoner of a mental dictatorship, where the concepts of liberty and autonomy are held captive as dissidents. Is this person "truly free" if we do not intervene? Or autonomous if we allow that mental dictatorship which may abruptly demand his or her execution? I agree with Szasz that the issue of suicide goes straight to the core of the human condition. This is so because of suicide's tragedy, absurdity, and the fears it produces about all that is uncertain with the human mind. But Szasz assumes that all suicide is the freely chosen act of a rational mind. With this stance, he has walked too far out onto his contrarian plank. The subject of suicide is too complex to resolve by confining it to the hammer-or-anvil test of autonomy versus paternalism. However, the fact that he is at odds here with nearly all suicidology research, most moral philosophers, and even the Supreme Court, would not likely faze the Szasz I knew. He took the subject of freedom more seriously than the most strident constitutional lawyers and remained true to his ideals his entire life.

References

Addington v. Texas. 1979. 441 U.S. 418.

Agerbo, Esben. 2005. "Midlife Suicide Risk, Partner's Psychiatric Illness, Spouse and Child Bereavement by Suicide or Other Modes of Death: A Gender Specific Study." *Journal of Epidemiology and Community Health* **59** (5) (May): 407–12.

Almeida, Daniel, and Gustavo Turecki. 2016. "A Slice of the Suicidal Brain: What Have Postmortem Molecular Studies Taught Us?" *Current Psychiatry Reports*, **18** (11) (November): 98. Accessed April 17, 2018. <link.springer.com/article/10.1007%2Fs11920-016-0736-8>

American Psychiatric Association (APA). 2003. *Practice Guideline for the Assessment and Treatment of Patients with Suicidal Behaviors*. Washington D.C.: American Psychiatric Association.

Appel, Jacob M. 2007. "A Suicide Right for the Mentally Ill? A Swiss Case Opens a New Debate." *Hastings Center Report* **37** (3) (May–June): 21–3.

Appelbaum, Paul S. 2007. "Assessment of Patients' Competence to Consent to Treatment." *New England Journal of Medicine* **357** (November 1): 1834–40.

Augustine. 1958. *City of God*, translated by Gerald G. Walsh, et al., edited by Vernon J. Bourke. Garden City, New York: Doubleday Image.

Baumeister, Roy F. 1990. "Suicide as Escape from Self." *Psychological Review* **97** (1) (January): 90–113.

Baumeister, Roy F., Alfred R. Mele, and Kathleen D. Vohs (eds.). 2010. *Free Will and Consciousness: How Might They Work?* New York: Oxford University Press.

Brooks, David. 2013. "Heroes of Uncertainty." *New York Times* **A19** (May 27).

Burke, Ainsley K., Hanga Galfalvy, Benjamin Everett, et al. 2010. "Effect of Exposure to Suicidal Behavior on Suicide Attempt in a High-Risk Sample of Offspring of Depressed

Parents." *Journal of the American Academy of Child and Adolescent Psychiatry* **49** (2) (February): 114–21.

Camus, Albert. 1955. *The Myth of Sisyphus and Other Essays*, translated by Justin O'Brien. New York: Vintage.

Centers for Disease Control and Prevention (CDC). 2013. "Suicide Among Adults Aged 35–64 Years—United States, 1999–2010." *Morbidity and Mortality Weekly Report (MMWR)* **62** (17) (May 3): 321–5.

Cerel, Julie, John R. Jordan, and Paul R. Duberstein. 2008. "The Impact of Suicide on the Family." *Crisis* **29** (1): 38–44.

Cruzan v. Director, Missouri Department of Health. 1990. 497 U.S. 261.

Curtin, Sally C., Margaret Warner, and Holly Hedegaard. 2016. "Increase in Suicide in the United States, 1999–2014." *NCHS Data Brief* (241) (April): 1–8.

Duffy, Olivia Anne. 2015. "The Supreme Court of Canada Ruling on Physician-Assisted Death: Implications for Psychiatry in Canada." *Canadian Journal of Psychiatry* **60** (12) (December): 591–6.

Durkheim, Émile. 1966. *Suicide: A Study in Sociology*, translated by John A. Spaulding and George Simpson. New York: Free Press.

Freud, Sigmund. 1950. *Totem and Taboo*, translated by James Strachey. New York: W.W. Norton.

Freud, Sigmund. 1961. *The Future of an Illusion*, translated by James Strachey. New York: W.W. Norton.

Furedi, Frank, Roger Kimball, Raymond Tallis, and Robert Whelan. 2009. *From Two Cultures to No Culture: C.P. Snow's "Two Cultures" Lecture Fifty Years On*. London: Civitas. Accessed April 18, 2018. <www.civitas.org.uk/pdf/TwoCulturesMar09.pdf>

Gay, Peter. 2006. *Freud: A Life for Our Time*. New York: W.W. Norton.

Grisso, Thomas, and Paul S. Appelbaum. 1998. *MacArthur Competence Assessment Tool for Treatment (MacCAT-T)*. Sarasota: Professional Resources Press.

Habermas, Jürgen. 1971. *Knowledge and Human Interests*, translated by Jeremy J. Shapiro. Boston: Beacon Press.

Hankoff, Leon D. 1982. "[Review]: *The Final Months: A Study of the Lives of 134 Persons Who Committed Suicide*, by Eli Robins." *JAMA* **247** (12) (March 26): 1765–6.

Harris, Sam. 2012. *Free Will*. New York: Free Press, Simon and Schuster.

Heron, Melonie. 2016. "Deaths: Leading Causes for 2013." *National Vital Statistics Reports* **65** (2) (February 16): 1–95.

Hewitt, Jeanette. 2013. "Why Are People with Mental Illness Excluded from the Rational Suicide Debate?" *International Journal of Law and Psychiatry* **36** (5–6) (September–December): 358–65.

Joiner, Thomas E. 2005. *Why People Die by Suicide*. Cambridge, Mass.: Harvard University Press.

Knoll, James L. 2008. "The Psychological Autopsy, Part I: Applications and Methods." *Journal of Psychiatric Practice* **14** (6) (November): 393–7.

Knoll, James L. 2009. "The Psychological Autopsy, Part II: Toward a Standardized Protocol." *Journal of Psychiatric Practice* **15** (1) (January): 52–9.

Kuramoto, Satoko Janet, Bo Runeson, Elizabeth A. Stuart, et al. 2013. "Time to Hospitalization for Suicide Attempt by the Timing of Parental Suicide During Offspring Early Development." *JAMA Psychiatry* **70** (2) (February): 149–57.

Laios, Konstantinos, Gerry Tsoukalas, M.-I. Kontaxaki, et al. 2014. "Suicide in Ancient Greece." *Psychiatriki* **25** (3) (July–September): 200–7.

Lifton, Robert Jay. 2011. *Witness to an Extreme Century: A Memoir.* New York: Free Press, Simon and Schuster.

Luft, Eric v.d. 2013. *The Value of Suicide.* Part I, "Suicide as a Practical Philosophical Problem"; Part II, Chapter 3, "Murdering God's Servant." North Syracuse, New York: Gegensatz Press.

Lykouras, Lefteris P., Elefteria-Fotini Poulakou-Rebelakou, et al. 2013. "Suicidal Behaviour in the Ancient Greek and Roman World." *Asian Journal of Psychiatry* **6** (6) (December): 548–51.

Maris, Ronald W., Alan Lee Berman, and Morton M. Silverman. 2000. *Comprehensive Textbook of Suicidology.* New York: Guilford.

Mayo, David J. 1986. "The Concept of Rational Suicide." *Journal of Medicine and Philosophy* **11** (2) (May): 143–55.

McMenamy, Jannette M., John R. Jordan, and Ann M. Mitchell. 2008. "What Do Suicide Survivors Tell Us They Need? Results of a Pilot Study." *Suicide and Life-Threatening Behavior* **38** (4): 375–89.

Miller, Franklin G. 2016. "[Review]: *Rational Suicide, Irrational Laws: Examining Current Approaches to Suicide in Policy and Law,* by Susan Stefan." *American Journal of Psychiatry* **173** (7) (July 1): 736–7.

Morse, Stephen J. 2007. "The Non-Problem of Free Will in Forensic Psychiatry and Psychology." *Behavioral Sciences and the Law* **25** (2): 203–20.

National Action Alliance for Suicide Prevention (NAASP). Survivors of Suicide Loss Task Force. 2015. *Responding to Grief, Trauma, and Distress after a Suicide: U.S. National Guidelines.* "Research on the Impact of Suicide," pp. 18–20. Accessed April 16, 2018. <actionallianceforsuicideprevention.org/sites/actionallianceforsuicideprevention.org/files/NationalGuidelines.pdf>

New York Codes, Rules, and Regulations. Mental Hygiene Law. Part 527. Rights of Patients. 527.8. Care and Treatment; Right to Object. 2018. Accessed April 18, 2018. <govt.westlaw.com/nycrr/Document/I50362336cd1711dda432a117e6e0f345?transitionType=Default&contextData=(sc.Default)>

Oates, Whitney J. (ed.). 1957. *The Stoic and Epicurean Philosophers: The Complete Extant Writings of Epicurus, Epictetus, Lucretius, Marcus Aurelius.* New York: Modern Library.

Oquendo, Maria A., Gregory M. Sullivan, Katherin Sudol, et al. 2014. "Toward a Biosignature for Suicide." *American Journal of Psychiatry* **171** (12) (December 1): 1259–77.

Pandey, Ghanshyam. 2013. "Biological Basis of Suicide and Suicidal Behavior." *Bipolar Disorders* **15** (5) (August): 524–41.

Pies, Ronald. 2014. "Suicide and Communal Values: Ethical Implications for Psychiatrists." *Medscape Psychiatry* (January 27). Accessed April 18, 2018. <www.medscape.com/viewarticle/819565_1>

Pies, Ronald. 2016. "Physician-Assisted Suicide and the Rise of the Consumer Movement." *Psychiatric Times,* **32** (8) (August): 40–3. Accessed April 17, 2018. <www.psychiatrictimes.com/couch-crisis/physician-assisted-suicide-and-rise-consumer-movement>

Plato. 1973. *The Collected Dialogues, Including the Letters,* edited by Edith Hamilton and Huntington Cairns. Princeton: Princeton University Press.

Preti, Antonio. 2011. "Animal Model and Neurobiology of Suicide." *Progress in Neuropsychopharmacology and Biological Psychiatry,* **35** (4) (June 1): 818–30.

Robertson, Michael. 2005. "Power and Knowledge in Psychiatry and the Troubling Case of Dr. Osheroff." *Australasian Psychiatry* **13** (4) (December): 343–50.

Robins, Eli. 1981. *The Final Months: A Study of the Lives of 134 Persons Who Committed Suicide.* New York: Oxford University Press.

Robinson, Edwin Arlington. 1897. "Richard Cory." Accessed April 18, 2018. <www.poetryfoundation.org/poems-and-poets/poems/detail/44982>

Schooler, Jonathan W. 2010. "What Science Tells Us about Free Will." In *Free Will and Consciousness: How Might They Work?* edited by R. Baumeister et al., pp. 191–218. Oxford: Oxford University Press.

Searle, John R. 2010. "Consciousness and the Problem of Free Will." In *Free Will and Consciousness: How Might They Work?* edited by R. Baumeister et al., pp. 121–34. Oxford: Oxford University Press.

Seiden, Richard H. 1978. "Where Are They Now? A Follow-Up Study of Suicide Attempters from the Golden Gate Bridge." *Suicide and Life-Threatening Behavior* **8** (4) (Winter): 203–16.

Shackelford, Todd K., and James R. Liddle. 2014. "Understanding the Mind from an Evolutionary Perspective: An Overview of Evolutionary Psychology." *Wiley Interdisciplinary Reviews: Cognitive Science* **5** (3) (May): 247–60.

Silverman, Morton M. 2006. "The Language of Suicidology." *Suicide and Life-Threatening Behavior* **36** (5) (October): 519–32.

Simon, Robert I. 2002. "Murder, Suicide, Accident, or Natural Death? Assessment of Suicide Risk Factors at the Time of Death." In *Retrospective Assessment of Mental States in Litigation: Predicting the Past*, edited by Robert I. Simon and Daniel W. Shuman, pp. 135–53. Washington, D.C.: American Psychiatric Publishing.

Spiwak, Rae, Jina Pagura, James M. Bolton, et al. 2011. "Childhood Exposure to Caregiver Suicidal Behavior and Risk for Adult Suicide Attempts: Findings from a National Survey." *Archives of Suicide Research* **15** (4): 313–26.

Szasz, Thomas S. 2002. *Fatal Freedom: The Ethics and Politics of Suicide, with a New Preface.* Syracuse: Syracuse University Press.

Szasz, Thomas S. 2011. *Suicide Prohibition: The Shame of Medicine.* Syracuse: Syracuse University Press.

Vacco v. Quill. 1997. 521 U.S. 793.

van Heeringen, Kees, and J. John Mann. 2014. "The Neurobiology of Suicide." *Lancet Psychiatry* **1** (1) (June): 63–72.

Varelius, Jukka. 2016. "On the Moral Acceptability of Physician-Assisted Dying for Non-Autonomous Psychiatric Patients." *Bioethics* **30** (4) (May): 227–33.

Washington v. Glucksberg. 1997. 521 U.S. 702.

Zinermon v. Burch. 1990. 494 U.S. 113, 110 S.Ct. 975.

Chapter 10

Myths, projections, and overextensions: The conceptual landscape of Thomas Szasz

Jennifer Church

10.1 Introduction

Thomas Szasz claimed that his writings belong to neither psychiatry nor antipsychiatry: "They belong to conceptual analysis, social-political criticism, civil liberties, and common sense" (Szasz, 2010, p. xxix).[1] Whether or not Szasz's self-description makes him more philosopher than psychiatrist, as many have suggested, it serves as an invitation to philosophically minded readers to take his conceptual analysis a step further, and to interrogate the normative basis for his politics.[2]

When, as a college student, I first read *The Myth of Mental Illness*, I had just heard that my cousin was schizophrenic and about to be committed to a mental institution. I read that up to 10 percent of Americans suffer from schizophrenia. An acquaintance who did mental health counseling told me that "schizophrenia" is defined as "unclear thinking." These factors—being a college student, being upset about my cousin, being skeptical about the statistics, recognizing the inadequacy of the definition—primed me to be sympathetic to Szasz's message. But I did not give much thought to what it means to claim that mental illness is a *myth*. As far as I was

---

[1] Also, in Szasz (1994): "My critique of psychiatry is two-pronged, partly conceptual, partly moral and political. At the core of my conceptual critique lies the distinction between the literal and metaphorical use of language—with mental illness as a metaphor. At the core of my moral-political critique lies the distinction between relating to grown persons as responsible adults (moral agents) and as irresponsible insane persons (quasi-infants or idiots)—the former possessing free will, the latter lacking this moral attribute because of 'mental illness'" (Szasz, 1994, p. 37; 2010, p. 278). Szasz goes on to complain that his critics have failed to address these issues, concentrating instead on his motives and on the benefits of psychiatry. This chapter thus addresses the two aspects of his work that he thinks are most important and most neglected.

[2] It is less clear how one might advocate for common sense in the context of widespread acceptance of the psychiatric terms and practices that Szasz rejects—a complication that Szasz himself notes (Szasz, 2010, p. x).

concerned, a myth was an influential but false story; so Szasz's book could just as well have been titled *The Influential but False Story of Mental Illness.*

It was only later, as I struggled with the increasingly popular term "social construction," and as I reconsidered the less than clear line that divides the imaginary from the real, that I returned to Szasz's critique of psychiatry and his notion of a myth. Szasz offers detailed explications of his use of the term "myth," yet many questions remain regarding his application of that term and its relevance to psychiatry. In what follows, I seek to distinguish cases in which psychiatric concepts and conventions have resulted in myths from cases in which psychiatric concepts and conventions have resulted in projections or overextensions. In the light of these distinctions, it is possible to ask whether Szasz's own reliance on the notion of an autonomous person might itself qualify as a myth, a projection, or an overextension.

10.2 What is a myth? What are the myths of psychiatry?

Szasz's claim that contemporary psychiatry rests on a "myth" owes much to Gilbert Ryle's view that contemporary philosophy of mind rests on a "myth." Both Ryle and Szasz were writing at a time when the methodology appropriate to the study of human beings was widely contested. Ryle's extremely influential *The Concept of Mind* (which opens with a chapter entitled "Descartes' Myth") was published in 1949 and Szasz's *The Myth of Mental Illness* in 1961. Szasz frequently includes passages from Ryle's writing in his books, including the following passage from *The Concept of Mind*, which he (mis)quotes in *Law, Liberty, and Psychiatry*: "A myth is, of course, not a fairy story. It is the presentation of facts belonging in one category in the idioms appropriate to another. To explode a myth is accordingly not to deny the facts but to re-allocate them" (Ryle, 1949, p. 8; Szasz, 1963, p. 11). Ryle objects to the way in which concepts that are appropriate to the domain of physical substances get applied, inappropriately and with bad results, to the domain of the mental—to the way we talk about knowledge, will, emotion, sensation, and imagination as well as "the mind" in general. Unlike Ryle's critique, which revolves largely around the contrast between objects and their functions, and between descriptive and expressive uses of language, Szasz's critique focuses primarily on the contrast between literal and metaphorical uses of language. He distinguishes himself from other critics of psychiatry as someone "willing to look at the problem through the resolving lens of literal/metaphorical meaning" (Szasz, 1987, p. 166). Likewise, in the new preface to *The Myth of Mental Illness*, Szasz describes his work as "an effort to recast mental illness and psychiatry from a medical into a linguistic-rhetorical phenomenon" (Szasz, 2010, p. xxiii). So, I want to begin by considering the notion of a metaphor before relating it back to the notion of a myth.

A metaphor is a descriptive use of a non-literal application of a term or phrase; so we can judge some use of a term to be metaphorical only insofar as we can recognize other uses to be literal. The clearest cases of this contrast arise when the literal use of a term meets physical criteria such as physical type (e.g., bear), physical function (e.g., cup), or physical relation (e.g., higher), while metaphorical use applies the same term to things that do not meet those physical criteria (e.g., bear market, cup half full, higher status).[3]

Certainly, the contrast between metaphorical and literal uses of words is what Szasz has in mind when he claims that "mental illness" is a metaphor. He regards the literal meaning of illness to be bodily illness: Thus, "the decisive initial step I take is to *define illness as the pathologist defines it—as a structural or functional abnormality of cells, tissues, organs, or bodies*" (Szasz, 1987, p. 12). He argues against the view that so-called mental illness can, in fact, be equated with such bodily abnormalities.[4] "Clearly, if disease means bodily disease, then mental diseases are metaphoric diseases, just as priests are metaphoric fathers. . . . Conceptually, psychiatry (except insofar as it addresses bona fide brain diseases) thus rests on a literalized metaphor" (Szasz, 1987, p. 37).

Often, a metaphor is recognized as a metaphor. When its users fail to recognize its metaphorical status, however, a metaphor is said to be "literalized." There are many cases, of course, in which we do not *notice* the metaphorical status of some use of a term but we quickly *acknowledge* its metaphorical status once it is brought to our attention. I might not notice the metaphorical nature of the term "sharp" when I speak of sharp minds, but I will quickly agree that minds are not literally sharp. Many instances of so-called "tired metaphors" are like this. There are also cases in which the metaphorical application of a word ceases to be metaphorical, gaining a literal meaning instead. Vigorously cheerful people are literally hearty, regardless of the state of their hearts. The cases that concern Szasz, however, are cases in which people mistake metaphorical truths for literal truths—for example, cases in which participants in the rite of communion interpret the phrase "the blood of Christ" as literally applicable to the liquid they are offered (Szasz, 1976, p. 36; 1987, p. 141).

Why is this so bad? The problems arise, primarily, from supposing that the methods and implications of one domain (the domain in which a given term applies literally) apply to some other domain (the domain in which the term applies only

---

[3] Defining metaphor is, of course, a topic of ongoing dispute. Recognizing the difficulty of defining metaphor, Szasz invokes Turbayne's 1962 claim that metaphor "involves the pretense that something is the case when it is not," and he cites dictionary lists of synonyms and antonyms—some more relevant than others: "The synonyms of literal are: Verbal, veritable, accurate, true, exact, precise, regular, real, actual, undeviating, veracious, undisputed. Among its antonyms we find, in addition to metaphorical, the following: Wrong, erring, misleading, mistaken, false, erroneous, deceiving, untrue, delusive, beguiling, fallacious, unsound, lying, distorted, unreal, allegorical, allusive, colloquial, symbolical, figurative, and mythical" (Szasz, 1987, p. 138).

[4] One influential line of defense against Szasz's argument points to the discovery of various neurological correlations (which are seldom straightforward or universal), and assumes (usually without argument) that the existence of such correlations indicates that mental disorders are equivalent to physical disorders. Another influential line of argument invokes the notion of a proper function, suggesting that mental disorders are like physical disorders insofar as both occur precisely when some system, mental or physical, is unable to fulfill its biologically determined function (Wakefield, 1992).

metaphorically). As though we could investigate Jesus's ancestry by analyzing DNA in the consecrated wine, and as though we could infer that there must be an enormous amount of Jesus's blood in the world. In the case of "mental illness," according to Szasz, a failure to recognize the metaphorical status of "mental illness" leads us to the inappropriate use of medical methods—drugs, surgery, electroshock, and a host of other tools, which are suited to physical ailments like broken bones, polio, or Lyme disease—and to suppose that sufferers are passive victims of a disease when they are not.

Szasz, of course, is acutely aware of the increasingly popular view that mental problems *are* brain problems. He is quick, however, to highlight the imperfections of suggested correlations between mental problems and physical problems[5] and, more importantly, quite willing to switch from talk of mental ailments to talk of physical ailments when and if reliable correlations can be established.[6] He insists that genuinely mental problems, however, are problems of a different kind—namely, ailments in one's ability to navigate the difficulties of living; that is, they are, in effect, moral rather than medical problems.[7] Normative judgments that belong in the domain of ethics are recast as descriptive judgments in the domain of science. "The pancreas may be said to have a natural function. But what is the natural function of the person? That is like asking what is the meaning of life, which is a religious-philosophical, not medical-scientific, question" (Szasz, 2010, p. xxiii). Moreover, "bodily illness stands in the same relation to mental illness as a defective television set stands to a bad television program. Of course, the word 'sick' is often used metaphorically. We call jokes 'sick,' economies 'sick,' sometimes even the whole world 'sick'; but only when we call minds 'sick' do we systematically mistake and strategically misinterpret metaphor for fact—and send for the doctor to 'cure' the 'illness.' It is as if a television viewer were to send for a television repairman because he dislikes the program he sees on the screen" (Szasz, 2007, p. 6).

The transition from metaphor to myth involves one more step. For literalizations of metaphors do not always result in myths. A child may misinterpret a metaphorical use of the term "branch"—in the phrase "a branch of the government," for

---

[5] "To be sure, it is possible to discover hitherto unidentified brain lesions. But that can be done only on the brains of specific patients. If certain never-before-seen lesions were identified in the brains of mental patients and considered to be lesions specifically identifying schizophrenia, then, given the way schizophrenia is in fact diagnosed, it is certain that many schizophrenics would not have such lesions, and that many nonschizophrenics would" (Szasz, 1987, p. 78).

[6] "If all the 'conditions' now called 'mental illnesses' proved to be brain diseases, there would be no need for the notion of mental illness and the term would become devoid of meaning. However, because the term refers to the *judgments of some persons about the (bad) behaviors of other persons*, the opposite is what actually happens: the history of psychiatry is the history of an ever-expanding list of 'mental disorders'" (Szasz, 2010, pp. xiii–xiv).

[7] This is just one of many examples of what Ryle would call a "category mistake." Cresswell (2008) recounts further examples. Szasz often describes the master mistake in psychiatry as the mistake of treating reasons as causes, and justifications as explanations (Szasz, 2010, pp. 149–51).

example—without that misinterpretation constituting myth. When the literalization of a metaphor supports a wide range of beliefs and practices that serve to sustain certain social arrangements, however, it becomes a myth. In Szasz's words, from the 2007 quote already given, the misinterpretation must be "systematic" and "strategic." So mental illness is a myth insofar as the metaphorical use of the term "illness" is mistaken for a literal use of that term, insofar as that mistake supports the systematic medicalization of our mental lives, and insofar as that system of errors serves certain social purposes—especially purposes having to do with the retention of power and the relinquishing of responsibility. (Social constructivist analyses also emphasize the systematic and strategic illusion of thinking that race and gender, for example, refer to physical properties, but they do not suppose that the mistake relies on the literalization of a *metaphor*.[8])

It is the medical and psychiatric establishment that most clearly gains from the myth of mental illness; psychiatrists and pharmacists and insurers all gain both money and power from medicalization of mental distress. But patients can also gain by perpetrating the myth of mental illness; for example, presenting oneself as mentally ill serves to absolve oneself of responsibility, and it gives one access to support services that would not otherwise be available. "Poor people, by definition, have no money and hence cannot pay, in real currency, for what they want. They therefore pay for it in the only currency they have, namely, pain, suffering, and the willingness to submit to medical and psychiatric authorities. And what is it they want and so obtain? Personal attention disguised as medical and psychiatric care; sedatives and stimulants disguised as treatment; and, finally, room and board disguised as hospitalization" (Szasz, 1976, pp. 128–9).

The master metaphor, according to Szasz, is the metaphor of mental illness. But there are many subsidiary metaphors whose literalization has also contributed to the medicalization of the mental. Consider the notion of a "conflict" or "clash" between ideas or values. Literal clashes occur between physical objects or forces; ideas and values can only clash metaphorically. But psychiatric theory, largely under the influence of Freud, has come to view these metaphorical clashes as literal clashes, leading to the positing of unconscious impulses—inner forces that can be investigated as physical phenomena (Szasz, 1987, p. 143). Similarly, the notion of being "stuck" in a certain pattern of behavior ceases to be treated as a metaphor and researchers end up looking for an inner mechanism that literally gets stuck.

There is a great irony to this pattern within psychiatric practice, since it is psychiatry, again largely under the influence of Freud, which has identified ways in which the literalization of metaphor underwrites two key mental disorders—hysteria and schizophrenia.[9] The classic hysteric takes a term that applies metaphorically to her

---

[8] According to race and gender constructivists, there are no literal applications of racial terms or gender terms. For further clarification of what I take the constructivist thesis to involve, see Church (2004).

[9] Hysteria was the most common diagnosis of mental illness in the late nineteenth and early twentieth centuries. Schizophrenia is a more common diagnosis now, still said to afflict about 10 percent of the population.

situation—a term like "crooked," "twisted," "unspeakable," or "blind" (as descriptions of dishonesty, deception, wickedness, or ignorance)—and she makes it apply literally to her own body, twisting her limbs, ceasing to speak, or ceasing to see; her body becomes the canvas on which she can express the ills of her situation.[10] A common contemporary case is that of Vietnamese and Cambodian women who are either "dumb" or "blind."

More generally, a "sick" situation is transformed into a "sick" body. Szasz suggests "that we view hysteria as a pretense of being ill" (Szasz, 1987, p. 177), and details several cases in which a person's "pain" is the literalized expression of a metaphorically painful situation. He describes, for example, "[a naval] corpsman who had completed more than twenty years of service with an excellent record . . . for whom all significant [painful] issues in his life were translated, so to speak, into the language of [bodily] pain and were then expressed in such a manner that neither the patient nor those to whom he addressed himself really knew what he was saying. . . . The persistence of the pain now becomes a 'complaint' and serves as retribution. This should be taken literally to mean that the patient is now complaining to (and against) those who he feels have let him down" (1957, pp. 99–100, 102). Likewise, Szasz follows Eugen Bleuler (who introduced the category of schizophrenia) in characterizing a schizophrenic as someone who interprets metaphors literally: "The difference between the use of such phrases [as 'I am Switzerland' or 'I am freedom'] in the healthy and in the schizophrenic rests on the fact that in the former it is a mere metaphor, whereas for the patients the dividing line between direct and indirect representation has been obscured. The result is that they frequently think of these metaphors in a literal sense" (Bleuler, 1950, p. 429; cited in Szasz, 1987, p. 149). Insofar as psychiatrists are themselves dependent on the literalization of metaphors, then, they share the defining symptoms of their hysterical and their schizophrenic patients.

Once the mythical status of a system of metaphors is recognized, whether these are the metaphors of a psychiatrist or the metaphors of a patient, it is possible to return one's focus to the ethical and political decisions that must be made in a given situation. Szasz does not favor the elimination of myths—"I believe that people are entitled to their mythologies" (Vatz and Weinberg, 1983, p. 171)—but he insists on the freedom of each of us to choose our own myths and the responsibility of each of us to take responsibility for the consequences of our myths. In the case of non-medical pain, for example, Szasz advocates "treating the client as a person responsible for his life rather than as a patient not responsible for his lesion, . . . treating pain as an idiom rather than as an illness, and . . . substituting his own dialectic and discursive language for the client's rhetoric and nondiscursive language. If such an enterprise is successful it is

---

[10] Freud (1915, p. 207) describes the classic case of a hysteric who "complained that *her eyes were not right, they were twisted*. This she herself explained by bringing forward a series of reproaches against her lover in coherent language. 'She could not understand him at all, he looked different every time; he was a hypocrite, an eye-twister, he had twisted her eyes; now she had twisted eyes; they were not her eyes any more; now she saw the world with different eyes.'" The German *verdrehen* means "to twist"; *Verdreher*, literally "twister," figuratively means "liar"; and *Augenverdreher*, literally "eye-twister," figuratively means "hypocrite" or "deceiver."

not because the therapist has succeeded in controlling the patient's pain, but because the patient has decided to become another kind of person" (Szasz, 1988, pp. li–lii).[11]

10.3 **What is a projection? What are the projections of psychiatry?**

The term "projection" is central to psychoanalytic theory; it refers to instances in which traits of one person or thing are attributed to some other person or thing. When a child, playing with her dolls, attributes her own anger to her doll, she is projecting it onto her doll. When a teacher flirting with a student insists that it is the student who is flirting with him, he is projecting his own intentions onto the student. In these cases, one's own mental states are assigned to someone else—typically, as a way of disowning them, of preserving one's own self-image and relocating responsibility; but the projecting child or teacher does not need to deny possession of the same trait. The opposite of projection is introjection, whereby traits of some other person or thing are attributed to oneself—typically, as a way of gaining power or boosting one's self-esteem, but also, at times, as a way of punishing oneself or avoiding confrontation by taking on extra responsibilities. Szasz discusses the conflicting goals of hysterics (2010, pp. 213–15).

Slightly different, but related, are cases in which the features of one person who is not oneself get attributed to another person who is not oneself. A student might attribute features of her mother to her teacher, or to her therapist. A worker might attribute features of a past employer to a present employer. These are often categorized as cases of "transference."[12] While transference can certainly be an important route to knowledge—for both patient and therapist—it rests on a mistake that, ultimately, ought to be recognized as such.

Unlike myths, projections do not mistake metaphorical attributions for literal attributions; instead, they mistake a merely possible subject of a literal attribution for the actual subject of a literal attribution. There is nothing so subtle as a "category mistake" (Ryle's term for the wrongful attribution of properties that belong to one kind of thing to another kind of thing). In the case of a projection, the designated subject *could* have had the property in question, but it does not.

Szasz describes several areas in which the institution of psychiatry, as well as individual psychiatrists, are guilty of such projections. One widespread example of

---

[11] Szasz offers this further elaboration of the linguistic focus: "The patient not only learns to speak the language of real illness, but, realizing and reflecting upon the problem of communication he faces with physicians, also undertakes an explicit study of his own problem. He learns both about his own communications and about those of physicians; in particular, he learns about the history, aims, and uses and abuses of each of these languages" (Szasz, 2010, p. 93).

[12] Szasz also uses the term "transference" when describing cases in which attributes of external objects get reassigned to one's own body (1988, p. 98, p. 132, pp. 137–8). Some such transfers involve the literalization of metaphors, as discussed in the previous section; others will simply shift from one literal attribution to another, as discussed in this section.

psychiatric projection is the attribution of distress to a patient when the distress actually belongs to those who have to deal with the patient. People may be socially deviant or socially incompetent without experiencing any mental distress. Many types of behavior that can lead to incarceration in a mental institution (e.g., nudity in public, shouted insults, lack of personal grooming, refusal to obey directions) are a cause of suffering in others, not in the person misbehaving.[13] But given our discomfort with infringing on the liberty of people who are not actually a threat to anyone else, it is convenient to project some of our discomfort onto those who make us uncomfortable; we can then claim to be acting for their own sake. Indeed, "certain personally or socially disapproved behaviors, especially when they eventuate in bodily harm to the individual who engages in them, are now conventionally classified as diseases: for example, Soviet psychiatrists find that persons who cannot—or do not—control their displeasure with the political system of their own country suffer from *creeping schizophrenia*, while American psychiatrists find that persons who do not control their greed when in a casino, suffer from *pathological gambling*" (Szasz, 1987, p. 14).

A more subtle and perhaps more pervasive form of projection occurs when psychiatrists project their own values and priorities onto their patients—assuming that everyone puts a premium on happiness, for example, or assuming that happiness requires physical health, friends, and family. There is a growing tendency to ground ethics in evolutionary theory, with various commentators supposing that the divide between descriptive claims and prescriptive claims (a divide that Szasz is intent on respecting) can be bridged by appealing to the sort of functioning that evolution has favored (Wakefield, 1992). One can doubt the inference from "X is a result of the evolution of species H" to "X is the best alternative for species H." However, certain options may not yet have been tested; other results may be accidental byproducts of the traits being selected for. Also, and more importantly for Szasz, there is no reason to think that any individual's priorities ought to conform to the priorities that have benefitted the species as a whole.[14] Still less should we assume that another individual's priorities ought to conform to one's own, since "we must decide whether we value freedom more than health or vice versa . . . I, placing freedom above health, advocate returning health and illness, mental health and mental illness, to their rightful owners—the so-called patients and mental patients, the persons who possess (or are said to suffer from) these conditions" (Szasz, 1987, p. 161).

What does this mean in practice? Szasz offers the following summary:

> Diseases may be treated. Game-playing behavior can only be changed. . . . In what directions, toward what sorts of game-playing behavior, does the patient want to change? In what direction does the therapist want him to change? As against the word 'change,' the word 'treatment' implies that the patient's present behavior is bad—because it is 'sick'; and that the direction in which the therapist wants him to change is better or good—because

---

[13] Hence "the idea of mental incompetence comprises certain conceptual-cognitive characteristics (of the agent diagnosed), and certain dispositional-justificatory decisions (of the agents making the diagnosis), the latter element generally greatly outweighing the former" (Szasz, 1987, p. 250).

[14] The same applies even if it is a gene pool, rather than a species, that is selected for.

it is 'healthier.' In this, the traditional psychiatric view, the physical defines what is good or bad, sick or healthy. In the individualistic, autonomous 'psychotherapy' which I prefer, the patient himself defines what is good or bad, sick or healthy. With this arrangement, the patient might set himself goals in conflict with the therapist's values: if the therapist does not accept this, he becomes 'resistant' to helping the patient—instead of the patient being 'resistant' because he fails to submit to the therapist. (Szasz, 2010, pp. 228–9)

This brings us to the difficult topic of agency, or the capacity to be a genuine actor, versus passivity—a topic to which I return in Section 10.5. In interpersonal interactions, especially when those interactions are stressful, attributions of agency can be difficult. Psychiatry, according to Szasz, systematically and strategically underestimates the agency of the so-called mentally ill. This too, I want to suggest, amounts to a projection error. There is no question that agency is something that can be attributed to people literally, and there is no question that psychiatrists recognize some degree of agency in their patients. The overriding experience of a psychiatrist confronting a hysterical or schizophrenic individual, however, is an experience of helplessness with regard to that individual. Normal words and actions fail to have their normal effects, and it is often impossible to imagine oneself in the shoes of that other. In such circumstances it is very tempting to regard other persons as less than persons and more like things—that is, as subject to forces outside their control rather than pursuing paths of their own devising. What this amounts to, however, is a projection of one's own helplessness, one's own lack of effective agency, onto another person—a projection that helps to restore one's own sense of control and helps justify one's disregard for the agency of the other.

Here again, we encounter a deep irony in the projective tendencies of psychiatry itself. Some of the most studied delusions (regarded as symptomatic of schizophrenia) are delusions regarding agency, and involve either projections or introjections: on the one hand, the projective delusion that one can control the movements of other people; on the other hand, the introjective delusion that other people (or gods, or computers) are controlling one's own thoughts. Insofar as psychiatry itself (and a psychiatrically-minded populace) depends on projections of passivity, it (and we) share in the symptoms of schizophrenia. While psychoanalysts are standardly taught to recognize instances of transference (countertransference), a part of Szasz's project, it might be said, is to teach them further to recognize how contemporary psychiatry itself, in theory and in practice, exemplifies various sorts of transference.

10.4 What is an overextension? What are the overextensions of psychiatry?

It is possible for a term to be overextended (e.g., "friends" meaning anyone accessible via Facebook), and it is possible for a practice to be overextended (e.g., sharing personal information), and the two often go together. In contrast to the notions of myth and projection, the notion of overextension points to attributions that are not so much mistaken—mistakenly taken as literal in the case of myth, and mistakenly attributed to one thing rather than the other in the case of projection—as they are sloppy or stretched to the point where they cease to be meaningful or effective.

Szasz often remarks on the sheer number of cases now categorized as mental illness. Instead of mental illness being a small subset of all possible illness, it has become a very large set containing many instances that have no medical basis at all.[15] Szasz diagnoses this expanding usage as stemming from the literalization of medical metaphors and, in particular, the metaphor of "illness." There are other ways in which a term or practice can expand, however—and it is worth noting some instances of these other expansions within the terminology and the practice of psychiatry.

The class of things deemed "irrational," for example, has continued to expand under the influence of contemporary psychiatry. Irrationality, or, more precisely, an incapacity for rationality, has been offered as the overarching criterion of mental illness (Fingarette, 1972; Moore, 1984; Szasz 1987, pp. 63, 246). DSM-V (APA, 2013) cites it as a defining component of specific mental illnesses such as schizophrenia, paranoia, and obsessive-compulsive and related disorders. But, as Szasz is quick to point out, what seems rational to one person may seem irrational to another, and mere failures of communication are often mistaken for instances of irrationality.[16] Psychiatry has a stake in broadening the meaning of irrationality, insofar as psychiatrists gain from certifying others as irrational. So, largely under the influence of psychiatry, a narrow definition of irrationality as the occurrence of internal inconsistencies or invalid inferences can be extended to cover all kinds of failure to fit into one's society.

Similarly, the class of conditions labeled "depression"—one of the most common psychiatric diagnoses—has also greatly expanded under the influence of contemporary psychiatry. Once restricted to states of inexplicable despondency, the category of depression has now expanded to cover inexplicable cases of prolonged sluggishness, sleep disorders, and anxiety. This expansion is largely due to psychiatrists' discovery that drugs that were able to relieve feelings of despondency (in some cases, for some period of time) were also able to relieve sluggishness, sleep disorders, and anxiety (in some cases, for some period of time). Kramer (1993) nicely documents this. Furthermore, in DSM-V (2013), wholly explicable cases of despondency—those that are due to a major loss (i.e., grief)—now fall under the category of depression (and now warrant drug treatment) whenever they last longer than what is deemed normal.

Over time, the boundaries of our concepts are bound to change, of course: sometimes covering more than before, sometimes less, sometimes just different. What makes the extension of a term an overextension is its tendency to obliterate important distinctions—the distinction between thinking irrationally and thinking differently, for example, or the distinction between depression and grief. This affects our practice as well as our thinking, for it enables psychiatrists to assume a managerial position with respect to more and more aspects of our lives and it justifies their use of a very narrow range of tools to address a very diverse set of conditions.

---

[15] Contrast his illustrations of the smaller box for mental illness within the larger box for all illness versus the larger box of mental illness totally separate from the smaller box of genuine illness (Szasz, 1987, pp. 53, 86).

[16] Gerrans (2014, p. 37) discusses doubts about equating madness or mental sickness with irrationality.

10.5 **Is autonomy a myth, a projection, or an overextension?**

> Personally, I support respect for the autonomy and integrity of one's self and others, but shall not make any attempt to justify these values here. I believe, however, that in a work of this kind it is necessary to make one's moral preferences explicit, to enable the reader to better judge and compensate for the author's biases.
>
> Szasz (2010, p. 166)

In this final section, I take up Szasz's invitation to "better judge and compensate for [his] biases." Given the importance of autonomy in Szasz's writing, it is appropriate to ask whether autonomy might itself be regarded as a myth, a projection, or an over-extension. We can, in brief, raise exactly the same questions about his concept of autonomy that he raises about the governing concepts of psychiatry.

First, though, a couple of clarifications: Szasz seems to assume that being autonomous is equivalent to having free will, and having free will means that one is responsible for one's actions.[17] There are many interesting and important distinctions to be made in this area, and I think that Szasz conflates several different things: making one's own decisions versus following one's own reasons; being guided by one's reasons versus being guided by one's own impulses; being responsible versus treating as responsible. For present purposes, however, I will ignore those distinctions. Another point of clarification concerns Szasz's view of the relation between mental health and autonomy. Since he rejects the categories of illness and health (versus distress and happiness) as applicable to the realm of the mental, he would view any attempt to equate mental health with autonomy (and mental illness with a lack of autonomy) as guilty of a category mistake.[18] But Szasz certainly recognizes that there are some individuals, many of whom are labeled "mentally ill," who are not even capable of being autonomous; individuals whose mental capacities are too limited or impaired to be capable of effective, rational thought. For such people—far fewer than psychiatry would have us suppose—Szasz is quite willing to advocate coercive, protective intervention.[19]

Is autonomy a myth? Certainly it has been called that—by friends and enemies alike. Some neo-Kantian philosophers emphasize the ethical importance of treating others *as though* they were autonomous (free, responsible), even though literal autonomy (freedom, responsibility) does not exist (Ameriks, 2000; Larmore, 2008). Stepping outside the confines of academia, certain government officials have acknowledged that autonomy may be dismissed by representatives from other countries as an American

---

[17] Szasz also seems to equate being autonomous with being free (Szasz, 1987, p. 161). Dworkin (1981) and Gracia (2012) offer nice overviews of a wide range of uses of the term "autonomy" in recent political, legal, and medical discourse.

[18] Edwards (1981) defends this equation.

[19] Szasz lists the unconscious and the intoxicated, and those who are acutely delirious or demented, as belonging to this class. He is quick to insist that the latter states, like the former, "are acute and chronic disturbances of brain function" (Szasz, 1987, p. 251)—capable of being diagnosed by clinical tests or autopsy. Such conditions, then, in his terms, are physical rather than mental.

myth.[20] Does Szasz's own understanding of myth, as detailed in Section 10.2, suggest something similar? The meaning of "autonomy" is "self-governing" or "self-ruled"—an autonomous entity being one that is the author of its own actions, not deferential to the dictates of others (Wallace, 2003). This definition relies on some key metaphors since the term "govern" applies literally to political relations between people, and the term "author" applies literally to relations between a writer and a text. If we fail to recognize the metaphorical nature of these terms when applied to an individual's psychological capacities, and if that failure has systematic and strategic import, then, by Szasz's own analysis, it becomes mythical.

Likewise, the notion of "free will" becomes part of the myth of an immaterial mind when a metaphorical application of the term "free" (to actions rather than people in a social situation) is treated as a literal description of certain parts of the mind, and when the term "will" is assigned a literal referent—namely, a special sort of action-guiding power that is not itself determined by other wills or external powers. Ryle (who clearly influenced Szasz) devotes a chapter of *The Concept of Mind* to "The Will" (1949, pp. 62–82), describing "the myth of volitions" as an extension of Descartes' "the myth of the ghost in the machine" (i.e., the myth which results from the assignment of a literal referent to the term "mind") and describing the myth of the "will" as resulting from the assignment of a literal referent to the term "will." On Ryle's analysis, a willed action is not an action with a special sort of causal history; it is, rather, an action by someone with a certain range of capacities. "When we say that someone could have avoided committing a lapse or error, or that it was his fault that he committed it, we mean that he knew how to do the right thing, or was competent to do so, but did not exercise his knowledge or competence" (Ryle, 1949, p. 70).

If Szasz follows Ryle's lead, rejecting the view that free will is a special kind of force, in favor of the view that it is indicative of a certain range of capacities (to think and act in ways that are reflectively integrated and not dictated by their social and physical surroundings), then his stated commitment to autonomy and personal integrity should translate into a commitment to enhancing people's ability to think and act in a reflectively integrated way. But why does this not allow interventions—coerced if necessary—that are designed to enhance people's autonomy? This, of course, is the stated aim of much of psychiatry—and the stated aim of much of childrearing. Szasz can, of course, dispute the success of such interventions (or the honesty of the stated intentions), pointing out the myriad ways in which psychiatric interventions, intentionally or not, work against autonomy. Many of his remarks point in a different direction, however: "it is not because I believe that so-called mentally ill persons are 'always autonomous' that I want to treat them as responsible moral agents: I clearly state that since somatic pathology per se is not a sufficient condition for depriving a bodily ill person of moral agency, it should not be a sufficient condition in the case of a mentally

[20] Michael Hayden, former director of the CIA, raised the following questions about his conversations with representatives from foreign countries: "What of my side of these dialogues did our partners dismiss as American mythology? When I talked about self-determination? Cultural pluralism? . . . I never figured that out, but the longer I did this, the more certain I was that it had to be going on" (Savage, 2016).

ill person either" (Szasz, 1987, p. 160). Here he appears to invoke "moral agency" as a value that ought to trump the value of autonomy. But what is the basis for moral agency if not autonomy, and what is autonomy if not the capacity to be a moral agent? Against the backdrop of Rylean analyses, it seems appropriate to wonder whether Szasz has here succumbed to the very mythologizing which he identifies elsewhere.

It is also appropriate to wonder whether Szasz's insistence on the autonomy of mental "patients" (i.e., his insistence that they are actually actors, not patients) involves a certain amount of projection on his part. There is perhaps a universal tendency to assume that one's own abilities are shared by others—especially when those abilities are mental rather than physical.[21] This can be a way of being generous (i.e., of emphasizing one's common humanity) or it can be a way of being intolerant or vindictive (i.e., insisting that others' problems are problems of their own devising, that others' failures are their own fault). Mistaken attributions of autonomy count as projections, however, only insofar as they serve to deflect responsibility from oneself onto another. Szasz is adept at identifying ways in which mental patients manage to deflect responsibility onto others. But is he likewise guilty of deflecting his own responsibilities onto his patients?

When Szasz defends game-playing models of patient behavior, he portrays patients as fully rational players of rule-governed games—and thus responsible for the unfortunate consequences of their choices. When the rules are stacked against certain patients—in the case of the poor, for example—Szasz has a tendency to invoke "the tragedy of living," as though there is nothing much anyone can do about the unfairness of life.[22] When he considers offering material support to those in distress, he echoes his economist friend who worries about calling any transfer of wealth "aid" (Szasz, 2010, p. xiii). When Szasz distinguishes his own critique of coercive psychiatry from those (like R.D. Laing) whom he calls "antipsychiatrists," he complains: "As the communists seek to raise the poor above the rich, so the anti-psychiatrists seek to raise the 'insane' above the 'sane'" (Vatz and Weinberg, 1983, pp. 171–2). There is a distinctly Nietzschean strain to his writing, here and elsewhere. This pattern, I am suggesting, indicates something more than a refusal to assign responsibility for the inevitable unfairnesses of life; it indicates a tendency to project responsibility onto the wrong parties.

We come, finally, to the worry that Szasz's recommendations rest on an overextension of the term "autonomy." Even if we agree that there are many people who are autonomous with respect to many aspects of their lives (which is not something everyone would agree to),[23] we seem to observe many people who are not autonomous

---

[21] For example, what would be a (cognitive) inference for us regarding external control of our thoughts might be a (precognitive) experience for the schizophrenic (Gerrans, 2014).

[22] Szasz claims "psychiatry is the denial of the reality of free will and of the tragic nature of life; this authenticated denial lets persons who seek a neuro-mythological explanation of human wickedness and who reject the inevitability of personal responsibility to medicalize life" (Szasz, 2010, p. 273).

[23] Feminists have taken a lead in recent critiques of the very idea or ideal of autonomy (Pateman, 1988; Kittay and Feder, 2003; Wallace, 2003; Kittay and Carlson, 2010; Radoilska, 2012; Church, 2013).

with respect to some aspect of their lives. The model of rational game-playing, contractual decision-making, and rule-book punishments seems applicable in some domains but not in others. Interestingly enough, Szasz seems to recognize that he is pushing the boundaries of these notions when he writes: "My opposition to deterministic explanations of human behavior does not imply any wish to minimize the effects, which are indeed significant, of past personal experiences. I wish only to maximize the scope of voluntaristic explanations—in other words, to reintroduce freedom, choice, and responsibility into the conceptual framework and vocabulary of psychiatry" (Szasz, 2010, p. 6).

Maximizing the scope of certain concepts at the expense of others is a familiar political and rhetorical practice, and Szasz is quick to see himself as engaged in a political and rhetorical dispute with contemporary psychiatry. He is less quick, perhaps, to see the dangers of overextending the scope of autonomy.

I conclude, then, that Szasz's concept of autonomy does indeed have elements of myth, projection, and overextension. Recognizing these elements leaves much of his critique of psychiatry intact, but it should lead to a more cautious assessment of Szasz's worldview and a more humble attitude when it comes to formulating psychiatric alternatives.

References

American Psychiatric Association (APA). 2013. *Diagnostic and Statistical Manual of Mental Disorders [DSM-V]*, 5th edn. Arlington, Virginia: American Psychiatric Association.

Ameriks, Karl. 2000. *Kant and the Fate of Autonomy: Problems in the Appropriation of the Critical Philosophy*. Cambridge: Cambridge University Press.

Bleuler, Eugen. 1950. *Dementia Praecox; or, The Group of Schizophrenias* [1911], translated by Joseph Zinkin. New York: International Universities Press.

Church, Jennifer. 2004. "Social Constructionist Models: Making Order Out of Disorder: On the Social Construction of Madness." In *The Philosophy of Psychiatry: A Companion*, edited by Jennifer Radden, pp. 393–406. Oxford: Oxford University Press.

Church, Jennifer. 2013. "Boundary Problems: Negotiating the Challenges of Responsibility and Loss." In *Oxford Handbook of the Philosophy of Psychiatry*, edited by K.W.M. Fulford et al., pp. 497–511. Oxford: Oxford University Press.

Cresswell, Mark. 2008. "Szasz and His Interlocutors: Reconsidering Thomas Szasz's 'Myth of Mental Illness' Thesis." *Journal for the Theory of Social Behaviour* **38** (1) (March): 23–44.

Dworkin, Gerald. 1981. "The Concept of Autonomy." *Grazer Philosophische Studien* **12**: 203–13.

Edwards, Rem B. 1981. "Mental Health as Rational Autonomy." *Journal of Medicine and Philosophy* **6** (3) (August): 309–22.

Fingarette, Herbert. 1972. *The Meaning of Criminal Insanity*. Berkeley: University of California Press.

Freud, Sigmund. 1915. "The Unconscious." In *The Standard Edition of the Complete Psychological Works of Sigmund Freud*, vol. **14**, pp. 159–215. London: Hogarth, 1957.

Gerrans, Philip. 2014. *The Measure of Madness: Philosophy of Mind, Cognitive Neuroscience, and Delusional Thought*. Cambridge, Mass.: MIT Press.

Gracia, Diego. 2012. "The Many Faces of Autonomy." *Theoretical Medicine and Bioethics* **33** (1) (February): 57–64.

Kittay, Eva Feder, and Ellen K. Feder (eds.). 2003. *The Subject of Care: Feminist Perspectives on Dependency*. Lanham, Maryland: Rowman and Littlefield.

Kittay, Eva Feder, and Licia Carlson (eds.). 2010. *Cognitive Disability and Its Challenge to Moral Philosophy*. Malden, Mass.: Wiley-Blackwell.

Kramer, Peter D. 1993. *Listening to Prozac: A Psychiatrist Explores Antidepressant Drugs and the Remaking of the Self*. New York: Viking Penguin.

Larmore, Charles. 2008. *The Autonomy of Morality*. Cambridge: Cambridge University Press.

Moore, Michael S. 1984. *Law and Psychiatry: Rethinking the Relationship*. Cambridge: Cambridge University Press.

Pateman, Carole. 1988. *The Sexual Contract*. Stanford, California: Stanford University Press.

Radoilska, Lubomira (ed.). 2012. *Autonomy and Mental Disorder*. Oxford: Oxford University Press.

Ryle, Gilbert. 1949. *The Concept of Mind*. London: Hutchinson's University Library; New York: Barnes and Noble.

Savage, Charlie. 2016. "General Hayden's Offensive: [Review of] *Playing to the Edge: American Intelligence in the Age of Terror* by Michael V. Hayden." *New York Review of Books* (May 26). Accessed April 12, 2018. <www.nybooks.com/articles/2016/05/26/general-haydens-offensive/>

Szasz, Thomas S. 1957. *Pain and Pleasure: A Study of Bodily Feelings*. New York: Basic Books.

Szasz, Thomas S. 1961. *The Myth of Mental Illness. Foundations of a Theory of Personal Conduct*. New York: Hoeber-Harper.

Szasz, Thomas S. 1963. *Law, Liberty, and Psychiatry: An Inquiry into the Social Uses of Mental Health Practices*. New York: Macmillan.

Szasz, Thomas S. 1976. *Heresies*. Garden City, New York: Doubleday Anchor.

Szasz, Thomas S. 1987. *Insanity: The Idea and Its Consequences*. New York: John Wiley & Sons.

Szasz, Thomas S. 1988. *Pain and Pleasure: A Study of Bodily Feelings*, 2nd edn. Syracuse: Syracuse University Press.

Szasz, Thomas S. 1994. "Mental Illness is Still a Myth." *Society* **31** (4) (May): 34–9.

Szasz, Thomas S. 2007. *The Medicalization of Everyday Life: Selected Essays*. Syracuse: Syracuse University Press.

Szasz, Thomas S. 2010. *The Myth of Mental Illness: Foundations of a Theory of Personal Conduct*, revised edn. New York: Harper Perennial.

Turbayne, Colin Murray. 1962. *The Myth of Metaphor*. New Haven: Yale University Press.

Vatz, Richard E., and Lee S. Weinberg (eds.). 1983. *Thomas Szasz: Primary Values and Major Contentions*. Buffalo: Prometheus.

Wakefield, Jerome C. 1992. "The Concept of Mental Disorder: On the Boundary Between Biological Facts and Social Values." *American Psychologist* **47** (3) (March): 373–88.

Wallace, Kathleen. 2003. "Autonomous 'I' of an Intersectional Self." *Journal of Speculative Philosophy* **17** (3): 176–91.

Chapter 11

The clinical wisdom
of Thomas Szasz

Mantosh J. Dewan and Eugene A. Kaplan

11.1 Introduction

Lost in the relentless focus on Szasz's more controversial views in *The Myth of Mental Illness* (1961) is a body of work that illuminates his contributions to clinical practice. Szasz offers insights that come from examining the essential ingredients of clinical practice through a prism of human relationships, a clear declaration of who has the power in that relationship, and a focus on promoting freedom—not just for the patient but also the therapist! In this chapter, we address five seminal contributions: (1) the physician-patient relationship, (2) the therapist-patient relationship, (3) the concept of transference, (4) pain and the context for understanding and treating psychosomatic symptoms, and (5) the psychology of schizophrenia.

11.2 The physician–patient relationship: models and their implications

Szasz, with his colleague Marc H. Hollender, notes that although the study of human relationships is central to psychoanalytic thought: "The concept of a relationship is a novel one in medicine" (Szasz and Hollender, 1956, p. 585). Further, he opines that psychoanalysis has had its most decisive effect on modern medicine by making physicians overtly aware of the possible significance of their relationships to patients. Although the three models of the patient–physician relationship which he elaborates embrace modes of interaction that are ubiquitous in human relationships, they gain specificity and relevance due to their interaction with technical procedures within a unique social context.

In the model of *activity-passivity*, the physician does something to an inert patient (e.g., during emergency surgery or involuntary treatment of a psychotic person). The physician is active; the patient, passive. Treatment occurs regardless of the patient's wishes or contribution. In a true sense, this is not an interaction, since the person acted upon is unable to contribute. This originated in—and is entirely appropriate for—the treatment of emergencies. Clinical interventions in this model are often lauded and have the potential for saving lives. However, even in his 1956 paper with Hollender and other early writings, Szasz is concerned that "treatment" (he used quotation marks) in this model could lead to abuse and harm to patients. All forms of coercion and abuse, such as involuntary hospitalization, became a major focus of his writing after *The Myth of Mental Illness*. He then argued that the prototype of this model is the relationship between parent and infant.

The model of *guidance-cooperation* underlies much of medical practice: The physician tells the patient what to do and the patient cooperates and "obeys orders"; for example, the patient takes medicine for an infection or anxiety, or accepts "advice" during supportive therapy. The prototype of this model is the relationship between parent and adolescent child. Although the prevalent model in the 1950s, it persists today (but to a lesser extent) despite concerted efforts to move practice toward Szasz's third model of mutual participation.

In the model of *mutual participation*, the physician helps the patient to help himself; for example, encouraging lifestyle changes for chronic disease or dynamic therapy for personality change in high-functioning patients. This relationship is akin to one between two consenting adults and is promoted today as informed collaboration (Shivale and Dewan, 2015) or the deliberative model (Emanuel and Emanuel, 1992).

Szasz asserts that all three models are appropriate and needed at different times and in different situations. While he favors mutual participation to be the norm, activity-passivity may still be the preferred and necessary model in an emergency. In most cases, the physician–patient relationship can and will change over time. If the needs of the physician or patient change but the physician–patient relationship does not accurately respond to this change, then there is a mismatch. For instance, in the model of mutual participation, if a patient is reluctant to take medication that the physician is convinced will be helpful, the well-meaning but frustrated physician may switch to the model of guidance-cooperation and order the patient to take medication. The patient, still in the model of mutual participation, may become overtly dissatisfied and see the physician as wrong, pushy, and uncaring; the physician, who has the power in this relationship, may label the patient "difficult" or "noncompliant" and enter this in the formal medical record.

Szasz suggests that, just as in psychoanalysis, physicians need to be schooled in the importance of the physician–patient relationship, sensitive to the inevitable tensions and distortions in it that adversely effect treatment, and skilled in addressing and repairing a rupture when it occurs.

11.3 The psychotherapist–patient relationship

Building on the model of mutual participation in the physician–patient relationship as his foundation, Szasz illuminates the importance and key elements of the psychotherapist–patient relationship in vivid terms. In *The Ethics of Psychoanalysis* (1965), he promotes "autonomous psychotherapy," which strictly rests on a human relationship between equals; that is, he eliminates the traditional power differential between therapist and patient. He describes the essence of psychotherapy as a noncoercive, helpful game that is played between therapist and patient and leads to the education (and thereby growth) of the patient. On autonomous psychotherapy, Szasz writes that the rules of the game and the principles underlying the aim and structure of the game can be formally taught. However, how to play a particular game cannot be formally taught and learned (e.g., how to be an analyst or an analysand). Players cannot be told how to play a game; that is their business. Szasz suggests that the very essence of games is that the players are free to play or not and, within the rules of the game, to play as they deem fit: "If a person is coerced—either to play against his will or to play in a certain fashion—then he is no longer a game-player (in the ordinary sense); although such a player may appear to others as though he were playing a game, he will actually be 'working,' not 'playing'" (Szasz, 1965, p. 215).

In emphasizing the "crucial role of freedom in game-playing" (1965, p. 215), Szasz insists that "both analyst and analysand must be left free to conduct themselves as they see fit, as long as they keep within the rules of the analytic game . . . The patient must, of course, be even freer to play the role of analysand as he sees fit than is the therapist to play the role of analyst. After all, the aim of the therapy is to observe and analyze the patient's game-playing strategies; if the analyst tells him how to behave, what is there to analyze?" (Szasz, 1965, p. 215).

In addition to learning the rules, the therapist must, of course, practice autonomous psychotherapy. Szasz endorses the traditional notion that the beginning therapist may profit from supervision. What is not traditional—and is typically Szaszian—is his view that the relationship between therapist and supervisor must also be "autonomous, that is, if the supervisor is the therapist's agent" (Szasz, 1965, p. 216). Therefore, the supervisor should not represent the faculty or an institution and can be terminated at the therapist's will.

In autonomous psychotherapy, the contract calls for the *therapist* to provide time and expert (talk) services in the office for a fixed fee. No other activity is—or can be—part of therapy. This sets very clean and unambiguous boundaries. Likewise, the contract calls for the *patient* to make the best use of this time and expertise, pay the bills, and decide when to terminate. Nothing else is expected or required of the patient.

Szasz has the following practical advice for therapists:

1. "Forget that you are a physician. If you are a psychiatrist, do not let your medical training get in your way. If you are not medically trained, do not secretly aspire to be a doctor. If . . . you propose to sell . . . analysis, you owe it to your clients and to yourself to be a competent analyst. Competence in another discipline—for example, in medicine—is not an excuse for incompetence in . . . psychoanalysis" (1965, p. 217).

2. "You are 'helpful' and 'therapeutic' if you fulfill your contract. Do not . . . comply with the patient's requests for nonanalytic services. You are not responsible for the patient's bodily health; he is. You need not show that you are humane, that you care for him, or that you are reliable by worrying about his physical health, his marriage, or his financial affairs. Your sole responsibility to the patient is to analyze him. If you do that competently, you are 'humane' and 'therapeutic'; if you do not, you have failed him, regardless of how great a 'humanitarian' you might be in other respects" (1965, p. 217).

3. "You must get to know your patient. You must see the patient often enough," with "continuity," "and over a long enough period to get to know him well" (1965, pp. 217–18).

4. Do not get "coerced by emergencies," which are among the major threats to autonomous psychotherapy. "Remember your contract" and trust your patient to take care of this as his responsibility. "It is unimportant whether the emergency is real or whether the patient is testing you" (1965, p. 218).

5. "Do not misconstrue the patient's feelings and ideas about you. What the patient feels and thinks about you is as 'real' as what anyone else feels and thinks. Though it may be reasonable to label some of his feelings and thoughts 'transference,' remember that, in doing so, conduct is being judged, not described" (1965, p. 219). (Szasz clarified that transference is more complex than the simple notion accepted by traditional psychoanalysis. In every relationship, there is a real and a transference element.)

6. "Your life and work . . . must be compatible with the practice of autonomous psychotherapy. If you practice autonomous psychotherapy, you will have to exhibit an attitude of 'live and let live' toward your patients. It will be difficult for you to do this if you are coerced and harassed by others or if, outside your analytic practice, you engage in activities that require you to coerce and harass others. For example, if you are a resident in a state hospital or a candidate in an analytic institute, how will you be able to leave your patients alone when your superiors do not leave you alone? Will you be able to let your patients become freer than you are yourself?" (1965, p. 219). (Recognizing the challenges of sustaining a full-time therapy practice, Szasz recommends combining a part-time practice with research, teaching, or writing.)

7. "Do not take notes. The psychoanalytic relationship is a personal encounter . . . Both of you play dual roles as participants in a relationship *and* as observers of it. What effect would note-taking have on your relationship with your mother, wife, or friend?" (1965, p. 220, original italics).

8. "You are responsible for your conduct, not for your patient's. This is the central principle of autonomous psychotherapy. You are not responsible for the patient, his health (mental or physical), or his conduct; for all this, the patient is responsible. But you are responsible for your conduct. You must be truthful; never deceive or mislead the patient by misinforming him or withholding information he needs. Do not communicate about him with third parties, whether or not you have his consent to do so. Make every effort to understand the patient by trying to feel and think as he does. Finally, be honest with yourself and critical of your own standards of conduct and of those of your society" (1965, p. 220).

Szasz uses patient, client, and analysand interchangeably. Although the rules of autonomous psychotherapy are derived from psychoanalysis, they are applicable to all therapies today. Perhaps they are best seen as aspirational; that is, they must be every therapist's firm guiding principles unless forced to diverge due to legal, insurance, or other requirements that now increasingly interfere with the practice of autonomous psychotherapy.

11.4 **The concept of transference**

In his later writings, Szasz is critical of Freud as well as of psychoanalysis (Szasz, 1978). However, his earlier writings contain a number of psychoanalytic gems. One particularly important paper (Szasz, 1963, 1994, 2004) on a central tenet of psychoanalysis, the concept of transference, was chosen as one of forty-five "classic" papers on psychoanalysis by Robert Langs (2004, pp. 25–36). Szasz writes: "Recognizing the phenomenon of transference, and creating the concept, was perhaps Freud's greatest single contribution. Without it, the psychotherapist could never have brought scientific detachment to a situation in which he participates as a person" (Szasz, 1963, p. 438; 1994, p. 181; 2004, p. 31). Therefore, the term must be understood clearly and used precisely.

Szasz examines transference and reality in the context of the power differential and as a conflict of opinion between therapist and patient. Freud's classic paradigm for transference is the phenomenon of transference love; that is, the female patient falling in love with the male therapist. Freud defined it as an illusion, as unwarranted by the treatment setting, and as a projection of the patient's unconscious relations with an earlier libidinal object onto the therapist. This is supported by numerous clinical examples in the literature. The therapist's task is to interpret and unmask these projections and expose their origins. The therapist's view is accepted as reality; the patient's view is seen as unreality or illusion—perspectives that need to be corrected and learned from. This is not so simple:

> Here is a more challenging situation: the analyst believes that he is kindly and sympathetic, but the patient thinks that he is arrogant and self-seeking. Who shall say now which is 'reality' and which is 'transference'? The point is that the analyst does not find the patient's reactions prelabelled, as it were; on the contrary, he must do the labeling himself . . . There is no denying, however, that the distinction between transference and reality is useful for psychoanalytic work . . . Practical utility and epistemological clarity are two different matters. Workmanlike use of the concept of transference should not blind us to the fact that the term is not a neutral description but rather the analyst's judgment of the patient's behavior. (Szasz, 1963, p. 433; 1994, p. 169; 2004, p. 26)

Typically, the female patient's declarations of love for the male analyst may be interpreted as unrealistic and due to transference. Transference, in this example, refers to the analyst's judgment.

Transference, Szasz claims, can also be used to describe a certain kind of experience which the analytic patient has, and which people in some other situations may also have. The analytic patient may think—with or without being told so by the analyst—that his love for or hatred toward or anxiety about the therapist's health is exaggerated or unwarranted. Essentially, the patient may be aware that the therapist is overly important to him. This phenomenon defines transference as experience and as self-judgment.

In fact, the analyst's judgment of whether the patient's behavior is transference (or not) may be validated by the patient; similarly, the patient's experience and self-judgment may be validated by the analyst. Since each of the two persons involved in therapy has a choice of two judgments, there can be four possible outcomes (Szasz, 1963, 1994, 2004):

1. Analyst and patient agree that the behavior is transference. The analyst can then interpret the transference, allowing the patient to experience and learn from it.

2. The analyst determines the patient's behavior as transference and labels it, for example, "transference love" or "eroticized transference." The patient does not see it as transference. Irrespective of who is correct, all such disagreements preclude analysis of the transference. Szasz suggests that the most common reasons for this impasse are that the analyst is mistaken in the judgment or that the patient, though exhibiting transference manifestations, is unaware of doing so.

3. Analyst and patient agree that the patient's behavior is reality-oriented and, therefore, further analysis is not needed. A caveat is that both analyst and patient may be mistaken.

4. The analyst considers the patient's behavior realistic, but the patient knows it is transference. This possibility, states Szasz, is rarely discussed in psychoanalysis despite its clinical import. The most common result is that the analyst "acts out." For example, the therapist may become sexually involved with the patient, when in fact the patient was only testing him; or he may stop analyzing, believing the patient to be too depressed, suicidal, or otherwise unanalyzable, when, again, the patient was merely "acting" difficult to test the analyst's perseverance. This sort of occurrence does not allow the analyst to make transference interpretations; it may give the patient an opportunity for self-analysis, either during the analysis or, more often, afterwards.

While some analysts have limited the phenomenon of transference to the analytic situation, Szasz endorses the view that transference plays a part in all human relations, such as the physician–patient relationship, marriage, and the work situation. The analytic relationship differs in two ways: first, it facilitates the development of relatively intense transference reactions in the patient; second, transferences are supposed to be studied and learned from, not acted upon.

Szasz also clarifies the distinction between transference and transference neurosis as being merely a matter of degree—and entirely arbitrary. He notes that, since we are looking for a quantitative difference but lack measuring instruments and standards of measurement for making quantitative estimates, this distinction between transference and transference neurosis remains arbitrary and impressionistic.

In an important insight with immediate clinical relevance, Szasz notes that the concept of transference serves two separate analytic purposes. First, it is an essential part of the patient's therapeutic experience, and second, it is a critical defense that protects the analyst from too intense an affective and real-life involvement with the patient. If the patient intensely loves or hates the analyst, and if the analyst can protect himself by viewing these attitudes as transferences, then, in effect, the analyst has convinced himself that the patient does not have these feelings and dispositions toward him but someone else. Unfortunately, warns Szasz, transference interpretations are so easily and frequently misused precisely because this simple maneuver provides ready-made protection by putting the patient at arm's length.

Szasz notes that Freud successfully used the concept of transference as defense to help his colleague, Josef Breuer, who was treating Anna O. for hysteria. As Szasz tells this story:

> So long as hysterical symptoms were undisturbed . . . patients were left free to express their personal problems through bodily signs and other indirect communications . . . Thus, as Breuer proceeded in translating Anna O.'s symptoms into the language of personal problems, he found it necessary to carry on a relationship with her without the protection previously afforded by the hysterical symptoms. For we ought not to forget that the defenses inherent in the hysterical symptoms (and in others as well) served not only the needs of the patient, but also of the physician. So long as the patient was unaware of disturbing affects and needs—especially aggressive and erotic—she could not openly disturb her physician with them. But once these inhibitions were lifted . . . it became necessary for the therapist to deal with the new situation: a sexually aroused attractive *woman*, rather than a pitifully disabled *patient*.(Szasz, 1963, p. 438; 1994, p. 183; 2004, pp. 31–2; original italics).

Breuer, as we know, could not cope with this new situation (Anna O. was not only highly intelligent, but extremely attractive in physique and personality) and fled from it. He and his wife literally left for Venice to spend a second honeymoon, which resulted in the conception of a daughter. Later, in addressing Breuer's disturbing experience with Anna O., Ernest Jones reports: "Freud told him of his own experience with a female patient suddenly flinging her arms around his neck in a transport of affection, and he explained to him his reasons for regarding such untoward occurrences as part of the transference phenomena characteristic of certain types of hysteria. This seems to have had a calming effect on Breuer, who evidently had taken his own experience of the kind more personally and perhaps even reproached himself for indiscretion in the handling of his patient" (Jones, 1953, p. 250). Szasz states:

> The notion of transference is reassuring to therapists precisely because it implies a denial (or mitigation) of the 'personal' in the analytic situation. When Freud explained transference to Breuer, Breuer drew from it the idea that Anna O.'s sexual overtures were 'really' meant for others, not for him: he was merely a symbolic substitute for the patient's 'real' love objects. . . . The concept of transference . . . introduced into medicine and psychology the notion of the *therapist as symbol*: this renders the *therapist as person* essentially invulnerable . . . Herein lies the danger. Just as the pre-Freudian physician was ineffective partly because he remained a fully 'real' person, so the psycho-analyst may be ineffective if he remains a fully 'symbolic' object. The analytic situation requires the therapist to function as both, and the patient to perceive him as both. Without these conditions, 'analysis' cannot take place. (Szasz, 1963, p. 442; 1994, pp. 190–1; 2004, p. 35)

"The use of the concept of transference in psychotherapy thus led to two different results. On the one hand, it enabled the analyst to work where he could not otherwise have worked; on the other hand, it exposed him to the danger of being 'wrong' vis-à-vis his patient—and of abusing the analytic relationship—without anyone being able to demonstrate this to him" (Szasz, 1963, p. 442; 1994, p. 192; 2004, p. 35). This harbors seeds of the destruction of psychoanalysis itself, states Szasz: "This hazard must be frankly recognized . . . Only the integrity of the analyst and of the analytic situation can safeguard from extinction the unique dialogue between analysand and analyst" (Szasz, 1963, p. 443; 1994, pp. 192–3; 2004, p. 36).

Szasz acknowledges the concept of transference to be Freud's greatest single contribution, but states that Freud's description is too simplistic and incomplete because it is based solely on the therapist's version of reality. By introducing the patient as an equal partner, Szasz clarifies that the experience and judgment of the patient must be valued and is necessary to make the correct determination about whether a phenomenon is "transference" or "reality." Depending on the concordance of views, it can be determined whether interpretation is warranted or feasible. He also alerts us to the danger of therapists "acting out" when they misinterpret the transference-based "testing" behavior of patients as reality—a topic that is rarely addressed. Szasz is at his best when he illuminates the obvious. He is the first to recognize and emphasize that, in the therapeutic relationship, the therapist has both a symbolic function (that can be interpreted and used as a psychological defense against the powerful affects of the patient) *and* a real relationship with the patient. His writing makes clear that the therapeutic situation is a complex, multilevel relationship, rich with possibilities and fraught with dangers.

One would think that a paper which modifies a basic tenet of psychoanalysis and is recognized as a "classic" (Bauer, 1994; Langs, 2004) would have had a major impact on the field. In fact, it has not.

11.5 Pain and the origins of psychosomatic symptoms

In the second edition of *Pain and Pleasure* (1975, 1988), Szasz updates his views and writes about the lack of clarity in our language, understanding, and treatment of patients complaining of pain, and the consequent pleasure and frustration that physicians experience in dealing with these patients. He makes the essential distinction between patients with pain and "painful persons," making explicit that the latter suffer from problems in living, should not be labeled as patients, and cannot be helped by procedures and medications. This is a clinically useful insight into our current era of the opioid epidemic.

The diagnosis of pain is another example of the power differential and the judgment of the physician trumping the experience of the patient. Szasz notes that physicians do not experience, and therefore cannot properly label, other people's pain. In reality, what physicians experience and classify are other people's complaints. When complaints of pain are considered legitimate, the physician labels it "organic," and the person is a legitimate patient and medically sick. However, persons complaining of illegitimate pains are regarded as illegitimate patients, as mentally sick or "psychogenic."

Szasz says that language is rarely used to create a pure description. Instead, its purpose is frequently to exert some kind of influence. Terms such as "organic" and "psychogenic" now must be recognized as "adjectives of a particular kind," akin to "normal" and "psychotic," "progressive" and "reactionary." Szasz clarifies that for the person experiencing pain, there is no such thing as "psychogenic pain" and no person would ever describe his or her own pain as "psychogenic," own conduct as "psychotic," or own political views as "reactionary." These terms are usually used by others to condemn. He views "organic pain" and "psychogenic pain," not as two kinds of pain in the sense in which English and French are two kinds of languages, but rather as expressions equivalent to "beautiful painting" and "ugly painting."

How can we understand persons with "psychogenic" pain? Szasz suggests that patients with chronic pain in the absence of bodily illness are often (but not always) "individuals who have made a *career* of suffering" (Szasz, 1988, p. xxiv, original italics). At one point they may have been functioning well, "but when their careers fail or no longer suffice to sustain them, they become 'painful persons' . . . or . . . 'hommes douloureux' . . . or . . . 'homini dolorosi'" (Szasz, 1988, p. xxiv). He cites Freud's account of Fraulein Elizabeth von R., who complained of pains without being demonstrably ill and who had not responded to medical treatment: "Here, then, was the unhappy story of this proud girl with her longing for love. Unreconciled to her fate, embittered by the failure of all her little schemes for reestablishing the family's former glories, with those she loved dead or gone away or estranged, unready to take refuge in the love of some unknown man—she had lived for eighteen months in almost complete seclusion, with nothing to occupy her but the care of her mother and her own pains" (Breuer and Freud, 1893–1895, pp. 143–4; Szasz, 1988, p. xxv). Szasz considers this "one of the finest and most important paragraphs in all of Freud's writing . . . Freud here reminds us, in plain and persuasive language, that playing the sick role may, for some people some time, be the most gratifying pursuit open to them" (Szasz, 1988, p. xxv).

Psychogenic pain, Szasz reminds readers, resembles older concepts of malingering, conversion hysteria, and hypochondriasis, wherein such patients are "like impostors." Although healthy, these patients deceive the physician (or even themselves) with faked illness. Szasz considers this view as substantially correct but incomplete because it neglects the "complementary deception of patients by physicians, which is the soil in which the patient's deception grows and flowers" (Szasz, 1988, p. xxxii). Instead of recognizing them as "painful persons," physicians provide the rich soil of extensive tests and medical diagnoses, sometimes driven by financial gain. Common examples today would include some "painful persons" who are misdiagnosed with low back syndrome, psychiatric disorders (e.g., somatic symptom disorder), or opioid misuse or overdose.

How should patients complaining of pain be approached? Szasz states that, although patients and physicians think they have countless options to fight pain, in fact, there is a choice of just four treatment categories: (1) a procedure (e.g., surgery, acupuncture), (2) medications, (3) psychotherapy, or (4) "the physician can decide and the patient can agree, or vice versa, that there is nothing specifically medical either one of them can do about the pain" (Szasz, 1975, pp. vi–vii). Further, "the choice they make is frequently fateful, and that it may be fatal—literally or metaphorically—is something both patients and physicians often realize only too late" (Szasz, 1975, p. vii). Presciently, Szasz warns us that the activist therapeutic posture, epitomized in "Don't just stand there, do something!" has no place in the management of chronic pain in the absence of demonstrable bodily disease. Both sufferers and would-be helpers might profit from inverting that phrase to "Don't do something, just stand there!"

With the best of intentions, treatment of pain is difficult. Surgical interventions are fraught with negative consequences. For instance, lobotomies eliminated pain, but some patients had markedly diminished levels of function. Today, surgery for non-specific low back pain frequently leads to the chronic disability and pain of "failed back surgery syndrome" (Baber and Erdek, 2016). The well-meaning encouragement to evaluate pain as another vital sign and to treat it aggressively, even when it had a significant subjective component, has contributed to the current opioid crisis.

What is a helpful psychotherapeutic approach? Szasz suggests that the therapist must choose from one of three choices when dealing with a "painful person." First, he may refuse to accept him as a patient. Second, he may accept him and undertake to "treat" him despite the patient's clearly stated desire to retain his painful identity. This frequently results in a growing antagonistic relationship, as the patient escalates his complaints of pain and as the therapist escalates his "therapeutic" assaults on him. Szasz tells us that these relationships are similar to "bad marriages, often end in divorce, the patient being referred to a neurosurgeon" (Szasz, 1988, p. li). Or, third, the therapist may accept someone for "treatment" but insist that the patient choose whether he or she wishes to remain the same or change. This is the application of the autonomous therapy approach to patients whose predominant problems involve pain. The therapist tries to avoid the impasses that arise with patients of this sort by treating each patient "as a person responsible for his life rather than as a patient not responsible for his lesion, by treating pain as an idiom rather than as an illness, and by substituting his own dialectic and discursive language for the client's rhetoric and nondiscursive language. If such an enterprise is successful, it is not because the therapist has succeeded in controlling the patient's pain, but because the patient has decided to become another kind of person" (Szasz, 1988, pp. li–lii). Essentially, the patient must find something real that is more personally meaningful than the trappings of pain. Szasz asserts:

> Severe, chronic illness does not necessarily lead to a career of pain, if the individual has something better to do with his life than to suffer. During his last years, Freud was afflicted with cancer of the oral cavity; he attended to his work, however, and not to his illness. When he was younger, and the significance of his work was less secure, he was hypochondriacal. On the other hand, people free of physical disease often suffer from the most intractable types of pain. In such cases, unless the patient can find something more interesting and worthwhile to attend to, the career of pain is apt to last till death. (Szasz, 1988, pp. xxviii–xxix)

Szasz's writings provide us with important, unique clinical insights and recommendations that are particularly relevant today. For patients, all pain is real and their experience needs to be respected. When there are complaints of pain in the absence of bodily illness—and particularly when this is chronic—start with "Don't do something, just stand there!" Do not keep ordering expensive tests, prescribing pain medications, or referring for surgical procedures (Baber and Erdek, 2016). Instead, carefully evaluate for a "painful person." Do not validate anyone's quest to become a legitimate patient or "help" by giving a medical or psychiatric diagnosis. Engage the person in working autonomously toward a more meaningful life, with activities that are more interesting and worthwhile to attend to than pain.

11.6 **The psychology of schizophrenia**

Another of Szasz's clinical insights borrows from psychoanalytic and philosophical understandings to build a fresh "formulation of the concept of 'schizophrenia' unburdened by the medical model of 'disease' and independent of whether its classic symptoms are manifest or not . . . The chief thesis of the essay lies in considering 'schizophrenia' as a state of (relative) deficiency of internal objects in the adult" (Szasz, 1956, p. 434). Rarely cited, Szasz's "psychology" (purposefully not "psychopathology") of schizophrenia provides a superb understanding of the development and inevitable troubles of the person with schizophrenia. Dewan (2016) presents an updated version that is faithful to Szasz's original ideas but also accounts for newer biological findings. Given that schizophrenia is a group of diseases, the deficit theory explains the condition of some (but not all) persons diagnosed with schizophrenia; there may or may not be overlap with one or more of the other putative disturbances, such as in the dopamine system or the immune system.

Szasz describes parallel processes for physical and psychological growth and development. A rich assortment of external objects must be eaten and assimilated to grow and develop the human body. Similarly, psychological growth and development requires that a rich array of external people and relationships be internalized and assimilated to create a vibrant, healthy psychological world of internal objects and object relationships. A fully grown adult who has been starved of food during childhood suffers from stunted growth and looks cachectic; he suffers from schizophrenia if he has been starved of healthy people and relationships and has a deficit of internal objects and object relationships.

In normal development, people ("objects" in object relations theory) are introjected through a biopsychosociocultural filter, through which this external person is evaluated and then internalized—both as a model of a person (object) and as a model for behavior (object relations). Therefore, the internal representation (or memory) of any particular object will differ from person to person based on the individuals' filters. Szasz proposes that normal psychological growth and development is the process of introjecting an abundance of people and interactions so that the inner world is filled with representations of countless people, rich and varied in their appearance and behavior. This rich inner world provides the person with numerous models of how to deal with real situations before they come up.

As a teenager or young adult, a person is ushered into a complex uncharted world where there are simultaneous pressures to leave home, move toward independence, find a job or get further education, and build adult relationships with love and sexual intimacy. Many of these experiences are new and anxiety-provoking. However, the normal adult manages them by using functional models from the vast repertoire of introjected people and behavioral models. They may not have done it, but they know how to do it (Dewan, 2016).

In a person who will develop schizophrenia, Szasz's "deficit" model asserts that there is a deviation, in several significant ways, from the normal introjection of numerous functional people and behavioral models. First, there is an abnormal biopsychosociocultural filter, which leads to a greater distortion of the introjected person, then to "bad" introjects being incomplete ("part objects") or malignant, full of the potential for internal conflict, and certainly less functional as models. Second, the premorbid predisposition to being withdrawn and schizoidal decreases the number of people with whom this person interacts, and therefore there are fewer introjects of people (i.e., a deficit of internal "objects"). Third, the abnormal filter also distorts the meaning of the behavior that this person witnesses, so that there are fewer functional behavioral models internalized (i.e., a deficit in internal behavioral models or object relations). For instance, if they are in a dysfunctional family and schizoidal, they may miss "corrective emotional experiences" that normal children get from supportive teachers, coaches, or other parents. The person who will develop schizophrenia therefore reaches young adulthood with a deficiency in number and maturity of internalized objects (which may be fragmented, malignant, or conflicted) and functional behavioral models. This is the deficit model of schizophrenia.

As a young adult, the person with these deficits is also thrown into a complex, uncharted world with the same simultaneous pressures that normal adults face: leave home, move toward independence, find a job or enter college, build an adult relationship with love and sexual intimacy, etc. The object-deficient person finds this not merely new and anxiety-provoking, but terrifying and catastrophic to become aware of his or her deficits and inability to manage the real world. The terror of this reality is dealt with by creating an alternative reality—that is, a restitutive psychosis which fills the deficit with a new reality constructed of delusions and hallucinations.

The psychological "meaning" of this restitutive psychosis is important from both a theoretical and a clinical point of view. Theoretically, the concept of restitutive psychosis is based on the well-accepted notion of defense mechanisms. Essentially, all defense mechanisms (including the psychotic-level defenses such as delusional denial, psychotic projection, and distortion) are utilized to convert a difficult and intolerable situation into a more tolerable (better) situation. Psychosis (perhaps the most difficult condition a human being can find himself in) is restitutive and *better* than the reality from which this person is fleeing (Dewan, 2016).

Years after Szasz described the deficit state, others elaborated on it (Gunderson and Mosher, 1975; Dewan, 2016) and empirical research has repeatedly validated the key elements: relative paucity of internal objects, their malignant transformation, and the prevalence of restitutive defenses in persons with schizophrenia (Bell et al., 1992; Blatt et al., 1990; Huprich and Greenberg 2003; Rosenberg et al., 1994). Despite this evidence, most texts on schizophrenia do not have a section on the psychology of the disorder and none acknowledge Szasz's contribution.

11.7 **Treatment implications**

Szasz summarizes:

> We conceive of the symptoms of 'schizophrenia' as restitutive manifestations which attempt to cover up a deficiency of internal objects. Substitutive 'internal objects,' which we called 'fantasy objects,' are thus created by the ego. This is made possible for the ego on the basis of whatever sources ('bad,' or inadequate) of internal objects it has available. Bodily feelings supply a most important source of 'objects' for the object-deficient ego

of the schizophrenic, and this accounts for the frequency of so called hypochondriacal preoccupations in these persons. The somatic and personal 'fantasy objects,' once manifest, clash with the 'objective' universe of the social norm and mobilize action toward, or oftener against, the patient. Rarely, this leads to psychotherapeutic efforts. More frequently, social action leads simply to the removal and incarceration of the manifestly offending ('offensive') individual. (Szasz, 1956, p. 433)

It is evident that this concept of schizophrenia as an object deficit state, and of psychosis as a restitutive response, have major clinical implications. First, the treatment of a person with deficits is to reduce and eliminate these deficits. This requires sophisticated and time-intensive use of a person (therapist) or persons to provide real, positive "prototype" experiences, so that the individual with schizophrenia can introject these experiences as a functional model of a person with a rich variety of real-world, functional behaviors. Szasz writes that

> to treat the schizophrenic, the therapist must have a need of his own to make contact with, and to devote himself to, the patient. This reciprocity of needs, and this alone, would make the therapist available to the patient as an object for introjection. However, this in itself is not enough. I would add to this, that the therapist must show the patient by example how he himself deals with the world (this includes his own impulses, as well as his orientations and techniques of relating to other people and inanimate objects). In this way the patient gains access to that prototypal experience from which he was deprived in childhood, namely, to learn how to deal with the world by introjecting adequate objects. (Szasz, 1956, p. 429)

Second, the deficit model would predict that merely getting the patient better by stamping out psychotic symptoms is counterproductive. From the patient's point of view, it merely sends him or her from a "better" restitutive psychotic condition back to a worse reality. In fact, a careful study showed that "some schizophrenics may prefer an ego-syntonic grandiose psychosis to a relative drug-induced normality" (Van Putten et al., 1976, p. 1443). This leads to another insight: A patient who is symptomatically better may be psychologically worse and therefore, logically, will not take "effective" medications. This psychological distress is usually reported in clinical drug trials as a side effect that causes "subjective distress," and studies have shown it to be "the most likely to affect willingness to take medications" (Velligan et al., 2009, p. 17). Understandably now, nonadherence is the rule.

In the treatment of persons with object deficits (schizophrenia), all proven treatments are helpful to the degree that they serve the primary objective—to improve reality by providing stable, real, positive relationships for the object-deficient person to introject.

> The primary effort is for the therapist to be a long-term, stable, reliable, clear, transparent person who skillfully resists being distorted by the many moods and projections of a psychotic person. The aim is for the patient to introject a functional image of a benign, caring person. In therapy, 'I' and 'you' rather than 'we' or 'us' can be used to facilitate a clear sense of 'self' and 'other' and to avoid the tensions inherent in the need-fear dilemma (needing closeness but being afraid of being engulfed or hurt). There needs to be constant vigilance and correction when the patient inevitably and repeatedly distorts himself or the therapist as is his wont. (Dewan, 2016, p. 566)

Persons with schizophrenia think in concrete terms. Therefore, the therapeutic relationship needs to be concrete and clear.

> For instance, on a beautiful day, it is not enough to talk about it; instead, concretely do (model) what normal people would on that day—go for a walk or sit outside in the sun for the duration of the session. Or, if a patient reports that he was thrown out of his apartment because he accused his neighbor of spying on him, do not ask him how he is going to get another apartment or refer him to the social worker. It is helpful to model behavior: 'You and I can look for what is available in the newspaper or online' and do so. (Dewan, 2016, p. 566)

Szasz makes an important distinction between a therapist's passive stance and active work with persons with schizophrenia. In the most passive stance, the therapist is like a drama critic who watches the opening performance and writes a review. The director is welcome to make changes based on this review—or ignore it. In work with persons with schizophrenia, the therapist needs to be more like the director—a real, active, invested, supportive collaborator who effectively tries to mold the actor's behavior (Szasz, 1963, 1994, 2004). In fact, the greater the deficit, the more involved in the patient's reality the therapist needs to be, sometimes crossing boundaries but being careful never to violate them. Thus, the therapist can talk about real-world solutions, actively help solve problems (e.g., finding an apartment with the patient), role play situations (e.g., social skills training), and encourage "homework," whereby behaviors rehearsed in session are repeatedly practiced in the real world (Dewan, 2016).

How should the therapist talk about "restitutive" psychotic symptoms? Delusions cannot be challenged or supported. However, the feeling created by the delusion is universal and can be a point of empathic connection.

Szasz is interested in understanding the condition of persons with object deficits, which "is in no way synonymous with 'illness'" (Szasz, 1956, p. 434), and he resists labeling them. He describes a form of psychotherapy that would logically address this deficit. However, since psychiatry is more impressed with the psychotic (and often "offensive") symptoms than with the deficits, the "apparent paradox of the 'therapeutic' use of destroying the highest centers of the brain" (Szasz, 1956, pp. 433–4) by lobotomy becomes understandable, but makes correcting object deficits impossible. He later claimed that schizophrenia was a social construct created by the therapeutic state to control and remove offensive persons from society. When challenged by new and replicable findings of brain abnormalities in patients with schizophrenia, Szasz (1976) argues that it must then be classified as a neurological disorder—it would still not qualify as a mental illness and should not be subject to a different set of "mental hygiene" laws, the most egregious of which allowed for involuntary hospitalization and forced treatment. None of his later views detract from his seminal contribution to the psychology of schizophrenia, which now has the backing of empirical evidence.

11.8 **Clinical wisdom: general considerations**

Although Szasz considered mental illness a "myth" and was opposed to the traditional practice of psychiatry, he was not "antipsychiatry" and—more importantly—was not against helping persons in distress. In fact, he was in favor of all the basic elements that physicians and therapists consider the bedrock of clinical practice. He urged that, whenever possible, they embrace the autonomy and freedom of both the physician and the patient; that they treat the patient as a person, with understanding and respect; that understanding is more important than diagnosis, and that this deeper understanding of persons and reality makes it easier to help people help themselves; that they need to be flexible and adapt to different models of the physician–patient relationship as required by changing circumstances; that they be real; and that they strive to be helpful.

Unfortunately—and to the detriment of the mental health field—even when his major contributions have been repeatedly validated by empirical evidence or acknowledged as "classics," they have had limited impact on clinical practice. Szasz himself may have contributed to this by not acknowledging or reconciling the ideas in his earlier writings with those in his prolific later publications. There are accounts of grateful individuals "practicing Szasz" (Breeding, 2014), but Szasz's papers are rarely cited, and his clinical wisdom has not made it into the mainstream.

References

Baber, Zafeer, and Michael A. Erdek. 2016. "Failed Back Surgery Syndrome: Current Perspectives." *Journal of Pain Research* **9**: 979–87.

Bauer, Gregory P. (ed.). 1994. *Essential Papers on Transference Analysis*. Northvale, New Jersey: Jason Aronson.

Bell, Morris, Paul Lysaker, and Robert Milstein. 1992. "Object Relations Deficits in Subtypes of Schizophrenia." *Journal of Clinical Psychology* **48** (4) (July): 433–44.

Blatt, Sidney J., Steven B. Tuber, and John S. Auerbach. 1990. "Representation of Interpersonal Interactions on the Rorschach and Level of Psychopathology." *Journal of Personality Assessment* **54**: 711–18.

Breeding, John. 2014. "Practicing Szasz: A Psychologist Reports on Thomas Szasz's Influence on His Work." *Sage Open* (October–December) 1–12. Accessed April 17, 2018. <journals. sagepub.com/doi/pdf/10.1177/2158244014551715>

Breuer, Josef, and Sigmund Freud. 1893–1895. "Studies on Hysteria." In *The Standard Edition of the Complete Psychological Works of Sigmund Freud, Volume 2*. London: Hogarth, 1955.

Dewan, Mantosh J. 2016. "The Psychology of Schizophrenia: Implications for Biological and Psychotherapeutic Treatments." *Journal of Nervous and Mental Disease* **204** (8) (August): 564–9.

Emanuel, Ezekiel J., and Linda L. Emanuel. 1992. "Four Models of the Physician-Patient Relationship." *JAMA* **267** (16): 2221–6.

Gunderson, John G., and Loren R. Mosher (eds.). 1975. *Psychotherapy of Schizophrenia*. New York: Jason Aronson.

Huprich, Steven K., and Roger P. Greenberg. 2003. "Advances in the Assessment of Object Relations in the 1990s." *Clinical Psychology Review* **23** (5): 665–98.

Jones, Ernest. 1953. *The Life and Work of Sigmund Freud, Volume 1, 1856–1900: The Formative Years and the Great Discoveries*. New York: Basic Books.

Langs, Robert J. (ed.). 2004. *Classics in Psychoanalytic Technique*, revised edn. Lanham, Maryland: Rowman and Littlefield.

Rosenberg, Stanley D., Sidney J. Blatt, Thomas E. Oxman, et al. 1994. "Assessment of Object Relatedness Through a Lexical Content Analysis of the TAT." *Journal of Personality Assessment* **63** (2) (October): 345–62.

Shivale, Swati, and Mantosh J. Dewan. 2015. "The Art and Science of Prescribing." *Journal of Family Practice* **64** (7) (July): 400–6. Accessed April 17, 2018. <www.mdedge.com/sites/default/files/issues/articles/JFP_06407_Article2.pdf>

Szasz, Thomas S. 1956. "A Contribution to the Psychology of Schizophrenia." *AMA Archives of Neurology and Psychiatry* **77** (4): 420–36.

Szasz, Thomas S. 1961. *The Myth of Mental Illness. Foundations of a Theory of Personal Conduct.* New York: Hoeber-Harper.

Szasz, Thomas S. 1963. "The Concept of Transference." *International Journal of Psychoanalysis* **44** (October): 432–43.

Szasz, Thomas S. 1965. *The Ethics of Psychoanalysis: The Theory and Method of Autonomous Psychotherapy.* New York: Basic Books.

Szasz, Thomas S. 1975. *Pain and Pleasure: A Study of Bodily Feelings*, 2nd edn. New York: Basic Books.

Szasz, Thomas S. 1976. *Schizophrenia: The Sacred Symbol of Psychiatry.* New York: Basic Books.

Szasz, Thomas S. 1978. "Sigmund Freud: The Jewish Avenger." In *The Myth of Psychotherapy: Mental Healing as Religion, Rhetoric, and Repression*, pp. 138–57. Garden City, New York: Doubleday Anchor.

Szasz, Thomas S. 1988. *Pain and Pleasure: A Study of Bodily Feelings*, 2nd edn. Syracuse: Syracuse University Press.

Szasz, Thomas S. 1994. "The Concept of Transference." In *Essential Papers on Transference Analysis*, edited by Gregory P. Bauer, pp. 165–94.

Szasz, Thomas S. 2004. "The Concept of Transference." In *Classics in Psychoanalytic Technique*, edited by Robert J. Langs, pp. 25–36.

Szasz, Thomas S., and Marc H. Hollender. 1956. "A Contribution to the Philosophy of Medicine: The Basic Models of the Doctor-Patient Relationship." *AMA Archives of Internal Medicine* **97** (5): 585–92.

Van Putten, Theodore, Evelyn Crumpton, and Coralee Yale. 1976. "Drug Refusal in Schizophrenia and the Wish to Be Crazy." *Archives of General Psychiatry* **33** (12): 1443–6.

Velligan, Dawn I., Peter J. Weiden, Martha Sajatovic, et al. 2009. "The Expert Consensus Guidelines Series: Adherence Problems in Patients with Serious Mental Illness." *Journal of Clinical Psychiatry* **70** (suppl. 4): 1–48.

Chapter 12

Thomas Szasz and the language of mental illness

Ronald W. Pies

> For philosophical problems arise when language *goes on holiday.*
>
> Ludwig Wittgenstein (1968, p. 19e, § 38)

12.1 Introduction

Imagine for a moment that within the next twenty years, neuroscientists find very spe-cific brain abnormalities that seem to account for all of the most serious psychiatric disorders. Let us say that this information is so precise that we can link schizophrenia, bipolar disorder, and major depression not only with abnormalities in specific regions of the brain, but also with highly specific neurochemical and genetic abnormalities. Would we then be able to eliminate the terms "mental illness," "mental disorder," and similar "mentalistic" terms from our clinical vocabulary? Would we be able to refer exclusively to "brain disease" when discussing, say, schizophrenia, bipolar disorder, or major depression?

I believe that Szasz would have answered yes to both questions—and that this would represent a serious conceptual error (Pies, 2015). For Szasz—who declared mental illness a "myth" and a "metaphorical illness"—psychiatry's (illegitimate) di-agnostic categories were only temporary stops on the road to the recognition of "real" and legitimate *bodily* diseases. Szasz argued that conditions once regarded as "mental illnesses" would rightly be reclassified as "brain diseases," insofar as scientific investigations would eventually uncover their neuropathology. The classic example was neurosyphilis. As its neuropathology became increasingly evident, Szasz claimed, tertiary syphilis ceased to be regarded as "madness" and came to be considered "brain disease." With each such neurological discovery, Szasz believed, "psychopathology" was appropriately reclassified as neuropathology. In principle, this process of reclas-sification could entirely eliminate the notion of "mental illness" and render the term meaningless.

Szasz himself put it this way: "In part, such a process of biological discoveries has characterized some of the history of medicine, one form of 'madness' after another being identified as the manifestation of one or another somatic disease, such as beri-beri, epilepsy, or neurosyphilis. The result of such a discovery is that *the illness ceases to be a form of psychopathology and is classified and treated as neuropathology. If all the 'conditions' now called 'mental illnesses' proved to be brain diseases, there would be no need for the notion of mental illness and the term would become devoid of meaning"* (Szasz, 2010, pp. xiii–xiv, italics added). I believe that in advancing this argument, Szasz fundamentally misread "the history of medicine" and misunderstood the philosophical and linguistic issues surrounding the terms "mental illness" and "brain disease."

Before developing my argument, however, I want to place these issues in the broader context of Szasz's nearly lifelong views on mental illness. I believe that Szasz's work, over a span of more than fifty years, eventuated in six primary claims or theses. I will first summarize these and offer some very brief rejoinders, prior to discussing my principle argument regarding the utility of the term, "mental illness."

12.2 Szasz's six main theses

12.2.1 Historical and ontological claims regarding the nature of "disease"

Szasz's principle historical claim about illness (or "disease," which he uses more or less synonymously with "illness") is: "Until the middle of the nineteenth century, and beyond, illness meant a bodily disorder whose typical manifestation was an alteration of bodily structure . . . [a] lesion, such as a misshapen extremity, ulcerated skin, or a fracture or wound" (Szasz, 2010, p. 11). Based on his understanding of the German pathologist Rudolf Virchow, Szasz further argues: "The accepted scientific method for demonstrating . . . diseases consisted, first, of identifying their morphological characteristic by post-mortem examination of organs and tissues; and second, of ascertaining, by means of systemic observations and experiments . . . their origins and causes" (Szasz, 1976, pp. 130–1). Furthermore, he asserts: "When the early (nineteenth century) psychiatrists spoke of mental disease or diseases of the mind, they understood, and often explicitly stated, that these expressions were figures of speech or metaphors" (Szasz, 1987, p. 140).

In addition to his historical claims, Szasz also makes a key *ontological* claim about disease; that is, a claim relating to *what disease actually is*, and not merely how it has been regarded: "Disease or illness can affect only the body. Hence, there *can be no such thing* as mental illness. . . . medical diagnoses are the names of genuine diseases, psychiatric diagnoses are stigmatizing labels" (2010, pp. ix, xii, italics added).

Historically, there has never been a single, universally accepted definition of "disease" or "illness," nor have these terms always been restricted to "bodily" conditions, lesions, or pathophysiology (Pies, 1979). Indeed, it is not clear that even Virchow would have made such a claim. Virchow, to be sure, viewed lesions and cellular dysfunction as the *basis* of *specific diseases*. But it is not clear that he saw such pathology as the *sine qua non* of "disease" in the broader, conceptual sense. Indeed, Szasz is in fundamental conflict with Virchow on a critical point: "Every 'ordinary' illness that persons have, cadavers also have" (Szasz, 1973, p. 87). But for Virchow, illness or disease is always a condition of the living organism; and whereas lesions or cytopathology may persist for some time after death (i.e., after *the illness of the person is terminated*) (Pies, 1979).

In any case, modern physicians have many varying understandings of the term "disease," some of which have little to do with cellular pathology and a great deal to do with suffering, incapacity, or impairment in various spheres of human endeavor.

12.2.2 Claims regarding "metaphoricity"

> Mental illness is a metaphor (metaphorical disease). . . . Individuals with mental diseases (bad behaviors), like societies with economic diseases (bad fiscal policies), are metaphorically sick.
>
> Szasz (1998)

Moreover, "if I say that mental illness is a metaphorical illness, I am not saying that it is some other kind of illness; I am saying that it is *not an illness at all*" (Szasz, 1987, p. 151, italics added).

A metaphor is generally understood as a locution involving an implied comparison of one kind of thing with another; for example, in the metaphor, "night's curtain," darkness is implicitly compared to an actual curtain. However, the term "metaphor" itself is highly contested in literary, linguistic, and philosophical theory (Pies, 2012; Ortony, 1993; Davidson, 2001; Lakoff and Johnson, 2003; Cools et al., 2013). Furthermore, Szasz seems unaware of the difference between metaphorical language and what modern philosophers would term "ordinary language." Thus, when we say, "Joe has a mental illness," there is no reason to suppose that we are "comparing" what Joe has to a "real" *bodily* illness or disease. Rather, we are using "illness" in a *literal* sense, even if we do not have in mind the same *kind* of illness as when we speak of, for example, "autoimmune illness." I take up these issues in more detail elsewhere.

But even if Szasz were right in claiming that the locution "mental illness" is a metaphor—and I believe he is wrong—this would not demonstrate that mental illness *does not exist*, or that it is "not an illness at all." Here, Szasz falls victim to a kind of positivist misunderstanding of metaphor, insofar as he seems to equate metaphoricity with falsity; that is, Szasz seems to think that if a locution X is metaphorical, then it has no ontological salience, no real-world referent. In effect, Szasz seems to believe that a metaphorical locution cannot accurately depict the actual state of affairs (i.e., the "what is") of a particular person. This is trivially fallacious. For even if the locution "mental illness" were a metaphor, it would not follow that those to whom the term "mental illness" is ascribed are merely "metaphorically sick." Here, Szasz conflates figures of speech (metaphors) with ontological realities. I am aware of the irony of my claim however, since Szasz has charged psychiatrists with precisely the same kind of confusion.

To put it differently: Metaphors are not false representations of the state of affairs in the world. Indeed, as the theologian Marcus Borg points out, "metaphors can be profoundly true . . . metaphor is not less than fact, but more" (2001, p. 41). Thus, if we say, "Night's curtain fell upon the village," we may indeed be speaking *metaphorically*, but not *falsely*—assuming that it did actually get dark in the village. Similarly, even if we were speaking metaphorically in saying "Joe suffers from mental illness"—that is, inviting the listener to entertain some sort of implied "comparison"—it would not follow that we were making a *false* statement, or one without ontological relevance. On the contrary, Joe might be suffering quite profoundly in the realm of the "mental." He might be extremely confused, distraught, incoherent, suicidal, and unable to function in his daily life. Joe would not be rendered "metaphorically sick" merely because we used a metaphor to describe his condition—he would be *actually* sick! Indeed, it is precisely Joe's sort of suffering and incapacity that has been the hallmark of "disease" for much of the history of medicine (Pies, 1979). The suffering of someone accurately diagnosed with a severe psychiatric illness is ontologically real, independent of the intentional or metaphorical properties of language. In short, we do not magically nullify actual disease simply because we use a metaphorical locution to describe the person's condition (Pies, 2012).

Finally, when Szasz describes mental illness as "a metaphorical illness," he appears, yet again, to be confusing *ontological* with *linguistic* claims. A metaphor is a locution—a figure of speech—and "metaphoricity" is an attribute of locutions, not of entities or putative entities, in the real world. We can no more speak logically of a "metaphorical illness" than we can of a "metaphorical table" or a "metaphorical apple." Thus, the term "metaphorical illness" appears to represent a Rylean "category mistake" on Szasz's part (Tanney, 2015).

12.2.3 The claim that the term, "mental illness," represents a "category error"

> The word 'disease' denotes a demonstrable biological process that affects the bodies of living organisms (plants, animals, and humans). The term 'mental illness' refers to the undesirable thoughts, feelings, and behaviors of persons. Classifying thoughts, feelings, and behaviors as diseases is a logical and semantic error, like classifying the whale as a fish. As the whale is not a fish, mental illness is not a disease.
>
> Szasz (1998)

It should be obvious that Szasz's first premise about what disease "denotes" merely begs the question; that is, it asserts, as a received truth, precisely what is at the heart of the fifty-year-old controversy that Szasz's work has engendered. As the philosopher Thomas Schramme tartly observes, "Szasz could be reproached for defining illness in such a way that leaves no space for mental illness from the outset" (2004, p. 112). I am not aware of any of Szasz's writings in which he seriously considers alternative (e.g., non-physicalist) concepts of "disease" or illness, such as that provided in the edition of Harrison's that I used as a resident: "The clinical method has as its object the collection of accurate data concerning all the diseases to which human beings are subject; namely, *all conditions that limit life in its powers, enjoyment, and duration*" (Harrison and Thorn, 1977, p. 1, italics added).

Whereas there is little or no scientific controversy as regards the necessary and sufficient criteria for what distinguishes a mammal (like a whale) from a fish, there is a great deal of controversy as to what the term "disease" denotes—so much so that the American Medical Association's Council on Science and Public Health was unable to say whether obesity is or is not a "disease." They concluded: "Without a single, clear, authoritative, and widely accepted definition of disease, it is difficult to determine conclusively whether or not obesity is a medical disease state" (AMA, 2013, p. 6).

12.2.4 "Analytic truth" claim about the term, "mental illness"

In his later writings, Szasz invoked the concept of "analyticity" in defending his claims regarding metaphor: "My claim that mental illnesses are fictitious illnesses is also not based on scientific research; it rests on the materialist-scientific definition of illness as a pathological alteration of cells, tissues, and organs. If we accept this scientific definition of disease, then it follows that mental illness is a metaphor, and that asserting that view is asserting an *analytic truth, not subject to empirical falsification*" (2010, p. xii, original italics).

As Szasz himself admits, his argument rests on whether or not we accept the definition of illness that he imputes to the "materialist-scientific" position. If we do not accept this premise, then the rest of his argument effectively falls apart. But, as previously noted, the "materialist-scientific" position—to the extent it can be defined—is far from universally accepted by physicians, or by philosophers of science. Moreover, terms like "science" and "scientific" are themselves highly contested and controversial. Furthermore, Szasz's claim that the statement "mental illness is a metaphor" asserts an *analytic* truth is deeply puzzling, since the statement does not conform to the usual structure of analytic truths as understood by most philosophers. Commonly cited analytic statements would include, for example: "All triangles have three angles" and "All bachelors are unmarried males." Indeed, the claim, "Mental illness is a metaphor," appears to be a *synthetic* claim; that is, one that requires "real-world" investigation into, for example, the nature of "illness" and "metaphor"—and not merely logical deduction. In any event, since the seminal work of philosopher Willard Van Orman Quine, the entire distinction between analytic and synthetic statements may have been seriously undermined, if not vitiated completely (Rocknak, 2013).

12.2.5 Counterfactual conditional claim about bodily illness versus mental illness

As usually defined: "Counterfactual conditionals are those in which the antecedent is false, and which assert that one event *would be*, or *would have been* the case if another event were, or would *have been* the case" (Merlino, n.d.). A simple example would be the folk saying, "If wishes were horses, then beggars would ride."

I believe that Szasz uses a modified counterfactual conditional claim (Aftab, 2014) in the following argument:

> When a person hears me say that there is no such thing as mental illness, he is likely to reply: 'But I know so-and-so who was diagnosed as mentally ill and turned out to have a brain tumor. In due time, with refinements in medical technology, psychiatrists will be able to show that all mental illnesses are bodily diseases.' This contingency does not falsify my contention that mental illness is a metaphor. It verifies it: The physician who discovers that a particular person diagnosed as mentally ill suffers from a brain disease discovers

that the patient was misdiagnosed. *The patient did not have a mental illness, he had, and has, a physical illness.* (Szasz, 2010, p. xiii, italics added)

In effect, Szasz's counterfactual conditional claim may be restated as follows: "If a so-called mental illness were shown to be a brain disease, then the condition would not be a mental illness (which would then constitute a misdiagnosis)."

The clear implication of this argument is that, for Szasz, mental illness and bodily illness (or brain disease) are mutually exclusive (disjunctive) categories. Accordingly, for Szasz, if we establish the presence of brain disease, we automatically and necessarily exclude the presence of mental illness. I believe this claim to be fallacious, and will deal with it in detail as a component of my main argument.

12.2.6 The claim regarding pathology texts and exclusion of "mental illness"

Every 'ordinary' illness that persons have, cadavers also have. A cadaver may thus be said to 'have' cancer, pneumonia, or myocardial infarction.

Szasz (1973, p. 87)

Szasz argues: "The pathologist uses the term 'disease' as a predicate of physical objects—cells, tissues, organs, and bodies. Textbooks of pathology describe disorders of the body, living or dead, not disorders of the person, mind, or behavior. René Leriche (1874–1955), the founder of modern vascular surgery, aptly observed: 'If one wants to define disease it must be dehumanized. . . . In disease, when all is said and done, the least important thing is man.' For the practice of pathology and for disease as a scientific concept, the person as potential sufferer is unimportant" (Szasz, 2010, p. xx).

Various versions of the observation that schizophrenia and other major mood disorders are not "listed" or discussed in pathology texts have appeared over the past several decades. Thus, psychologist Jeffrey Schaler writes: "If 'mental illness' is really a brain disease, it would be listed as such in standard textbooks on pathology. It is not listed as a brain disease because it does not meet the nosological criteria for disease classification" (1998). I have dealt with this erroneous claim in detail elsewhere (Pies, 2008) and will not repeat the counterarguments here. Suffice it to say that there is no obvious reason why pathologists should serve as the sole authorized arbiters of what constitutes a "real" disease, as opposed to, say, family practitioners or gynecologists. But more to the point, many modern pathology texts refer to and discuss conditions that are widely regarded as psychiatric illnesses, such as schizophrenia (Pies, 2008).

On a more fundamental level, Szasz's claim that "Every 'ordinary' illness that persons have, cadavers also have" (1973, p. 87) is not merely risible but is completely at odds with the position of Szasz's supposed mentor, Virchow, for whom disease is predicated only of *living* organisms—cadavers may show cytopathology, but not "disease." Indeed, if cadavers could have illnesses just as "persons" have them, as Szasz claims, then we ought to be able to say, with a straight face, "This cadaver seems *extremely ill*" or "That cadaver is only *mildly ill*." This consequence of Szasz's view is so obviously untenable, it requires no further comment. As for the notion that a "scientific" view of disease precludes reference to the "person," this flies in the face of nearly all medical writing in the area of psychosomatic and consultation-liaison psychiatry, not to mention existential psychiatry. To suggest that these disciplines are not "scientific" is to impose a procrustean positivism that has been widely discredited by philosophers of science. Finally, medical ethicists would likely raise serious objections to any view of disease claiming, as Szasz seems to believe, that "the person as potential sufferer is unimportant" (Szasz, 2010, p. xx).

12.3 Szasz's views on the term, "mental illness"

Let us return now to Szasz's claims summarized at the beginning of this chapter; specifically, to his historical claim that a condition "*ceases to be a form of psychopathology and is classified and treated as neuropathology*" once the condition's neuropathological foundations are discovered. Contrary to the implications of this claim, the term "mental illness" has not disappeared or become meaningless, with respect to conditions for which specific neuropathology has been ascertained. Thus, Alzheimer's disease and other forms of dementia are widely considered instantiations of "mental illness," notwithstanding their well-characterized neuropathology.

Indeed, DSM-V classifies Alzheimer's disease and other dementias as mental disorders. In part, this is because DSM-V does not regard neuropathology—which Szasz seems to impute solely to "brain disease"—as a disqualifying factor for the existence of a mental disorder. Also, more classical "psychiatric" symptoms, such as depression or delusions, often appear in Alzheimer's disease and related dementias, generally prompting psychiatric involvement. Indeed, psychopathology does not evaporate upon the discovery of neuropathology. These are complementary, not contradictory or disjunctive terms. Just as some mental illnesses, such as schizophrenia, may be considered "brain diseases," some brain diseases—such as Alzheimer's disease—may manifest as "mental illness." This relationship was made evident by Orth and Trimble (2006).

Furthermore, the term, "mental illness," is a useful and established element of what philosophers like Wittgenstein (1958, 1968) called "ordinary language." As Wittgenstein put it, "ordinary language is all right" (1958, p. 28). Wittgenstein also claims that "a word hasn't got a meaning given to it, as it were, by a power independent of us, so that there could be a kind of scientific investigation into what the word *really* means" (1958, p. 28, original italics). Yet the whole of Szasz's critique seems predicated on just such a positivist fallacy.

The locution, "mental illness," remains a useful, albeit imperfect, shorthand term to describe a particular kind of suffering and incapacity, usually affecting cognition, emotion, reasoning, and behavior. DSM-V implicitly recognizes this, in its definition of "mental disorder" as "a syndrome characterized by clinically significant disturbance in an individual's cognition, emotion regulation, or behavior that reflects a dysfunction in the psychological, biological, or developmental processes underlying mental functioning" (APA, 2013, p. 20).

12.4 **Neuropsychiatric conditions**

Even if all mental illnesses were conclusively and causally linked to specific brain pathologies, I maintain that we would still need "mental language" in our ordinary discourse, and in our work with patients (Brown, 1991). We will probably always require a vocabulary of psychopathology, and the vocabulary of psychotherapy will always retain a "mentalistic" orientation. We will never greet a depressed patient by asking, "And how is your prefrontal cortex this morning, Mrs. Jones?"—just as we will probably never substitute the expression, "I changed my brain" for "I changed my mind." This claim is not predicated on any dualistic metaphysics, in which "mind" and "brain" denote two ontologically discrete entities or "substances"; it is merely to state a practical truth about how ordinary language actually functions.

Consider Alzheimer's disease. While we do not fully understand its causes, we do know, and can reliably detect, the basic neuropathology of Alzheimer's disease (i.e., the presence of amyloid plaques and neurofibrillary tangles in the brain). Nevertheless, neurologists and psychiatrists have long referred to the *psycho*pathology of Alzheimer's disease. David Boyd (1936) described "the psychopathology of Alzheimer's Disease," using terms such as "mental failure" and "mental disorganization." He focused mainly on cognitive deficits, such as the "slowness of mental reactions" in afflicted patients. However, we now recognize that psychopathology in Alzheimer's disease often includes *delusions, hallucinations, and depression.* Dementia expert Davangere Devanand produced a video lecture on precisely this topic (2013).

These psychological phenomena have important implications for the emotional states of patients, and for caregivers of those afflicted with Alzheimer's. That we can identify neuropathology in the brains of these patients in no way eliminates "psychopathology," as Szasz's argument seems to require. Nor does the identification of brain lesions render the term "mental illness" meaningless when referring to Alzheimer's disease or other dementias. Recall that DSM-V, psychiatry's manual of *mental* disorders, includes Alzheimer's disease and other forms of dementia under the rubric, "neurocognitive disorders."

12.5 **Is "mental illness" a useful term?**

To use the vocabulary of "mental illness" or "mental disease" is not, as Szasz seems to think, to posit some metaphysical or actual entity called "mind," which is held to be "ill" or "diseased." When we say, "Smith is mentally ill" or "Smith's mind is sick," we are not making an *ontological* claim which requires that some nonmaterial entity called "mind" actually contain a lesion or physiological defect of some sort—an implausible notion, to be sure. Neither are we using a *metaphor* (i.e., an implied comparison), whereby we invite the listener, as Lakoff and Johnson put it, to experience *"one kind of thing in terms of another"* (2003, p. 5, original italics). On the contrary, when we speak of a "sick mind," we are simply using an alternate but quite *literal* meaning of "sick," commonly found in many English dictionaries. For example, among the online *Merriam-Webster Medical Dictionary* definitions of "sick" is "mentally or emotionally unsound or disordered." Similarly, when we use the term "illness" in juxtaposition to the term, "mental," we are using "illness" in a straightforward, literal sense, in accordance with ordinary language (i.e., as "an unhealthy condition of body or *mind*"; *Merriam-Webster*, italics added).

Furthermore, the attribution of "mental illness" or "sickness of mind" does not require us to have identified a physiological abnormality or lesion of any kind. As Michael Moore points out: "In so using mental illness one is thus committed to no funny, nonmaterial substances that are in some nonspatial way injured or impaired. . . . To say that someone's mind is ill is only to say that his capacity for rational action is diminished . . . Being in a state properly called 'ill,' then, does not depend on one's knowing, or even in the first instance of there being, any particular physiological condition. It depends on one's being in a state characterized roughly by pain, incapacitation, and the prospect of a hastened death" (1975, p. 1490; 1984, pp. 168, 170).

Similarly, as Schramme tells us: "One can surely postulate a bodily basis of mental phenomena, but still talk of mental illness. This possibility would be ruled out only if mental phenomena could be exhaustively *explained* by the underlying bodily processes; i.e. reduced to brain disease. . . . it suffices to state that even if mental illness has a bodily basis, it will not follow necessarily that referral to mental illness will be confusing, misleading, and unnecessary" (2004, p. 113, italics added). Here, Schramme uses the crucial term, "explained." *Explanation*, in a purely physical and causal sense, differs from *understanding*, in a meaningful and "human" sense. The philosopher of history Wilhelm Dilthey, and later, the psychiatrist Karl Jaspers—both following standard German usage whose technical philosophical aspect goes back at least as far as Immanuel Kant, the founder of critical philosophy—use the terms *erklären* ("causal explanation") and *verstehen* ("meaning-based understanding") to describe these modes of knowing (Jaspers, 1997, p. 27).

These two levels of discourse are not contradictory, but complementary, and represent two different modes of knowledge. The relationship of *erklären* to *verstehen* is roughly analogous to that of neuropathology to psychopathology. *Verstehen* requires a language of subjectivity and personhood. For example, we might someday be able to give a causal account (*erklären*), in purely neurophysiological terms, of such subjective experiences as loneliness, alienation, or depersonalization. In principle, we might be able to say, for example, "When Mr. Jones experienced loneliness, it was because neuronal network A1762 was activated in his lateral hippocampus." But with regard to communicating a deep and useful understanding of Mr. Jones, this causal account would be of little value. To have an understanding of his loneliness, we would need to know, for example, that he had just been evicted from his apartment and was alone and homeless on the streets, or that his wife had just left him. Thus, when we apply the term "mental illness" to someone who, say, believes that Russian spies have implanted a radio transmitter in their brain, we are beginning to speak at the level of *verstehen*. We are only beginning, because we would need to know much more about the structure of the person's inner world, his object relations, and so on—what some philosophers call "phenomenology." For example, was the patient always mistrustful of others? What was his relationship to his parents? Was he traumatized early in life or very recently? In short, we are trying to understand, as Jaspers says, "*how one psychic event emerges from another*" (Jaspers, 1997, p. 27, original italics).

To be sure, there are several serious drawbacks to the term "mental illness." It perpetuates and reinforces spurious Cartesian distinctions between mind and body, "mental" and "physical." It is often inaccurately conflated with "psychosis" or "insanity" and misleadingly linked to a high risk of violence. All too often, "mental illness" may be misused as a prejudicial label, or as an excuse for discriminating against someone in hiring. This is especially true when popular media refer to "*the* mentally ill," as if persons with psychiatric disorders comprised a homogeneous group. In general, therefore, it is preferable to refer to specific conditions, such as bipolar disorder or schizophrenia, rather than to speak generically of "mental illness."

Nevertheless, terms like "mental illness," "mental disease," and "mental disorder" retain significant meaning and utility, in both ordinary language and professional communication. These or related terms are likely to persist because they serve three important functions of language: *communication, condensation, and classification.* "Mental illness" readily communicates a set of observational conclusions—often made by family members or other lay persons—regarding the impairment of a person's agential capacities (Daly, 1991, 2013). Moreover, the locution "mental illness" condenses a multitude of ancient, transcultural beliefs, holding that *minds* may indeed be "ill"; and it classifies a form of human suffering and incapacity as one involving disordered emotion, cognition, reasoning, and behavior.

12.6 **Conclusion**

The Szaszian claim that the terms "neuropathology" and "psychopathology" are mutually exclusive is not supported by current formulations of illness and disease. Rather, these are complementary terms, and constitute elements of two distinct but complementary discourses (*erklären* and *verstehen*, respectively). For all its drawbacks, the term, "mental illness," as DSM-V defines it, still serves a useful communicative function, on the level of *verstehen.* Just as some mental illnesses may be conceived as brain diseases, some brain diseases, such as the dementias, may also manifest as mental illnesses; that is, as clinically significant disturbances in cognition, emotion, reasoning, or behavior, leading to substantial suffering and incapacity. Although biological abnormalities often underlie and causally explain such disturbances (*erklären*), the attribution of "mental illness" to an individual does not require precise knowledge of its biological underpinnings. Nevertheless, the locution, "mental illness," is ordinarily not a metaphor; rather, it employs "illness" in the straightforward, literal sense of "an unhealthy condition of body or mind" (*Merriam-Webster*). Finally, no matter how well we understand the brain, we will never eliminate either the vocabulary of mind or the need for those who can interpret it with empathy and understanding.

References

Aftab, Awais. 2014. "Mental Illness vs. Brain Disorders: From Szasz to DSM-5." *Psychiatric Times* (February 28). Accessed April 13, 2018. <www.psychiatrictimes.com/dsm-5-0/mental-illness-vs-brain-disorders-szasz-dsm-5>

American Medical Association (AMA). 2013. "Report of the Council on Science and Public Health: Is Obesity a Disease?" Accessed April 13, 2018. <www.ama-assn.org/sites/default/

files/media-browser/public/about-ama/councils/Council Reports/council-on-science-public-health/a13csaph3.pdf>

American Psychiatric Association (APA). 2013. *Diagnostic and Statistical Manual of Mental Disorders [DSM-V]*, 5th edn. Arlington, Virginia: American Psychiatric Association.

Borg, Marcus J. 2001. *Reading the Bible Again for the First Time: Taking the Bible Seriously but Not Literally*. San Francisco: HarperCollins.

Boyd, David A. 1936. "A Contribution to the Psychopathology of Alzheimer's Disease." *American Journal of Psychiatry* **93** (1) (July): 155–75.

Brown, Robin Gordon. 1991. "Thomas Szasz, Mental Illness and Psychotherapy." *British Journal of Psychotherapy* **7** (3) (March): 283–94.

Cools, Arthur, Walter Van Herck, and Koenraad Verrycken (eds.). 2013. *Metaphors in Modern and Contemporary Philosophy*. Brussels: University Press Antwerp (UPA).

Daly, Robert W. 1991. "A Theory of Madness." *Psychiatry* **54** (4) (November): 368–85.

Daly, Robert W. 2013. "'Sanity' and the Origins of Psychiatry." *Association for the Advancement of Philosophy and Psychiatry Bulletin* **20** (1): 2–17.

Davidson, Donald. 2001. "What Metaphors Mean." In *Inquiries Into Truth and Interpretation*, 2nd edn., pp. 245–64. Oxford: Clarendon Press.

Devanand, Davangere P. 2013. "Psychopathology and Its Treatment in Alzheimer's Disease." Columbia University Psychiatry Grand Rounds (February1); SUNY Downstate Medical Center Psychiatry Grand Rounds (April 24). Accessed November 30, 2014. http://www.downstate.edu/psychiatry/pdf/Psychiatry-Grand-Rounds-04-2013.pdf

Harrison, Tinsley Randolph, and George Widmer Thorn (eds.). 1977. *Harrison's Principles of Internal Medicine*, 8th edn. New York: McGraw-Hill.

Jaspers, Karl. 1997. *General Psychopathology, Volume I*, translated by J. Hoenig and Marian W. Hamilton. Baltimore: Johns Hopkins University Press.

Lakoff, George, and Mark Johnson. 2003. *Metaphors We Live By*. Chicago: University of Chicago Press.

Merlino, Scott. n.d. "Three Reasons to Distrust 'Coulda, Woulda, Shoulda' Thinking." Accessed April 13, 2018. <www.csus.edu/indiv/m/merlinos/counterfactuals.html>

Merriam-Webster Medical Dictionary. n.d. "Illness." Accessed April 13, 2018. <www.merriam-webster.com/dictionary/illness#medicalDictionary>

Merriam-Webster Medical Dictionary. n.d. "Sick." Accessed April 13, 2018. <www.merriam-webster.com/dictionary/sick#medicalDictionary>

Moore, Michael S. 1975. "Some Myths About 'Mental Illness." *Archives of General Psychiatry* **32** (12) (December): 1483–97.

Moore, Michael S. 1984. *Law and Psychiatry: Rethinking the Relationship*. Cambridge: Cambridge University Press.

Orth, Michael, and Michael R. Trimble. 2006. "Friedrich Nietzsche's Mental Illness: General Paralysis of the Insane vs. Frontotemporal Dementia." *Acta Psychiatrica Scandinavica* **114** (6) (December): 439–45.

Ortony, Andrew. (ed.). 1993. *Metaphor and Thought*, 2nd edn. Cambridge: Cambridge University Press.

Pies, Ronald. 1979. "On Myths and Countermyths: More on Szaszian Fallacies." *Archives of General Psychiatry* **36** (2) (February): 139–44.

Pies, Ronald. 2008. "Psychiatric Diagnosis and the Pathologist's View of Schizophrenia." *Psychiatry (Edgmont)* **5** (7) (July): 62–5.

Pies, Ronald. 2012. "Mental Illness is No Metaphor: Five Uneasy Pieces." *Psychiatric Times* (September 14). Accessed April 13, 2018. <www.psychiatrictimes.com/addiction/mental-illness-no-metaphor-five-uneasy-pieces>

Pies, Ronald. 2015. "Mind-Language in the Age of the Brain: Is 'Mental Illness' a Useful Term?" *Journal of Psychiatric Practice* **21** (1) (January): 79–83.

Rocknak, Stefanie. 2013. "Willard Van Orman Quine: The Analytic/Synthetic Distinction." *Internet Encyclopedia of Philosophy*. Accessed April 13, 2018. <www.iep.utm.edu/quine-an>

Schaler, Jeffrey. 1998. "Mental-Health Parity [Letter to the Editor]." *Philadelphia Inquirer*, **A12** (August 22). Accessed April 13, 2018. <www.schaler.net/philly082298.html>

Schramme, Thomas. 2004. "The Legacy of Antipsychiatry." In *Philosophy and Psychiatry*, edited by Thomas Schramme and Johannes Thome, pp. 94–119. Berlin: Walter de Gruyter.

Szasz, Thomas S. 1973. *The Second Sin*. Garden City, New York: Doubleday Anchor.

Szasz, Thomas S. 1976. *Schizophrenia: The Sacred Symbol of Psychiatry*. New York: Basic Books.

Szasz, Thomas S. 1987. *Insanity: The Idea and its Consequences*. New York: John Wiley & Sons.

Szasz, Thomas S. 1998. "Thomas Szasz's Summary Statement and Manifesto." Accessed April 13, 2018. <www.szasz.com/manifesto.html>

Szasz, Thomas S. 2010. *The Myth of Mental Illness: Foundations of a Theory of Personal Conduct*, revised edn. New York: Harper Perennial.

Tanney, Julia. 2015. "Gilbert Ryle." *Stanford Encyclopedia of Philosophy Archive*. Accesed April 13, 2018. <plato.stanford.edu/archives/spr2015/entries/ryle>

Wittgenstein, Ludwig. 1958. *The Blue and Brown Books: Preliminary Studies for the Philosophical Investigations*. New York: Harper & Row.

Wittgenstein, Ludwig. 1968. *Philosophical Investigations*, translated by G.E.M. Anscombe. Oxford: Basil Blackwell.

Part III

Szasz's larger impact

Chapter 13

The myth and reality of mental illness

Allen Frances

13.1 Introduction

Tom Szasz's landmark book, *The Myth of Mental Illness*, published more than half a century ago, contained a crusading bill of rights for psychiatric patients. He argued passionately for the dignity and freedom of choice of mentally ill inmates warehoused, often for life, in state psychiatric hospitals that were aptly named "snake pits." Szasz was probably the greatest defender of patient rights since Philippe Pinel, a founder of modern psychiatry who, two centuries ago, started the profession off on the right foot by releasing the mentally ill from their chains—although it is worth noting that Szasz had little respect for Pinel, seeing him as incorrigibly paternalistic (as he once told our coeditor Eric v.d. Luft in conversation). Szasz was trying to protect not only the specific individuals involved, but also, more generally, the inviolable integrity of basic constitutional principles that he knew to be both precious and fragile.

Childhood experiences in Hungary, under a succession of horribly repressive Fascist, Nazi, and Communist regimes, had turned Szasz into a radical libertarian and a staunch defender of the categorical imperative to protect at all costs the right of the mentally ill to make their own decisions—even if part of the cost was that they often made bad decisions.

I was much impressed by *The Myth of Mental Illness*, which I first read in the midst of my misspent residency training in psychiatry. I was mostly treating people who did not want to be in the hospital and who really did not belong there. We were being taught to overdiagnose relatively normal people as "schizophrenic" and then to overmedicate them into zombiehood. I still feel terribly ashamed of this and am grateful to those of my long-suffering patients who have generously forgiven me. Szasz's defense of personal freedom and patient dignity was a breath of fresh air and a welcome corrective to the patronizing smugness that characterized so many of my teachers in their interactions with our patients. At this point I had not yet met him, but felt that I knew him through his book and also his frequent television appearances. He became a kind of mentor *in absentia*.

Not surprisingly, I chose an almost Szaszian environment for my first job after training. It was open-door, egalitarian, noncoercive, and very cautious in the use of medication. Soon, however, my experiences made clear how unrealistic was any strict adherence to Szasz's dogmatic mental health libertarianism. Daily contact with extremely difficult patients pulled me down from Szasz's ivory tower, his idealistic perch, and thrust me instead into the muddy waters of desperate clinical reality—the kind that confronts any psychiatrist working in a busy emergency room or an acute in-patient setting. Without medication, the severely ill lived in chaos, despair, danger, dis-organization, and decline. What would Szasz do for someone suffering from the "myth" of schizophrenia who has compelling command verbal hallucinations ordering him to murder his son, who has had no insight or reality testing, and who feels compelled to follow the commands. Suppose that he is brandishing a gun and says he must use it. This is not myth—this is clinical reality, and it brings us face to face with the perils, but occasional absolute necessity, of involuntary treatment.

Szasz in his own career never had to face these challenging clinical experiences and never really came to understand the substantial challenge they presented to his ide-ology. During the early years of his residency in Chicago, he refused on principle to see involuntary, severely ill inpatients, and focused instead on his psychoanalytic training with relatively healthy outpatients. When faced with an ultimatum from his depart-ment chair to work on an inpatient unit with involuntary patients, Szasz refused, on libertarian principle, and chose instead to move to Syracuse, where he remained for the rest of his life, teaching and working in an exclusively outpatient practice. He never had any hands-on decision-making responsibility with desperate or vulnerable patients, who were unable to care for themselves, had markedly impaired judgment, or were at considerable risk of harming themselves or others. Markedly impaired psy-chiatric patients are not living a theoretical myth; they are trapped in a painful clinical reality that forces psychiatrists to face the real pitfalls, and sometimes inevitability, of involuntary treatment.

Several years later, in the mid-1970s, I had dinner with Szasz. He was a brilliant con-versationalist, but also a good listener and a very kind man. Also touchingly honest, I posed to him a hypothetical situation in which his son was having a transient psy-chotic episode, was hearing voices commanding that he kill himself, felt compelled to act on the commands, and refused any treatment or advice. I asked: "As a father, Tom, would you stand by your libertarian principles or would you feel compelled to protect your son from himself, even if this required a very temporary coercion?" Tom smiled ruefully and said: "I am a father first and protector of human rights second."

Many of Szasz's most vehement followers would respond quite differently—shouting a resounding, impassioned, all-inclusive "Never!" to any psychiatric coercion; not ever, not even under the most seemingly urgent of circumstances. Szasz was wiser than the radical Szaszians who followed him.

13.2 **Is mental illness reality, construct, or myth?**

Szasz based his case against coercion on the argument that mental disorder is myth, not disease, and therefore should not be grounds for depriving anyone of free choice. Psychiatric disorders were no more than "myth" because they have no established bio-logical causation. If the definition of "disease" requires a well-understood etiology and pathology, then schizophrenia—along with most conditions treated by physicians—would certainly not be considered a disease.

But Szasz's definition of disease was too strict and arbitrary. Despite all the powerful tools at our disposal, science is still in the early stages of discovering the causes and mechanisms of most of the things that physicians treat. We are often in the dark about how treatments work and why they sometimes do not. Medicine is still based much more on trial and error empiricism than any deep understanding of cellular mechanics. Szasz's overly idealized view of medical science led to his degrading of psychiatric disorders, rather than seeing them as part of the continuum of medical disorders. We do know less about schizophrenia than about lupus, Parkinson's, or migraine, but we really do not know much about the pathogenesis of any of these or of many other medical conditions. This does not mean we cannot accurately diagnose and effectively treat them. Until we learn more, clinical constructs in psychiatry and medicine count as wonderfully useful, if only temporary, heuristics.

I agree completely with Szasz that mental disorders are not diseases and that treating them as such can sometimes have noxious legal consequences. But I strongly disagree that mental disorders are worthless "myths." The "myth" issue is perhaps best understood by comparing the epistemologies of my old friends, the three umpires:

First umpire: "There are balls and strikes, and I call them as they are."

Second umpire: "There are balls and strikes, and I call them as I see them."

Third umpire: "There ain't any balls or strikes until I call them."

Szasz correctly made mincemeat of the naive realism of the first umpire. Humans are not gifted with the tools to see reality straight on, and mental disorders most certainly are not diseases. But the third umpire (a true Szaszian) also blows the call—just because mental disorders are not diseases does not make them "myths." The second umpire has better vision—mental disorders are constructs, nothing more, but also nothing less. Schizophrenia is certainly not a disease; but equally it is not a myth. The construct "schizophrenia" helps to further communication, prediction, and decision-making—even if (as Szasz correctly points out) the term has only descriptive, and not explanatory, power.

Almost certainly, schizophrenia will not turn out to have a unitary cause. Eugen Bleuler (who first coined the term more than one hundred years ago) intuited this and described the "group" of the schizophrenias. Even the term "group" does not do full justice to the great heterogeneity likely to characterize the causality of a psychiatric disorder. Brain functioning is ridiculously complex and things can go wrong in all sorts of different ways. As with breast cancer, there will likely be dozens, perhaps hundreds, of different pathways to the final common descriptive construct that we call "schizophrenia." This inherent heterogeneity is also probably true of neurodegenerative processes that get lumped under useful but also temporary rubrics like "Alzheimer's disease" or "Parkinson's disease."

It will be the work of many decades to tease out the multiple causes of most medical conditions. The psychiatric disorders will be the toughest to crack. The human brain is the most complicated thing in the known universe—far more complicated than any other organ of the body. It will yield its many secrets only very slowly and in small bites. But the secrets are there to be found along the steady (if frustratingly slow) path of scientific discovery. Psychiatric disorder is not the stuff of "myth," nor of the nihilistic solipsism expressed in: "There ain't any balls or strikes until I call them."

Indeed, schizophrenia can be considered "myth" only by those who have not had much clinical or life experience getting to know well the unfortunate people who bear its burdens. Though not a discrete "disease entity" (like, say, tertiary syphilis or pulmonary tuberculosis), schizophrenia certainly produces severe, profound, and prolonged "*dis*-ease"—that is, suffering and incapacity. The patterns of its presentation are clearly recognizable, can be reliably diagnosed, run in families, have brain imaging correlates, predict its course, and respond to specific treatments. Schizophrenia is real enough—and no "myth" or psychiatric invention for those who suffer from it or for their loved ones. As constructs, psychiatric disorders should neither be reified nor given more weight than they can carry—but also should not be given less credit than they deserve as useful predictors of prognosis and treatment.

Admittedly, psychiatric disorders are imperfect constructs. There are no objective biological or psychological tests; presentations and course are heterogeneous; and boundaries are fuzzy. Psychiatric disorders are often diagnosed far too loosely, and medications are often prescribed carelessly, without proper indications or concern for dangerous side effects. The diagnostic evaluation is fallible when done quickly or inexpertly. It relies on information gathered from the patient and other informants, family history, and the findings on the mental status exam—after also ruling out the many psychiatric, substance use, and medical conditions that can mimic any condition. Definitive diagnosis may require following the patient and observing his course over a period of months or years. But the procedures used in diagnosing psychiatric disorders are not very different from those of a neurologist diagnosing "migraine headache" or an internist diagnosing lupus or many other medical conditions. Reliable, accurate, and useful diagnosis of psychiatric disorders is possible when care is taken.

With all its limitations, the diagnosis of psychiatric disorders does convey a great deal of information that is vital to clinical decision-making. Mental disorders do not have to be well-defined "diseases" (in the pathoanatomical sense) to be useful. It is enough if their recognition guides treatment, predicts prognosis, and helps to reduce our patients' suffering and incapacity. Most medical diagnosis does no more. Szasz was disappointed in psychiatric diagnosis because he expected too much from it and did not fully appreciate the limits of all medical diagnosis.

13.3 **The worst coercion is not psychiatric—it is prison or homelessness**

The risks of psychiatric coercion are familiar, longstanding, and are still being realized around the world (even in our own freedom-loving country). It was abusive protopsychiatry in medieval times when doctors of the church exorcised the demons, which they presumed were causing mental illness, through the diagnostic and treatment techniques of torture and drowning. In Soviet times, coercive psychiatry was used to suppress political dissenters by calling them crazy and parking them for long stretches in mental hospitals. China reputedly is running its own "psychiatric gulags" to quiet the vociferous economic complaints of peasants cheated by greedy local party officials. One has to question the well-meaning Australian practice of anesthetizing and intubating psychotic Aboriginals so that they can be flown to distant places for hospital treatment.

We in the United States are shamed by a massive misuse of psychiatry to preventively detain sexual criminals. Twenty states and the federal government have passed "sexually violent predator" statutes that allow for the often lifelong detention of rapists, beginning after they have already served their full prison sentences. The fig leaf of Supreme Court approval for the constitutionality of this seemingly double jeopardy violation of due process is provided by the requirement that the sexually violent predator have a mental disorder. But the judicial spirit of this necessary mandate to preserve constitutional protections is being violated, in forensic practice, by ignorant or unscrupulous psychologists willing to testify that the mere act of being a rapist qualifies the offender as mentally disordered and therefore subject to indefinite involuntary psychiatric commitment. Before heaping what would be completely appropriate condemnation on abusive practices in other countries, we should get our own house in order.

That said, the current looming threat to those with severe mental disorder is not psychiatric coercion but, rather, imprisonment or homelessness. There are now only about 65,000 beds in psychiatric hospitals, usually occupied for stays of only days to weeks. At least ten times this number of people live in prisons or on the street—and often for years or even lifetimes. Coercive psychiatric treatment is frequently the only way to prevent a patient from becoming a prisoner.

A patient's reaction to involuntary treatment varies greatly, depending on the person, the circumstances, when the request or demand is made, how it is done, and the family's attitude. A minority of patients remain angry about commitment after they have gotten better—sometimes feeling abused and humiliated for life. Another minority feels relief—unwilling to volunteer for treatment, but they are happy enough to go along with it. The majority are unhappy at the moment when involuntary treatment is imposed, but later understand its necessity once they have recovered from their acute symptoms.

Coercive treatment in the U.S. is often a last resort made necessary because we do such a lousy job of providing expectant treatment, decent housing, social outlets, and meaningful work. Psychiatry in the Nordic countries and Italy can be much less coercive than in the U.S., precisely because it is much better funded and occurs in a social context of much greater respect for patients and their families. We would need much less end-stage coercive treatment if, early on, we provided much greater access to good treatment.

Szasz performed a great service when, fifty years ago, he first began exposing the risks and excesses of coercive psychiatry and began the fight for patient empowerment, freedom, and dignity. He was reacting against the degrading snake-pit conditions of the state mental hospital system that then warehoused more than 650,000 patients, usually involuntarily and often inappropriately. But that system no longer exists. With only about 65,000 psychiatric beds left, the problem has become how to find a way into the hospital, not how to find a way out.

Deinstitutionalization has thrown our mentally ill from frying pan into the fire. What started as a humanistically motivated civil rights crusade quickly degenerated into a callous exercise in cost-cutting and neglect. The money saved by closing hospitals rarely followed the patients into the community, where it could have provided support for decent, independent living. Instead, we have created a vicious revolving door—discharging our mentally ill patients from hospitals, which were and are admittedly far less than ideal, and subjecting them to totally inappropriate, dreadfully Dickensian, prison environments or relegating them to living on the streets. This is a barbaric throwback to more primitive times and a shameful contrast to the more humane, enlightened, and cost-effective community treatment available in most of the rest of the developed world. Things have gotten worse as a result of the steady erosion of state revenues—in recent years, billions of dollars have been cut from what were already stingy and draconian mental health budgets.

Mental health services in the U.S. are a failed mess: underfunded, disorganized, inaccessible, misallocated, dispirited, and driven by commercial interest. We have hundreds of thousands of the severely ill in prison for nuisance crimes that easily could have been avoided had they received adequate treatment and housing. Sleeping on a stoop, stealing a Coke, or shouting on a street can get a person arrested. Once arrested, not being able to make bail or not fitting in well with jail routine leads to prolonged incarceration and, too frequently, crazy-making solitary confinement. The U.S. today is probably the worst place and worst time ever to suffer from a severe mental illness.

Neo-Szaszians are fighting the last war when they now rail against the outdated paper tiger of psychiatric coercion. Psychiatric hospitalization is now rare, short-term, and is usually a well-meaning attempt to help the person avoid the real, modern-day, coercive threats of imprisonment and homelessness.

Decriminalizing mental illness and deprisoning the mentally ill should be an appealing common banner. When discussing specifics, there is much more common-ground agreement about when psychiatric coercion makes sense than when discussing this hot-button issue in the abstract. It greatly oversimplifies a complex clinical and legal conundrum to assert categorically that involuntary treatment should be completely eliminated. "Coercive psychiatry" can be either a horrible abuse or a life-saving salvation—depending completely on the specific circumstances.

13.4 Finding common ground

Is there possible middle ground between lofty principles defending individual freedom and the difficult reality that an acutely psychotic person does not really express anything resembling "free choice" when obeying a command hallucination to jump out the window? The academic perch is very different from the clinical trench. I am fully mindful that involuntary treatment is a slippery slope that can easily lead to grave abuse. Witness the loose diagnostic practice in sexually violent predator cases in the United States. But I am also convinced there are dangerous clinical situations in which it would be irresponsible to let things freely follow what would be an obviously disastrous course. Physicians should first do no harm, but also cannot shirk unpleasant responsibility.

There will never be any compromise acceptable to the most die-hard defenders of psychiatry or to its most fanatic critics. Some inflexible psychiatrists are blind biological reductionists who assume that genes are destiny and that there is a pill for every problem. Some inflexible antipsychiatrists are blind ideologues who see only the limits and harms of mental health treatment, not its necessity or any of its benefits. I have spent a good deal of frustrating time trying to open the minds of extremists at both ends—rarely making much headway.

Common ground can be based on the recognition that one size cannot possibly fit all. Finding common ground has never been more important. There is an urgency to the needs of the severely ill that gets lost in ideological zealotry. It is silly arguing whether psychiatry is all good or all bad while severely ill people are languishing in prisons or on the street. We simply cannot afford a civil war among the various advocates of the mentally ill at a time when strong and united advocacy is so desperately needed. We must work together if we are to help regain freedom for those who have been inappropriately imprisoned. We must provide adequate housing to reduce the risks and indignities of homelessness. We must provide medication for those who really need it and avoid medicating those who do not. We must provide psychosocial support and treatment in the community for patients and their families.

Debates should be specific and practical, not polarized, polarizing, or ideological. Many psychiatrists err by being too quick to write prescriptions. Antipsychiatrists err in the opposite direction, thinking that because they have personally done better without medications, no one else ever needs them. Reasonable people can agree that we need to re-educate both physicians and the public that medications have harms, not just benefits, and should be reserved only for narrow indications and only when they are really necessary. It is ludicrous that 20 percent of our population takes a psychoactive pill every day, and it is equally ludicrous that anyone should be sent to jail for symptoms that would have responded to medication if the waiting time for an appointment had been one day, not two months. Our neglect of the severely ill is deeply entrenched, largely because there are few and fairly powerless advocates for the most disadvantaged. It makes no sense for them to be battling each other, rather than joining forces to fight for patient welfare.

Coercion is an even more contentious topic, but one that also has a common-sense common ground. Szasz could see the occasional need for coercion, and I will bet that anyone who spends any time in an emergency room will soon find dogmatic ideological opposition melting in the face of desperate presentations. While it is never comfortable to force someone to accept treatment, on rare occasions it is the only safe and responsible thing to do, and occasionally it can be life-saving. Involuntary commitment should never be done casually, but should also not be casually rejected on questionable theoretical or ideological grounds. Involuntary commitment should never be a careless decision, should always be a last choice, should usually be very brief, should be carefully monitored to prevent abuse, and, if so, may often be appreciated by the patient after the fact. Commitment is a judicial decision under very restrictive "emergency" criteria—usually imminent danger to self or others. It is a necessary last option that cannot be wished away by armchair idealists who can suggest no realistic alternative—because there really is none. "Coercive psychiatry," however unpleasant, must be available as a necessary last resort when nothing else will do. This is an imperfect world which sometimes requires choosing among lesser evils.

How do we thread the needle between an arbitrary abuse of psychiatric power and the avoidance of an unpleasant but necessary responsibility? Always work to gain the patient's trust and cooperation so that the need for involuntary treatment will be reduced to a bare minimum. Always discharge the patient as soon as he is ready or convert him to voluntary status as soon as he is willing. Build in tight monitoring and quality control assurances that involuntary commitment is done only when absolutely necessary and is terminated just as soon as is feasible. Perhaps best of all, give patients who have a track record of needing involuntary treatment, the opportunity to sign an advance directive when they are well—permitting it in the future should they again need it.

13.5 **Conclusions**

So where does all this leave us? Is it possible to reconcile Szaszian extreme libertarianism with common-sense psychiatry? Throughout my career, I have advocated for an antipaternalistic psychiatry—for engaging the patient as a full partner in all decision-making, whenever this is possible; for avoiding overdiagnosis and overtreatment; for normalizing; and for accepting individual differences. I have not seen much value in psychiatric hospitalization, except when the risks of outpatient care become too great to assume. I have discharged many hundreds of patients from emergency rooms and hospitals when the risks were real, but worth taking.

However, even though I admired Tom Szasz personally, respected his principled stance, and found great value in his cautions against the real and potential abuses of psychiatric power, I think that he and his followers go too far. Insulated from clinical reality, they present an inflexible, impractical, and extremist position that creates its own set of serious dangers (e.g., committing violent acts or winding up in jail) for the very people whom they are trying to defend. Individual freedom of choice is one of our highest values and is to be preserved at almost all costs—except in rare and extreme situations when it clashes with the even more pressing value of preserving the life and liberty of those who have lost the capacity to make free choices. I could be wrong (and it is not really a fair argument), but I am pretty sure that Tom Szasz would have been less extreme and dogmatic if he had allowed himself to have clinical experience dealing with real life-and-death situations rather than playing with abstractions.

Fortunately, there are many reasonable people in both camps who may differ markedly in their overall assessment of psychiatry, but still can agree that it is certainly not all good or all bad. With open-mindedness as a starting point, common ground can usually be found; seemingly divergent abstract opinions seem not so divergent when the discussion involves how to deal with practical problems. I very much regret that Tom Szasz is no longer around. I would like to have him here to lead the movement to free the severely ill from prisons, just as fifty years ago, he helped to free them from hospitals.

Chapter 14

Reform and revolution in the context of critical psychiatry and service user/survivor movements

Nancy Nyquist Potter

14.1 Introduction

This chapter argues that one of the outcomes of Thomas Szasz's work on mental illness as a myth is the rise of the field of critical psychiatry, a stance that seeks to bridge an apparent chasm between psychiatry as a form of social control and a necessary psychopharmacological intervention for the mentally ill. During the time of Szasz's early writing, psychiatry provoked a number of shifts in how psychiatric theory and practice are viewed today. The shift toward critical psychiatry was not prompted solely by the work of Szasz, but he has been influential in focusing psychiatric academic work. Additionally, his antipsychiatry position came at a time of some significant and visible reports of abuses of psychiatry in the United States during the 1950s and 1960s, and were likely to have helped to coalesce some of the protests.

I am not an historian and so do not aim to give an historical account of some rather seismic shifts in both popular culture and in psychiatry itself. I address some of the tenets and challenges to both critical psychiatry and to the rise of service user/survivor movements. I first identify some of the central ideas of critical psychiatry. Yet critical psychiatry, as an outgrowth of critical theory, all too often maddeningly fails to see madness as political (Rose, 2016). I say "maddeningly" because, even if one were to accept that mental disorders exist as biological kinds, this does not remove or address the myriad questions of value, including questions of how science is conceptualized and practiced. But that is a topic for elsewhere.

In this chapter, Section 14.2 focuses on one aspect of critical psychiatry networks: that of the voices and experiences of users/survivors. While I cannot do justice to the significant contributions to psychiatry that service users' critiques have played, I focus on four themes emerging from voices of users/survivors who have been diagnosed, perhaps institutionalized, and medicated: (1) the production of knowledge, knowers, and not-knowers; (2) questions of voice, marginalization, and identity; (3) visual representations that reproduce stereotypes and stigma; and (4) the production of the political subject. Bear in mind that these various movements and challenges should not be viewed as necessarily antithetical. Some people highlight the ways that psychiatry has both harmed and helped them, while others advocate a complete rejection of the language, ontology, and epistemology of psychiatry. In the conclusion, I argue that, by taking patients' experiences into consideration, a deeper challenge to Szasz's position on individualism presents itself—in particular, with respect to good epistemic and ethical practices in psychiatry, or alternatively, with respect to fundamental reconceptualizations of what it means to live with mental distress. I suggest that, while critical psychiatry is more likely to work for reform from within, user/survivor movements may aim for something more like revolution. Even this is not a tidy mapping, though.

14.2 **Critical psychiatry**

Critical psychiatry has developed as a way to challenge the current psychiatric industry while avoiding the polarization that antipsychiatry often provokes (Double, 2002). Szasz gives the illusion of clarity about putative physical/mental distinctions by appealing to binary thinking which, in reality, is much more complex and messy than it appears. Critics from critical theory as well as from critical psychiatry argue that distinctions such as biology/social science; freedom/coercion; individual/state; bodily illness/mental illness; free market/socialism—distinctions that Szasz insisted mapped easily onto reality—conceal political, ethical, ontological, and epistemic complexities (Bracken and Thomas, 2010, p. 222). Critical psychiatry takes on some of these realities of human suffering as people encounter the domain of mental health in various societies and cultures. It aims at reforming practices and, ideally, promotes a shift in the ontological and epistemic commitments of its practitioners.

A number of foci can be identified in critical psychiatry. Philip Thomas and Patrick Bracken (2004) identify four themes: (1) the questioning of traditional assumptions about mind, meaning, and knowledge; (2) a reconceptualization of the relationship between medicine and service users, driven from the ground up; (3) a call for psychiatrists to learn different ways to engage with and grasp the experiences of service users; and (4) active campaigning to limit the control of corporations, especially pharmaceutical companies, over the direction of psychiatry. Another call for reform is to transform psychiatry on a parallel with democratic values such as the right of patients to be fully involved in their care. The idea is that, just as in an ideal democracy, all citizens are participants with a voice not only through representation, but also through active decision-making. Democracy in practice should conceptualize and treat people with mental distress as genuine participants in the diagnosis, treatment, and interpretation of their own voices and experiences. This should include what counts as important issues to take up and who gets to decide them.

Another important reform that critical psychiatry emphasizes is the role of psychiatry in addressing the broader context in which distress and suffering occur. As Thomas and Bracken (2004, p. 361) explain, service users make meaning of their experiences in terms of the social and cultural contexts of their lives, and so many of them find biomedical interpretations unhelpful or even harmful. But it is not enough to understand that people living with mental illnesses are situated in particular social, cultural, and economic contexts: "Overcoming poverty, exclusion, and discrimination, and working for the provision of decent housing and opportunities for employment, are presented as important aspects of health policy" (Thomas and Bracken, 2004, p. 361).

The point here, made vivid by David Ingleby's anthology (2004), is that mental illness is a political, not merely a biological, or even a biopsychosocial, issue (Ingleby, 2004; Rose, 2016). One of Ingleby's arguments is that science censors explanatory theories that are not causal. Kenneth Kendler (2008) argues that earlier scientific models relied on a physics-like law model and that psychiatry needs to move away from laws to a multilevel mechanistic model as the explanatory goal of our science. Yet even a broader explanatory model can miss the shift that Ingleby's work suggests. According to Thomas and Bracken, Ingleby proposes an interpretive approach to psychiatry, an approach that "takes for granted that human beings engage in meaningful behaviour that transcends causal explanation and objectivity" (Thomas and Bracken, 2004, p. 364). Work in the area of medical anthropology suggests that context, culture, and differing discursive practices call for an emphasis on an interpretive model of mental distress (Jenkins, 1996). Such models open up our understanding of people's experiences of mental distress in recognizing the ways that interpretation is always localized in cultural and social situatedness, and thus that understanding needs always to consider "the body in context" (Lock and Scheper-Hughes, 1996). This accepts and invites persons living with mental distress to be part of the interpretive process— as, indeed, they necessarily are (though in many causal models they are diminished participants). I return to this point in Section 14.4.

14.3 The production of knowledge, knowers, and not-knowers

Bracken and Thomas optimistically state: "Because psychiatry deals specifically with 'mental' suffering, its efforts are always centrally involved with the meaningful world of human reality" (Bracken and Thomas, 2010, p. 219). While in one sense this is true— psychiatry must engage in meaning-making—it is much less clear that that meaning-making is within the control of users/survivors themselves. Jijian Voronka says that "those who had hitherto been objects of study (subaltern, disabled, queer, racialized, diasporic) critiqued the ways in which scholarship had historically been produced *on* them—rather than *with* or *from* them—and in this way sustained Western hegemonic epistemologies" (Voronka, 2016, p. 190; italics added). This problem is as true for user/survivor voices as it has been in feminist, anticolonialist, and critical race theory's scholarship. As Jayasree Kalathil and Nev Jones point out: "Service users and survivors continue to represent a tiny fraction of the overall research and evaluation workforce in academia, service delivery, organizations, and the community" (Kalathil and Jones, 2016, p. 183).

Few service users and survivors are involved in knowledge production and, when they are, they typically are not treated as full participants. By this I mean that, despite the idea of democratic reform and co-participation in knowledge production, users/survivors hardly ever are treated as knowers, without qualification. Knowing agents, by definition and by tradition, are objective, rational, and value-neutral, whereas longstanding assumptions and stereotypes about mental capacity in service users tend to reproduce what Miranda Fricker (2007) calls "epistemic injustice" and Kristie Dotson (2011) calls "epistemic violence".

Fricker calls attention to one form that epistemic injustice takes—testimonial injustice—where the "hearers fail to exercise any critical awareness regarding the prejudice that is distorting their perception of the speaker" (Fricker, 2007, p. 89). To be epistemically unjust means that the listener could have done otherwise and that his or her failure to attend appropriately to the speaker results in distorted beliefs. It occurs when the listener holds (often socially based) biases and prejudices that influence his or her assessment of the speaker's telling. It is ethically unjust because it is unfair; the listener does not accord the speaker the credibility that is warranted. The fictional Marge Sherwood,[1] then, can be understood to be excluded from what Fricker calls "trustful conversation" (Fricker, 2007, p. 52).

Trustful conversation is one of the ways that the mind steadies itself, and when someone is repeatedly denied testimonial justice—that is, when she or he has a history of not being given uptake—it "gnaws away at a person's intellectual confidence, or never lets it develop in the first place" (Fricker, 2007, p. 50) and damages her or his epistemic function in general (Potter, 2016). This is only one way in which people are damaged by testimonial injustice, but since so much of ordinary life depends on who we believe and what we come to believe in—including people's testimony about economic deprivation and experiences of racism, homophobia, and transphobia—testimonial justice can be said to be a primary virtue to pursue.

Dotson (2011) deepens and broadens our understanding of what sorts of failures to listen well can result in epistemic harm. She explains that successful communication entails reciprocal dependence of audience and speaker. Audiences are dependent on speakers to give them good information and to be trustworthy, but speakers depend on audiences giving uptake to their speech in order for their communication to be successful (Potter, 2016). Epistemic violence can be seen in attempts to eliminate knowledge possessed by marginal subjects; it is a form of violence in that it does damage to a given group's ability to speak and be heard (Dotson, 2011). Epistemic violence is a harm done to speakers where there is the failure of an audience to communicatively reciprocate, either intentionally or unintentionally, in linguistic exchanges owing to pernicious ignorance. Pernicious ignorance, Dotson (2011) argues, is a reliable ignorance or incompetence in listening that concerns a maladjusted sensitivity to the truth with respect to some domain of knowledge. Such insensitivity is due to the existence of epistemic difference, which is the gap between different worldviews caused by differing social situations (e.g., economic, sexual, cultural, material) that produce differing understandings of the world, differing knowledges of reality.

While Dotson suggests that epistemic violence occurs through pernicious and intentional actions and attitudes, she does include microaggressions (microinvalidations, microinsults) as well. Microaggressions are brief and commonplace daily verbal, behavioral, or environmental indignities, whether intentional or unintentional, that

---

[1] Fricker analyzes Patricia Highsmith's novel, The Talented Mr. Ripley (2008), at the point where Marge's fiance has gone missing and she expresses suspicion and distrust about Tom who she believes may have murdered him. The men in the conversation blow her off and Fricker suggests that her testimony is not given uptake because of an identity-prejudicial credibility deficit.

communicate hostile, derogatory, or negative slights and insults toward members of marginalized groups (Nadal, 2008). I consider people with mental distress to be vulnerable to either epistemic injustice or violence and other forms of microaggressions. Such harms affect the voices and visual communications of people with mental distress as well as our ability to interpret and understand one another.

14.4 **Voice and identity**

One crucial problem that reform measures of critical psychiatry aim to address is the propensity to reproduce structural and interpersonal harms on users/survivors. The next two sections develop some of the reasons why many users/survivors call for more fundamental change than reform can bring about. This section discusses the interplay between knowledge production and voice.

To treat users/survivors as not-knowers, silencing their testimony and speaking for them, are ways of "interpreting them" and telling their stories about them and for them—sometimes in ways they cannot recognize. This severely undermines efforts to democratize psychiatry.The oppressive nature of speaking about the Other is described by bell hooks: "No need to hear your voice when I can talk about you better than you can talk about yourself. No need to hear your voice. Only tell me about your pain. I want to know your story. And then I will tell it back to you in a new way. Tell it back to you in such a way that it has become mine, my own. Re-writing you, I write myself anew. I am still author, authority. I am still the colonizer, the speaking subject, and you are now at the center of my talk" (hooks, 1990, p. 343; 2015, p. 54; quoted by Russo, 2016, p. 220).

No well-developed philosophy of voice can be found in extant literature, but I will gesture toward what I mean by voice and silence. "Voice is a complex element of thinking and its experience" (Dumm, 2008, p. 70; quoted by Norval, 2009, p. 313). We become subjects when we can affirm, negotiate, and contest the episteme and micropractices that shape and limit our lives. Silencing, as we saw from Dotson, can take the form of quieting or smothering; it also can be proactive. Proactive silence is an actor's silence motivated not by resignation or defensiveness, but by other-directed feelings of concern for the social group and a desire to enhance or bring about cooperation (Van Dyne et al., 2003).

A full analysis of voice is beyond the scope of this chapter, so I focus on experiences that people have of being silenced and of frustrated, misunderstood, or misinterpreted voice. In silences and absences that are not able to be represented (Norval, 2009; Spivak, 1988), what is at stake is the very possibility of speaking, of visual, embodied communicating, and of being heard on one's own terms. The worry is that these silences can play out in academic psychiatry and some community services, as well as in treatment. Consider the following case: One night, a thirty-year-old transperson (male to female) of color, whom I will call "Eleanor," visited emergency psychiatry, where she had been seen a number of times previously. The file identified her as male; however, she requested that she be referred to with the female pronoun, as she was transgender. She reported feelings of depression and anxiety, and presented to emergency psychiatry with suicidal ideation. She repeatedly expressed that she feared for her safety in the shelters, while the attending and the resident continued to refer to her with male pronouns, even though she had asked to be addressed as female. The health-care team believed that she thought hospitalization was a way to avoid spending another night in a shelter. They assessed her as not being a danger to herself and not needing crisis intervention. Therefore, she was discharged.

I suggest that this is a situation of silencing—a form of testimonial quieting and eventual smothering—in that Eleanor's knowledge of danger and her needs are not acknowledged and her identity not affirmed. I also see microaggressions, in that her repeated requests to be addressed in ways consistent with her gender identity are invalidated. Eleanor is not heard on her own terms; the health-care team's interpretation of her situation seems to be incorrect, and thus she is put in harm's way again. It is not clear that the outcome would have been hospitalization, but the process could have been much different—and better—for Eleanor. Development of this theme would take me too far off the topic of this chapter.

As I have suggested, the emergence, or silencing, of voice can facilitate movement into subjectivity, or the crushing, or thwarting, or deformity of it. This is not to say that each individual has one core ontological subjectivity to be brought into existence. As I will discuss, subjectivities are in ebb and flow with one another, and we shift, transform, contest, and affirm our subjectivity in continual engagement with others and they with us. Still, in order better to understand another idea from critical psychiatry—and to understand why many of us enact epistemic injustice, violence, or microaggressions—we need at least a sketch of how representations of self and other are formed and created.

14.5 Visual representations that reproduce stereotypes and stigma

This section explains in more detail why many service users/survivors call for a deeper change in mental health theory and practice, beginning with a discussion of stereotypes. A stereotype is a cognitive mechanism that allows us quickly to categorize things into groupings and to organize the plethora of stimuli bombarding us. Prima facie, a stereotype is neither good nor bad, but the deployment of stereotypes is complex; they play a crucial role in how individuals think about, feel about, and decide to act toward others (Cudd, 2006, p. 69). Ann Cudd defines them as "generalizations that we make about persons based on characteristics that we believe they share with some identifiable group (2006, p. 69). Thus, the formation of stereotypes is a type of categorizing.

The cognitive act of stereotyping involves a complex series of inferences about characteristics that individuals believe set people in one group apart from people in other groups. As such, they form the foundation of our beliefs about groups (Cudd, 2006). A negative stereotype is a false or misleading generalization that is intransigent with respect to evidence to the contrary, unless we invest (sometimes significant) effort into it. It is a generalizing, fixed, false belief. In other words, stereotypes do not only help us make quick and efficient judgments; they buffer us from anxieties and fears by creating an external Other who is "bad" or "dangerous" to us. We tend to favor in-groups and disadvantage out-groups of the stereotype, while simultaneously creating and maintaining those very in-groups and out-groups, often without realizing what we are doing.

Patrick Corrigan states that commonly held stereotypes about people with mental illness include that such people are dangerous, that they are incompetent (i.e., incapable of independent living or real work), and that they are to blame—and thus are responsible—for the onset and continuation of their mental distress because of weak character (Corrigan, 2004). Here, too, it is important to note that just because we experience social absorption of stereotypes does not mean that we endorse them. We may actively be trying to expunge learned beliefs in stereotypes. But they can be insidious and stealthy, so that even mental health workers unwittingly may hold discriminatory attitudes and beliefs that impede creating the space for service users/survivors' voices to be heard properly. A full explication of what it means to "hear another properly" is beyond the scope of this chapter.

Regardless of whether we are victims of stereotyping or are doing the stereotyping—and most of us are both to varying degrees—we circulate and continue to reproduce them to the detriment of the mentally distressed. Additionally, stereotypes in conjunction with public representations can undermine attempts to challenge and reconceptualize the mad. The difficulty in challenging representations of the mad comes from the tenacity of stereotyping, especially when they appear in popular outlets such as movies and social media.

Flick Grey analyzed billboards intended to give hope to those living with distress and suffering by representing sympathetic people who would help them find their way to a better place. Grey introduces the idea of "benevolent othering," which, like hostile othering, "involves simplistic and self-serving representations that gloss over the complexity and diversity of people's lives, constructing a self-affirming image of 'benevolent subjects' as superior and masterful (just as hostile forms of othering serve to justify colonialism)" (Grey, 2016, p. 243). Billboards portray the distressed or struggling person as needy, thereby discursively producing a benevolent subject position (Grey, 2016, p. 244). In other words, they depict the person living with distress as a not-knower—she does not know how to care for herself, how to seek help, what to do about her feelings or where they come from—and this ignorance requires that a (good and helpful) knower come along to raise her up. To be sure, most of us feel confused and uncertain sometimes, but the contrast between the "mentally ill" person and her savior is stark, and the images, coupled with the written copy, construct the person ontologically and politically in quite particular ways. "Mind's billboards are normative and 'enthralled by respectability' . . . Overwhelmingly white and middle class, slim, productive, and mildly content (perhaps looking too happy could be mistaken for mania). The implication is that everyone expresses distress—and recovery— in the same ways, regardless of gender, class, ethnicity, or individual temperament and worldview" (Grey, 2016, p. 245). Grey's point, I think, is that the representation of the benevolent rescuer holds up a standard that is unattainable and is, in fact, a markedly privileged one. Hence, the depicted images and accompanying words work to increase distance between the "normal" and the "mad." As Grey explains, the counterpart of respectable recovery evokes " 'degraded others': People who *do not* recover to become slim, perky, middle-class self-improvers, people for whom schizophrenia *is* a 'life-sentence'—people who are chronically impaired by their experiences or disabled by their environment, people who commit suicide or people whose life expectancy has been significantly lowered by psychotropic medications and their attendant physical health problems—as well as people for whom recovery imperatives do not resonate and people whose experiences of extreme states do not entail curling up into a 'sad' ball (in which they seem respectable, passive, unthreatening, helpless, and lacking in agency)" (Grey, 2016, p. 245, original italics).

Representations that hold up a standard of recovery as respectability especially exclude people whose lives fall outside dominant structures of reasoning, discourse, and social positioning—such as people in prison systems, homeless shelters, halfway houses, and the streets, as well as those who actively repudiate the whole apparatus of the psychiatric and psychopharmacology industries (Kalathil and Jones, 2016, p. 187; see also Hopper, Kim, John Jost, et al. 1997.).

Grey argues that these billboards serve the function of domesticating national space. That is, representations of mad folks on billboards attempt to domesticate them by making viewers feel at home while "dominating others in the process" (Grey, 2016, p. 246). In addition to the homogenizing and othering that occurs in many billboards, this sort of discursive production of subjectivity situates service users as welcome to participate in research, community service, or mental health committees as long as they stay in their place—that is, do not challenge the at-homeness of psychiatry or claim themselves as knowers or legitimate meaning-makers regarding diagnosis, treatment, or medication (Grey, 2016, p. 247).

For these reasons, and because the epistemic and ontological commitments of psychiatry ordain it to a social institution that potentially is oppressive and harmful, many users/survivors call for more fundamental change than reform can bring about. Timothy Kelly (2016) points out that revolutionary change, then, seems to require two projects working in tandem. One is a commitment to valuing situated knowledges and an understanding of the ways that subjugated knowledges are suppressed or erased through the production of dominant (scientific) knowledge. The second is a political need for voice and experience to coalesce as a collective identity (e.g., "service users"). However, as Voronka (2016) and Jasna Russo (2016) argue, the second project gives rise to tensions between individual and collective experiences: "That is, in constructing a unitary voice or narrative, do we necessarily obscure the heterogeneities of experience?" (Kelly, 2016, p. 230). Here, I focus on the difficulty of creating political movements while avoiding the conservatism that comes with treating people who live with distress and suffering as sharing a set of common (essential) characteristics.

Voronka discusses ontological and epistemological problems that user/survivor movements face when they try to form a cohesive group; if such cohesion reifies "people with lived experience" as an undisputed whole category, it risks assuming an essence of the experience of living with madness that belies the complexities and differences of people within varied locales. The political worry is that, by attending to individual differences, such a focus can undermine the power of movements. While it seems politically necessary to present identities as an essential category that is held together by an essential shared experience of being diagnosed, treated, and produced as mad by psychiatric institutions, it is not inevitable that collectivities preclude a recognition of difference (Rose, 2016). Furthermore, as Voronka's writing makes clear, essentializing "people with lived experience" does not map onto people's actual experiences. A white woman from a privileged family who hears voices is likely to experience her illness, or madness, quite differently from a Black woman from impoverished Chicago who hears voices, even though they both experience what are called, in DSM classification, psychoses at times. Not only might their access to adequate health care, but also their developmental trajectory, differ quite dramatically. Such differences, made manifest in and through the material body in varying locales and times, seem to produce quite different actual lived experiences. The point is that theoretical claims about the essential properties of X do not seem to ring true in actual life when it comes to experiencing mental distress. A thorny question presses about the extent to which we can say that any of us share experiences or characteristics sufficient to declare that there is some "essence of experience" that binds us together; but as this is not the primary subject of this chapter, I leave readers to study the works of Voronka (2016), Lugones and Spelman (1983), and others for articulations of this problem.

14.6 Conclusion: binaries and the production of the political subject

One thing that makes Szasz's binary framework problematic (biology/social science; freedom/coercion; individual/state; bodily illness/mental illness; free market/socialism) is that human experience is always historically, culturally, and linguistically situated (Bracken and Thomas, 2010, p. 222). An entailment of this fact is that the unit of discourse—the individual, for Szasz—is in fact intersectional. The construct of intersectionality highlights the ways that identities are neither purely individual nor devoid of social markers of structurally imbricated subjectivities. Additionally, intersectionality necessarily points to ways in which systematic hardship, discrimination, stigma, and meaning are hegemonically shaped. Ann Garry gives a useful definition of intersectionality: "Oppression and privilege by race, ethnicity, gender, sexual orientation, class, nationality, and so on do not act independently of each other in our individual lives or in our social structures; instead, each kind of oppression or privilege is shaped by and works through the others. These compounded, intermeshed systems of oppression and privilege in our social structures help to produce (a) our social relations, (b) our experiences of our own identity, and (c) the limitations of shared interests even among members of 'the same' oppressed or privileged group" (Garry, 2011, p. 827).

Garry provides a way to understand claims about intersectionality as a reality of people's lives. However, it is important to appreciate that the idea of intersectionality was introduced by Black African-American women, in particular Kimberlé Williams Crenshaw, as metaphor and methodology rather than ontology (Carastathis, 2014). Intersectionality calls us out on binary thinking.

Put another way, subjectivities are produced—and produced in tension with power and resistance, as well as with each other, and in flux and movement. As Voronka writes: "My willful embodiment of lived experience as resistance can actually work to retrench dominant notions of the mentally ill figure. What I say or do, or how I act can have me at once understood as mad, recovered, mentally ill, and more" (Voronka, 2016, p. 198). Therefore, it behooves us to pay attention to how this functions in the creation of identities of the mentally ill, what sorts of subjectivities we might want to produce, and who is harmed and benefitted by different representations and interpretations of identities, differences, and voices.

Szasz was a champion of individualism. I want to make two concluding remarks about that view: First, for people whose lived experiences include distress, suffering, and, sometimes, painful encounters with psychiatry, it is neither true that they all share some core commonality nor true that they are radical individual subjects. They comprise a heterogeneous group—with outliers, including the profoundly marginalized. Their stories, while not strictly speaking "their own," emerge from positionalities and knowledges that many or even most others may not share. As Michel Foucault (1995) argues, our subjectivities are both the site of structural subjection and of becoming subjects—through mechanisms of power/knowledge—which produce shifting and varied subjectivities. Because of this duality in the functions of power, subjects are never fully subjected; they can be, and are, resisters. This leads me to the second point: Resistance is much more difficult to do individually, especially when one is marked as mentally ill. Marginalized people are most often disenfranchised with respect to participation in knowledge production and to voice. Those experiencing mental distress—and those who are taken to be mentally ill—are easily separated out from the "normal," and silenced. This does not mean that individuals are not and cannot be successfully resistant and defiant, but we most often need collectivities in order to provoke change and to be more effective than individuals alone can be. While some will call for reformative changes within psychiatry, others advocate something akin to revolution itself: the abolition of psychiatry as we know it. We need both kinds of movements in order for the historic and ongoing harms of psychiatry to be reduced or eliminated.

References

Bracken, Patrick, and Philip Thomas. 2010. "From Szasz to Foucault: On the Role of Critical Psychiatry." *Philosophy, Psychiatry, and Psychology* **17** (3) (September): 219–28.

Carastathis, Anna. 2014. "The Concept of Intersectionality in Feminist Theory." *Philosophy Compass* **9** (5) (May): 304–14.

Corrigan, Patrick W. 2004. "How Stigma Interferes with Mental Health Care." *American Psychologist* **59** (7) (October): 614–25.

Cudd, Ann E. 2006. *Analyzing Oppression*. Oxford: Oxford University Press.

Dotson, Kristie. 2011. "Tracking Epistemic Violence, Tracking Practices of Silencing." *Hypatia* **26** (2) (Spring): 236–57.

Double, Duncan. 2002. "The Limits of Psychiatry." *BMJ* **324** (7342): 900–4.

Dumm, Thomas L. 2008. "Connolly's Voice." In *The New Pluralism. William Connolly and the Contemporary Global Condition*, edited by David Campbell and Morton Schoolman, pp. 62–84. Durham, North Carolina: Duke University Press.

Foucault, Michel. 1995. *Discipline and Punish: The Birth of the Prison*, translated by Alan Sheridan. New York: Vintage.

Fricker, Miranda. 2007. *Epistemic Injustice: Power and the Ethics of Knowing*. Oxford: Oxford University Press.

Garry, Ann. 2011. "Intersectionality, Metaphors, and the Multiplicity of Gender." *Hypatia* **26** (4) (Fall): 826–50.

Grey, Flick. 2016. "Benevolent Othering: Speaking Positively About Mental Health Service Users." *Philosophy, Psychiatry, and Psychology* **23** (3–4) (September–December): 241–51.

Highsmith, Patricia. 2008. "The talented Mr. Ripley." New York: W.W. Norton & Co.

hooks, bell (pseudonym of Gloria Jean Watkins). 2015. "Choosing the Margin as a Space of Radical Openness." In *Women, Knowledge, and Reality: Explorations in Feminist Philosophy*, 2nd edn., edited by Ann Garry and Marilyn Pearsall, pp. 48–55. New York: Routledge.

hooks, bell (pseudonym of Gloria Jean Watkins). 1990. "Marginality as a Site of Resistance." In *Out There: Marginalization and Contemporary Cultures*, edited by Russell Ferguson et al., pp. 341–3. Cambridge, Mass.: MIT Press.

Hopper, Kim, John Jost, et al. 1997. "Homelessness, Severe Mental Illness, and the Institutional Circuit." *Psychiatric Services* **48** (5) (May): 659–65.

Ingleby, David. 2004. *Critical Psychiatry: The Politics of Mental Health*, 2nd edn. London: Free Association Books.

Jenkins, Janis H. 1996. "Culture, Emotion, and Psychiatric Disorder." In *Handbook of Medical Anthropology: Contemporary Theory and Method*, revised edn., edited by Carolyn F. Sargent and Thomas M. Johnson, pp. 71–87. Westport, Conn.: Greenwood.

Jones, Nev, and **Mona Shattell**. 2016. "Taking Stock of the Challenges and Tensions Involved in Peer Leadership in Participatory Research about Psychosis and a Call to do Better." *Issues in Mental Health Nursing* **37** (6): 440–2.

Kalathil, Jayasree, and **Nev Jones**. 2016. "Unsettling Disciplines: Madness, Identity, Research, Knowledge." *Philosophy, Psychiatry, and Psychology* **23** (3–4) (September–December): 183–8.

Kelly, Timothy. 2016. "Heterogeneities of Experience, Positionality, and Method in User/Survivor Research." *Philosophy, Psychiatry, and Psychology* **23** (3–4) (September–December): 229–32.

Kendler, Kenneth S. 2008. "Explanatory Models for Psychiatric Illness." *American Journal of Psychiatry* **165** (6) (June): 695–702.

Lock, Margaret, and **Nancy Scheper-Hughes**. 1996. "A Critical-Interpretive Approach in Medical Anthropology: Rituals and Routines of Discipline and Dissent." In *Handbook of Medical Anthropology: Contemporary Theory and Method*, revised edn., edited by Carolyn F. Sargent and Thomas M. Johnson, pp. 41–70. Westport, Conn.: Greenwood.

Lugones, María C., and **Elizabeth V. Spelman**. 1983. "Have We Got a Theory For You! Feminist Theory, Cultural Imperialism, and the Demand for 'The Woman's Voice.'" *Women's Studies International Forum* **6** (6): 573–81.

Nadal, Kevin L. 2008. "Preventing Racial, Ethnic, Gender, Sexual Minority, Disability, and Religious Microaggressions: Recommendations for Promoting Positive Mental Health." *Prevention in Counseling Psychology: Theory, Research, Practice and Training* **2** (1) (December): 22–27. Accessed April 22, 2018 <www.div17.org/preventionsection/Prevention_Pub_08.pdf>

Norval, Aletta. 2009. "Democracy, Pluralization, and Voice." *Ethics and Global Politics* **2** (4): 297–320.

Potter, Nancy Nyquist. 2016. *The Virtue of Defiance and Psychiatric Engagement*. Oxford: Oxford University Press.

Rose, Diana. 2016. "Experience, Madness, Theory, and Politics." *Philosophy, Psychiatry, and Psychology* **23** (3–4) (September–December): 207–10.

Russo, Jasna. 2016. "In Dialogue with Conventional Narrative Research in Psychiatry and Mental Health." *Philosophy, Psychiatry, and Psychology* **23** (3–4) (September–December): 215–28.

Spivak, Gayatri Chakravorty. 1988. "Can the Subaltern Speak?" In *Marxism and the Interpretation of Culture*, edited by Cary Nelson and Lawrence Grossberg, pp. 271–314. Urbana: University of Illinois Press.

Thomas, Philip, and Patrick Bracken. 2004. "Critical Psychiatry in Practice." *Advances in Psychiatric Treatment* **10** (5) (September): 361–70.

Van Dyne, Linn, Soon Ang, and Isabel C. Botero. 2003. "Conceptualizing Employee Silence and Employee Voice as Multidimensional Constructs." *Journal of Management Studies* **40** (6) (September): 1359–92.

Voronka, Jijian. 2016. "The Politics of 'People with Lived Experience': Experiential Authority and the Risks of Strategic Essentialism." *Philosophy, Psychiatry, and Psychology* **23** (3–4) (September–December): 189–201.

Chapter 15

Thomas Szasz and the insanity defense

Neil Pickering

Many modern psychotherapists have adopted, as their credo, Socrates'
declaration that the unexamined life is not worth living. But for modern man
this is not enough. We should pledge ourselves to the proposition that the
irresponsible life is not worth living either.

Szasz (1963, p. 255)

15.1 Introduction

Szasz was opposed to the insanity defense. Throughout his career he wrote in opposition to it in books and articles. He appeared in court on one occasion to rebut defense psychiatrists who had given their opinion that a defendant was insane and so
not guilty. There is no doubt, also, that his opposition to the insanity defense was consistent with his overall view of life (as illustrated in the opening quotation) and with
his well-known claim that mental illness is a myth.

This chapter considers the persuasiveness of Szasz's arguments against the insanity
defense. A persuasive argument will be deemed to be one which draws its conclusion
from the narrowest and most plausible premises—that is, the argument which successfully infers its conclusion from a set of grounds most likely to be accepted by a wide
group. There will be no attempt to defend these criteria for persuasiveness of argument; they will be an assumption of the chapter.

Three broad arguments identifiable in Szasz's oeuvre will be tested for their persuasiveness, in the following order:

1. The moral argument against the insanity defense.
2. The argument that the insanity defense relies on a nonexistent entity—namely,
   mental illness.
3. The argument that the sciences of psychiatry cannot offer any reason to believe that
   a person lacks responsibility.

As will emerge, the last of these is by far the most persuasive argument that Szasz has
on the tests proposed. I shall suggest that it supports Szasz's conclusion, and relies only

upon a narrow agreement about what the sciences of psychiatry can offer, which are also widely accepted premises.

Before proceeding, two further things should be noted. First, while I suggest that the third argument is Szasz's best, it does not necessarily represent the primary logic of Szasz's actual position. That logic comes from the idea that humans are invariably morally responsible for their acts, and that only accidents and coercion really excuse humans from this responsibility. This underlies his whole approach, including his belief that mental illness is a myth. Second, at no point in this chapter will there be an attempt to analyze the insanity defense in legal terms. Rather, the legal terms in various versions of the defense will be treated as ordinary language terms.

15.2 Moral opposition to the insanity defense

Szasz acknowledges that his opposition to the insanity defense involves rejecting a proposition which "seems self-evident and commendable" (Szasz, 1963, p. 132) and compelling (Szasz, 1958). This proposition is "our collective conscience does not allow punishment where it cannot impose blame" (Durham v. United States, 1954, at 13, p. 76) or that someone must be morally "responsible for his act before we, society, can punish him" (Szasz, 1958, p. 192). As Stephen Morse puts it, "the moral basis of the insanity defense is that there can be no just punishment without desert and no desert without responsibility" (Morse, 1985, p. 783; cf. Hathaway, 2009). Szasz believes that this proposition is neither self-evident, nor commendable, and should be re-examined. This also suggests where Szasz stands on the question of whether versions of the insanity defense from premodern times (before the idea of mental illness had been developed) were based on any basic human sense of what is just. The answer is plainly that he does not think so (see Chapter 1, this volume).

In Szasz's work, three rather different kinds of reason for objecting on moral grounds to the insanity defense are to be found. The first is derived from the ethical principle of truth telling; the second is an empirical argument based on evidence about the actual fate of those who successfully use the insanity defense; and the third is more directly moral, namely, that despite appearances, the insanity defense is neither humanitarian nor liberal.

15.2.1 The argument from truth telling

The argument from truth telling is that a person who is considering using the defense, or is offered it by her or his lawyer, should be told that it is by no means what it appears to be. When a person is "acquitted" by the defense, she or he in fact frequently ends up being confined (i.e., imprisoned) anyway. Szasz—ever with an eye for historically challenging fact—refers us to the case of Daniel M'Naghten, the defendant after whom the M'Naghten rules are named. He was acquitted of the murder of Edward Drummond by reason of insanity (Daniel M'Naghten's Case, 1843; Quen, 1968). Subsequently, judges in the House of Lords set out the criteria upon which the insanity defense should rely: the M'Naghten rules (Quen, 1968). But what happened to M'Naghten after his acquittal? Szasz tells us that "M'Naghten died in Broadmoor in

1865, having been incarcerated for the last twenty-two years of his life" (Szasz, 1967, p. 271; 1991, p. 98). So much for acquittal.

John Hinckley Jr., who attempted to assassinate Ronald Reagan, and injured three others in the process, was also acquitted by reason of insanity. Reagan's press secretary, James Brady, died in 2014 and his death was ruled to have resulted from his injury; but Hinckley, having been acquitted of all charges, was not held responsible. Hinckley was finally released from the care of St. Elizabeths Hospital (a psychiatric facility in Washington, D.C.) on August 5, 2016, having been under care since 1982, though he had extensive periods of parole in the later years (John Hinckley Jr., 2018). The term, "acquittal," in the context of the insanity defense, does not seem to mean what it usually means—that a person should walk from the court a free person.

This seems a reasonable point to make. However, it is not a principled objection to the insanity defense. For example, Szasz asks, "what would happen in jurisdictions where commitment follows automatically upon acquittal by reason of insanity, if the defendant clearly understood this choice [i.e., prison for a set period or incarceration in a mental hospital for a nonset period] . . . I venture to predict that such pleas would become very infrequent, and perhaps would disappear altogether" (Szasz, 1967, p. 280; 1991, p. 109). Perhaps they would, but this is not the main thing about the insanity defense which Szasz aims at establishing. The primary truth in Szasz's mind is that the defense is inherently immoral. To argue that it is a bad defense because it involves a lie about the meaning of the term, "acquittal," seems to risk burying this greater truth. After all, Szasz does not think that the insanity defense is a legitimate basis for acquittal.

15.2.2 **The empirical argument**

The empirical argument is that, as a matter of fact, the insanity plea has "dire consequences for the defendant" (Szasz, 1967, p. 280; 1991, p. 109) and that this consequence of the insanity defense makes it immoral. The immorality of these consequences is related partly to the fact that those who use the defense are pragmatically worse off that they would have been had they not used it; and partly to the fact that a person who once uses it loses rights and moral standing. Szasz suggests: "There is evidence that, from the subject's point of view, confinement in a mental hospital is more unpleasant than imprisonment in jail" (Szasz, 1967, p. 277; 1991, p. 105). In support of this claim he cites Hugh McGee: "One of my clients . . . who has served in the prison systems of Florida, Georgia, Virginia, and Maryland, and on road gangs, too, of those states, told me dead seriously that he would rather serve a year in any of them than 6 months in old Howard Hall" at St. Elizabeths Hospital (Szasz, 1967, p. 277; 1991, p. 105, quoting McGee, 1961, p. 659). Szasz also quotes McGee as claiming that keeping a person in a maximum security ward amounts not only to "an unconstitutional deprivation of liberty but also . . . to cruel and inhuman punishment." The person kept in the maximum security ward "loses more rights than a criminal in the penitentiary" (Szasz, 1967, p. 277; 1991, p. 105, citing McGee, 1963, p. 215).

This appears a powerful argument, as it appeals to the widely accepted idea of equality of treatment and rights of all people, including those who use the insanity plea. But while there is considerable rhetorical capital to be made from this appeal, Szasz cannot safely deploy it as an argument against the insanity defense. Suppose that the reverse were true; that is, that it was better for a person to be acquitted under the insanity defense than found guilty through the usual justice system, as is sometimes alleged (Morse, 1985). If this allegation were true, if in fact it were beneficial for an accused to use the insanity defense, would Szasz see that as an argument in support of the retention of the defense? No—the evidence for how well people happen to do after using the defense is neither here nor there, at least if we approach the issue from Szasz's point of view. This version of the moral argument does not capture the real basis of Szasz's moral objection to it.

15.2.3 The insanity defense and human autonomy

We turn now to the third, moral argument—this is the most direct of the three. It is that the insanity defense is neither humanitarian nor liberal: "Neither the M'Naghten rule, nor the Durham rule, nor the American Law Institute rule is 'humanitarian'—for all diminish personal responsibility and thus impair human dignity; nor is any of them 'liberal'—for none promotes individual freedom under the rule of law" (Szasz, 1967, p. 282; 1991, p. 111). Weinberg and Vatz correctly identify Szasz's argument: "Szasz believes that only when we eliminate the idea that mental 'illness' may be an excusing condition for crime will we be treating all people as human beings, autonomous and responsible for their actions" (Weinberg and Vatz, 1982, p. 421).

But there seems to be a problem with this as an argument for the abolition of the insanity defense. For though it appears to focus only upon eliminating mental illness as an excusing condition for crime, in fact it must eliminate all excusing conditions which work by implying a reduction of autonomy. This seems to amount to denying that autonomy can ever be reduced. This is because the problem with the appeal to insanity, which the argument identifies, is precisely that it implies failing to recognize autonomy; and if this is a problem for insanity, it ought to be a problem for any other appeal that works the same way. Now, if all appeals to excuses that work by implying that the person had reduced autonomy are given up, then, logically speaking, the argument against the insanity defense works a fortiori. That is, if a person can never be innocent of a crime that she or he has committed by reason of reduced autonomy, then of course that person can never be innocent of a crime by reason of reduced autonomy attributed to insanity. But, the a fortiori logic of the position lacks persuasive strength, for the stronger or wider claim (i.e., that no one is ever nonautonomous) seems less likely to be acceptable than the weaker and narrower claim which it supports (i.e., that people are not ever nonautonomous by reason of insanity). However, Szasz advances arguments intended to support the wider claim. The remainder of this section assesses these.

Descriptive autonomy

Szasz supports the wider and stronger claim on the grounds that it is a descriptive truth about human beings that they are responsible for their actions—the "descriptive sense of autonomy" claim, as Weinberg and Vatz (1982, p. 421) call it. As Szasz puts it: "I would insist that, to some extent at least, all people do shape their own destinies, no matter how much they might bewail the superior forces of alien wills" (Szasz, 1974, p. 155). Presumably Szasz believes that to whatever extent this is, it is sufficient to make the person responsible for their acts. Weinberg and Vatz set out the claim explicitly: "Szasz is committed to the principle of autonomy in two senses. He believes in autonomy in the *normative* sense that people ought to be free to make choices about their lives, and believes in autonomy in the *descriptive* sense that when people act without physical coercion, such actions should be inferred to represent freely chosen behavior" (Weinberg and Vatz, 1982, p. 423) This position seems to share some parallels with Hobbes's notion of liberty (Mill, 1995).

The connection to the moral claim upon which Szasz relies is: "Only if we accept descriptive autonomy can we protect normative autonomy" (Weinberg and Vatz, 1982, p. 423). However, the claim that accepting descriptive autonomy is necessary to protect normative autonomy is not a strong argument for the truth of descriptive autonomy. The truth of a descriptive claim cannot be founded on the basis of the good consequences that would follow if it were true. The ecological health of the earth would be much improved if the oceans were not being polluted; but it is an uncomfortable truth that the oceans are being polluted nonetheless. The descriptive autonomy claim has to stand on its own merits, whatever they may be.

Descriptive autonomy assessed

The merits of the descriptive autonomy claim can be assessed by looking at how well it survives objections, and by looking at what is in favor of it. There are two sorts of objections to it. First is the objection that those with mental illnesses may behave in ways which clearly show the strong—perhaps irresistible—forces of their mental state on their actions. In short, this objection is that there are undoubted examples where people's behaviors are clearly symptomatic, just as a feverish person's are symptomatic of an infection. This is an objection which Szasz explicitly rejects. For example, he argues that "'symptomatic' behavior also obeys the principles of rule-following actions" (Szasz, 1974, p. 150). That is, the behaviors described as "symptomatic" are not in fact any different from behaviors that are not symptomatic. If the term, "symptomatic," is supposed to imply that these behaviors are structured and influenced in some special way, then (according to Szasz) this is a false implication. However, Szasz's rejection of the argument that people are sometimes clearly not autonomous seems to rely on his position that people always are autonomous, rather than to offer it independent support. (But we shall return to the claim that there is no difference between behaviors which are alleged to be symptomatic of a mental illness and those which are not, as Szasz offers a quite different argument in support of it.)

The second objection is that Szasz relies on a very attenuated notion of autonomy. In effect, he takes autonomy to consist in freedom from coercive pressure. But this narrow view of autonomy is open to challenge. If autonomy is not simply freedom from coercive pressure, then it may presumably be undermined even in cases where a person remains free from coercion. Suppose, for example, that a person may lack autonomy if her or his actions, while not coerced, are inconsistent with this person's "attitudes, values, dispositions and life plans" (Miller, 1981, p. 24). That is, the person may act nonautonomously by acting inauthentically. This may raise serious concerns about whether the action reflects the genuine desires of the person, and may suggest that, after all, this person is not in fact autonomous. In short, it would be wrong to attribute autonomy to this person, descriptively speaking, even though the person is not coerced. To link this to the present concern, it might be that mental illnesses are perceived to undermine autonomy in this sense, while not being coercive.

On behalf of Szasz, and in defense of his narrow version of autonomy, Weinberg and Vatz (1982) offer a counterargument. They argue that judgments that a person is acting inauthentically are often unreliable, or involve a hidden value judgment in the observer. The point about the unreliability of such judgments is wholly epistemic—it relates to whether people can know something about another. We may think that we know what a person's "attitudes, values, dispositions, and life plans" (Levine, 1988, p. 272) are—but we can easily be wrong. The problem with Weinberg and Vatz's response, which is, in effect, that it is impossible "to find the mind's construction in the face" (Shakespeare, *Macbeth*, I.iv.12), is that it flies in the face of ordinary experience in a very large number of cases. In fact, we often know what other people are like—sometimes better than they do themselves. The second point—that judgments about authenticity rely on hidden value judgments—is partly epistemic as well. The value judgment implicit in this case is that people ought to behave in line with their previous attitudes and values. But this seems to impose the value of consistency upon the person, who may not value it at all. Yet, while this seems true, it also seems to be a significant issue if the person suddenly actually does alter all his or her attitudes and values. In such cases, explanations may be found—for example, Saul's sudden change of attitudes and values may be attributable to his seeing God on the road to Damascus (Acts 9:3–18). But where such a narrative is lacking, or where it is unconvincing, perhaps, concerns about authenticity seem reasonable, and this seems to undermine the account of autonomy which Weinberg and Vatz (1982) attribute to Szasz.

Their defense of Szasz's thin notion of autonomy against objections may be rather ineffective. But perhaps something can be said in a positive way about Szasz's approach to autonomy. Weinberg and Vatz canvas two arguments. The first is that to expand autonomy beyond autonomy as free action opens the concept of responsibility up to abuses (e.g., the insanity defense). But, at least in the present case, such an argument appears to be circular, for it is the question of whether the insanity defense represents an abuse of autonomy which is at stake. More validly, Weinberg and Vatz propose that Szasz's descriptive autonomy "comes close to defining the nature of human beings" (1982, p. 422). In Szasz's own words, "the concept of personal responsibility is central to the concept of man as moral agent. Without it, individual freedom . . . becomes a 'denial of reality', a veritable 'psychotic delusion' to endow man with a grandeur he does not in fact possess" (Szasz, 1970, p. 11).

While this claim is not implausible, it is certainly a large claim. Claims about human nature typically are. Moreover, it might be argued that the claim that humans are by nature autonomous is not inconsistent with holding that some people are unable to exercise their autonomy. Perhaps the worry about this argument is that it implies that someone who is said to be unable to exercise autonomy is, in effect, defined as not fully human—or as Szasz puts it, has impaired dignity (Szasz, 1967, p. 282; 1991, p. 111). However, this worry appears to arise only if descriptive autonomy is accepted, rather than being an independent reason for supporting it. For it is only if humans are descriptively autonomous that failing to uphold their autonomy normatively has the implication of treating them as less than human. Many people hold quite consistently that those with mental illness may be said to lack autonomy, and do in some sense lack the dignity of commanding their own affairs, but that they retain the human right to care and treatment, the latter of which may be aimed at returning their autonomy to them (Edwards, 1982).

Szasz's moral argument, then, is not entirely convincing in any of its forms. The argument that the insanity defense involves misleading people about what the term, "acquittal," means seems to miss the main point of Szasz's objection to the insanity defense. The empirical argument that the insanity defense has dire consequences for the person who appeals to it is subject to empirical refutation—and so is not ideal for Szasz's purposes. These arguments do not appear logically to entail Szasz's views (which is the first requirement if they are to be persuasive). The argument that the insanity defense involves treating some people as nonautonomous (as nonagents) does not seem to follow from the claim that it is human nature to be autonomous—in short, it too has logical shortcomings. But in any case, it seems to ask far too much of someone to base their objections to the insanity defense on such a metaphysically vast and controversial foundation. It does not do well on any of the criteria for persuasiveness assumed in this chapter.

15.3 **The "mental illness does not exist" objection**

I shall most often use the term, "mental illness," rather than "mental disease" or "mental disorder." However, for the purposes of this chapter, these terms can be taken to be interchangeable.

Szasz's best-known claim is that mental illness is a myth—that there are no mental illnesses—as in the title of his 1961 book (Szasz, 1974). This seems to lead directly to a rejection of the insanity defense: "All tests of criminal responsibility rest on the premise that people 'have' conditions called 'mental diseases' which 'cause' them to commit criminal acts. The value of these tests thus hinges on the soundness of this underlying concept" (Szasz, 1967, pp. 272–3; 1991, p. 100).

The first problem that this argument against the insanity defense runs into is obviously the widely accepted counterclaim that there is such a thing as mental illness. Szasz argues that the things we call mental illnesses are patterns of behavior disvalued by most in society, and which society wishes to control. In contrast, defenders of the notion of mental illness argue, amongst other things, that mental illnesses are natural kinds or have a natural element, typically biological dysfunction (Boorse, 1976; Wakefield, 1992). The question of whether mental illnesses may be natural kinds will arise in Section 15.4. This chapter is not the place to join that debate, for there is another route of objection to Szasz's approach, which is not to assert that mental illness exists, but to deny that its existence matters one way or the other to the insanity defense.

On the surface, the claim that mental illness is not relevant to the insanity defense seems not very plausible, for most versions of the insanity defense do appear to make mental illness an essential part of the definition of insanity. For example, the M'Naghten rules state: "To establish a defence on the ground of insanity, it must be clearly proved that, at the time of the committing of the act, the party accused was labouring under such a defect of reason, from disease of the mind, as not to know the nature and quality of the act he was doing; or, if he did know it, that he did not know he was doing what was wrong" (Daniel M'Naghten's case, 1843, at 210, p. 722). The Durham rules version reads: "An accused is not criminally responsible if his unlawful act was the product of mental disease or mental defect" (Durham v. United States, 1954, at 862).

Despite the appearance that mental illness is required, a version of an argument framed by Germund Hesslow (1993) may show that this is merely an appearance. Hesslow does not offer the form of argument which I shall deploy here in the case of the insanity defense. His argument with respect to the insanity defense is that there is no point in punishing a person who is insane because that person cannot learn from punishment, and that is the point of punishment. Hesslow extends this argument to children and others who are similarly unable to learn, and claims that it is this inability to learn from punishment, rather than anything to do with mental illness, which explains our approach. The argument is that the state of insanity which leads to a person being exculpated can be set out quite independently of the presence of mental disease. This is not so easy to see in the Durham wording, but is plain enough in the M'Naghten rules, in which the insanity is described as not knowing the nature and quality of the act the person was doing, or, if knowing that, not knowing what he was doing was wrong. These words capture the exculpating state of mind, and no reference to mental disease is required in order to state it.

The general form of Hesslow's (1993) argument is that we do not need to appeal to disease in a number of cases where it is often supposed that we need to appeal to it (e.g., to establish whether a person's condition should be treated, or whether a person should be offered insurance). Hesslow argues, in each case, that it is not enough that a person has a disease to get treatment (as we do not treat or get offered insurance for all diseases) and it is not necessary (given that we treat and can get insurance for some non-diseases). Given that disease is neither sufficient nor necessary, he argues that disease is irrelevant, or more precisely, attempting to conceptualize disease definitively is a waste of time. Adapted for present purposes, if mental illness is neither sufficient (i.e., not enough in and of itself to be a basis for judging whether someone is or was insane) nor necessary (i.e., not a requirement for the insanity defense), then it is not relevant to the question of sanity or insanity. It follows—at least insofar as this chapter is concerned—that whether mental illness exists or not is not relevant to the question either. If this is right, then Szasz's "mental illness is a myth" objection to the insanity defense is beside the point.

The nonsufficiency claim is in fact widely accepted; that is, it is widely agreed that solely having a mental illness in itself does not fulfill the requirements of the insanity defense. This is written into both the M'Naghten and Durham versions of the defense. In the M'Naghten case, it is not enough that a person has a mental disease, but it must cause the exculpatory state of nonknowing. In the Durham wording, there must be a causal connection between the behavior and the disease. Szasz makes this point too. The following text is taken from his testimony at the trial of Darlin June Cromer (People v. Cromer, 1980; Finney, 1982). Cromer had been charged with the torture and murder of Reginald Williams, a five-year-old Black child. Cromer's defense wanted to use the insanity plea to get her acquitted and Szasz (A) appeared for the prosecution to rebut the defense psychiatrists' claim that Cromer was insane. The questioner (Q) is the prosecutor, Deputy District Attorney Albert Meloling:

Q: Is there anything in the definition of a psychotic which necessarily means that a psychotic is not responsible for what they do?

A: Well, as people who have studied this area know very well, that's long been a matter of debate in psychiatry and all the authoritative opinion has been to the point that terms like psychotic, schizophrenic, and so forth have no point-to-point relationship to irresponsibility.

The person can be called schizophrenic or psychotic and can be considered to be and held to be responsible. So it is quite irrelevant to talk about whether the person is psychotic because it doesn't mean he or she is not responsible . . .

Q: You said that the question of whether or not a person was suffering from schizophrenia is really not relevant to the question of whether or not they are responsible?

A: That is correct . . . responsibility . . . in the sense in which I was using the term, whether the person knew what they were doing and therefore has free will, can control their actions, and so forth, is sort of independent from whether or not they may be diagnosed as schizophrenic. (Finney, 1982, pp. 13–14)

Quite a number of others have supported the claim that having a mental illness does not equate to being nonresponsible (Feinberg, 1970; Mitchell, 1999).

The widely accepted argument that mental illness is not a sufficient basis for a defense of insanity does not on its own show that disease is not relevant to the insanity defense, and hence that the argument from the nonexistence of mental illness will not work. But from the point of view of this chapter, the second claim—that mental disease is not necessary either—is potentially damaging to Szasz's argument. If the state of mind which exculpates a person—the insane state of not knowing, as given in the M'Naghten rules—can be described without mention of mental illness, then mental illness is clearly not necessary to the defense. This claim, if true, would circumvent Szasz's argument that the insanity defense is mistaken because it relies on a nonexistent thing (mental illness). It would lead to the counterclaim that it does not rely upon that thing's existence. Indeed, this counterclaim is consistent with Szasz's view that there is no such thing as mental illness. Thus, it threatens Szasz's position by showing that his conclusion (that the insanity defense is a mistake) does not necessarily follow from his premise (that there is no such thing as mental illness).

Some responses are available to Szasz. Suppose, for instance, that the causal role of disease in the M'Naghten version of the insanity defense were removed, leaving only the words which describe the insane state of mind. The insanity defense would then be that not knowing that something is wrong or not knowing what oneself does is a basis for a plea of insanity. But this is not a suitable basis for a defense, since it seems to constitute a state of ignorance of the law, and as Szasz points out: "In the Anglo-American (and also Roman) philosophy of law, ignorance of the law is no excuse. . . .

the well-being of a free society is based on the assumption that every adult knows what he may and what he may not do. *Legal responsibility is an expectation:* first, that people will learn the laws of the land; second, that they will try to adhere to them. Thus, if they break the law, we consider them 'blameworthy.' If . . . mental illness is similar to ignorance (as indeed it is)—then again it is not a condition that excuses violation of the law" (Szasz, 1963, pp. 132–3, original italics). Szasz's claim would, I think, be widely accepted, except for the last move, where he says that mental illness is similar to ignorance.

The reasoning that says that the insanity is in the nonknowing state of mind also runs into the objection that this is consistent with a person simply not believing that a particular killing was wrong. Since knowledge is widely defined as nonflukily justified true belief, we can infer that, if a person does not believe what he or she did was wrong, then that person cannot know that it was wrong. The famous Gettier (1963) examples suggest that knowledge cannot be defined purely as justified true belief. Yet the insanity defense does not stretch to claims that the murderer believed that the victim deserved to die and so it was not wrong to kill him or her.

What seems to be missing, if the words which refer to the causal role of disease are removed, is any sense of how a person came to be ignorant of the law (in the M'Naghten rules sense). While it makes sense to say that the state of mind which exculpates is not coterminous with any particular mental disorder, it also makes sense to ask whether the insane state of mind has any causal relationship with mental disorder (or indeed is the result of any number of other conditions, such as brain injury, being very young, and so on). On Szasz's behalf, Weinberg and Vatz (1982) contrast the defense that a person was too young to know what he or she did was wrong with the insanity defense. According to them, Szasz argues that, in the former case, the defense is based upon the infancy or youth of the individual, not on the immaturity of his or her thoughts. But in the case of the insanity defense, it is based on the claimed insanity of the thoughts, and there is no equivalent to the independent judgment of infancy. If the apparent insanity is the result of any of these other conditions, then the state of ignorance of right and wrong seems to arise in a potentially excusable (i.e., nonculpable) way. Mitchell (1999) argues that, in some cases at least, a person who was insane at the time of a crime is culpable for being insane, and so should not be excused on the ground of that insanity. The general thought is that it is unjust for a person to use a defense where he or she has "effectively created the conditions of his own defence" (Mitchell, 1999, p. 600). An example might be someone who deliberately fails to take medication for a psychotic condition, and then kills while in the psychotic state.

If this is accepted, then mental illness does seem to come back into the picture and play a potentially significant role in it. With such a role comes Szasz's claim that there is no such thing as mental illness. For, insofar as the existence of mental illness is a part of the picture in which the insanity defense operates, its nonexistence would disrupt that picture. Even if mental illness is neither sufficient nor necessary to the use of the insanity defense, the question of its presence or absence becomes material.

So the argument comes back, after all, to the contention that without mental illness, the insanity defense cannot work. But on the tests which I have proposed for the strength of Szasz's arguments, the claim that there is no such thing as mental illness seems to fail by not being widely accepted. Szasz is not quite a lone voice in denying the existence of mental illness, but his voice is clearly not with the vast majority. Additionally, his arguments against mental illness have been well known for many years, but have not persuaded many people. Insofar as the persuasiveness of his arguments against the insanity defense relies upon the persuasive force of his argument that mental illness is a myth, they clearly lack such persuasiveness.

15.4 The sciences of psychiatry and psychology do not help to determine guilt

The arguments in this section spring from quite a different source than those considered so far which are built upon premises which are more dramatic, or have a larger scope, than the conclusion that they support. But the ones to be considered in this section are not premised on large and controversial metaphysical or conceptual claims. Rather, they arise in the light of the question of what a psychiatrist, qua scientist, can add to the discussion of whether someone is guilty. In practice, the insanity defense relies, or so it may be said, upon scientists to pronounce upon this matter. The insanity defense can operate only where the scientists' pronouncements are material. Szasz argues, in a number of ways, that scientists' pronouncements cannot be material in the way required.

Before proceeding to look more closely at this argument, two caveats will be entered. First, this approach lacks the broad sweep of the first two arguments. Even if correct, this argument can show only that scientists cannot do the work expected of them by the courts in cases of the insanity defense. Scientists cannot determine whether a behavior had any causal connection with a scientifically describable state of the human mind, such that the latter might excuse the former; they cannot contribute to a judgment of innocence or guilt.

Second, and related to the first caveat, it may be argued that psychiatrists do not appear in court as scientists. It may be suggested they appear as practitioners of psychiatry, who offer their considerable, but not solely scientific, expertise and experience to the jury to help them in their deliberations as to guilt or innocence. As such, they represent experts whose role is socially legitimated (i.e., conventionally regarded as pertinent and useful to a jury's deliberations). (I owe this important point to one of the anonymous referees of this chapter. Interestingly, the referee noted that the psychiatrist may be seen to be very like a member of the jury. I suspect that Szasz would be inclined to agree, but with the rider that the psychiatrist would be welcome in court as—but only as—a member of a jury.)

But there are two problems with this second caveat. First, the social legitimation of the role of psychiatrist appears to be part and parcel of the defense. Thus, the defense and the social legitimacy of those involved in it stand or fall together. Second, if some independent support for the psychiatrist's role in court were to be found, it would seem likely to be predicated upon the scientific credentials of psychiatry. It is the relevance of these credentials which is at stake here.

Szasz's claim, then, is that scientific pronouncements related to the insanity defense are not material. For this claim, Szasz offers a number of distinct arguments—not all equally plausible. First, he argues that, since the scientific terms of psychiatry are all theoretical, no causal claims can be based upon them. Second, he argues that a scientific explanation might mean that we understand why a person did something, but does not mean that we forgive (or acquit) the doing of it. Third, he suggests that any scientific explanation of behaviors will either underdetermine the behavior or lead to the absurd claim that behaviors are determined by each and every psychological and nonpsychological influence. As will emerge, the first two arguments are not persuasive: but the third has considerable persuasive characteristics.

15.4.1 Scientific explanations are theories: theories cannot cause behavior

The argument that mental illnesses are explanatory theories and cannot be causes is based upon Gilbert Ryle's notion of a category mistake. To illustrate his idea, Ryle invented the example of the person visiting the University of Oxford or Cambridge for the first time, and being shown around, seeing the libraries, colleges, fields, and other features. Ryle imagines the person then asking: "But where is the university?" (Ryle, 1973, p. 18). Asking this question seems to suggest that the person has misunderstood something. The mistake that the person has made is to assume that the university is in the same category as the buildings, etc. (i.e., that it is another physical thing). But the university is not another building; rather, it is constituted (at least in part) by the buildings. The category mistake argument applied to the present case might be: "Schizophrenia is in the class of explanatory theories, and is not a member of the class of causes." The parallel is not exact, at least when it comes to Ryle's example, in which what is seen (the buildings) are in fact constituents of a more abstract existence (the university). For Szasz: "The word 'disease' always denotes a theory, not a fact . . . Thus, if the more complex term 'mental disease' means anything at all, it too refers to a theory, not to a fact" (Szasz, 1963, p. 133).

Szasz illustrates this argument in his early *Columbia Law Review* article:

> Let us take a simple hypothetical example, purely for the purposes of making clear the logical fallacies inherent in the principles of the *Durham* decision. Suppose a man 'goes berserk,' pulls out a gun in broad daylight, and shoots down several people who are sightseeing in front of the White House. When arrested and questioned about his deed, he explains that he was protecting the President from communist assassins who were about to throw an atomic bomb on the White House lawn. . . . Today, psychiatrists would testify (a) that the murderer suffers from schizophrenia, and (b) that schizophrenia was the 'cause' of his act. But was it? I suggest that 'schizophrenia' is a theory by means of which we seek to explain, to ourselves and others, how it is that such a thing as this happened. (Szasz, 1958, pp. 191, original italics)

He acknowledges that the theories or explanations of psychiatrists about how this happened are likely to be quite sophisticated, compared with those of laypeople:

> Similarly, the theoretical physicist has a more sophisticated theory of how electricity flows in a wire than does the layman. Indeed, the former may express his theory in mathematical equations whereas the latter pictures the process as consisting of electrons, visualized as little balls rolling along on little copper rails. In any case, does the theory of electric flow in

a wire *cause* the light bulb to glow and the radio to play? Clearly, this question itself is improper. Similarly, I maintain that it is utter nonsense to ask, much less to answer, whether in the hypothetical case cited the murderer's 'schizophrenia' was the cause of his criminal act. An explanation or a theory can never be a cause. (Szasz, 1958, p. 191, original italics)

It seems virtually self-evident that Szasz's claim that theories do not cause the events about which they theorize is correct. For example, if it were the theory of gravity that caused massive objects to be attracted to one another, then none of them would have been attracted to one another prior to 1665–1667 or so, the period during which Newton is standardly reputed to have come up with the theory (White, 1997, pp. 85–6). But this is absurd. However, if schizophrenia, or indeed mental illness, are terms that refer to theories about behavior, then neither can be referring to a cause of behavior.

The most obvious response to Szasz here is to accuse him of making a category mistake himself. It is not those who claim that schizophrenia can cause criminal behaviors who are confusing theory and reality. It is Szasz, ignoring the fact that schizophrenia and other such concepts are used to refer to something in the world, who is making a category error. For it is that to which they refer which does the causing, not the concept which refers to them. There are some complex issues hereabouts in the philosophy of science, and in the theory of reference, which are beyond the scope of this chapter. In brief, though, it seems reasonable to claim that concepts and words as used in science are intended to refer to things with causal powers, and this is sufficient to undermine Szasz's argument.

15.4.2 **Scientific explanations give us understanding—but not forgiveness**

The argument considered in this section is that scientific explanations give us understanding of why people act as they do, but do not ground a claim that we should forgive people's criminal or immoral acts. This argument is in serious tension with the previous argument. In saying that scientific theoretical explanations help us to understand, Szasz presumably means that they help us to understand the causal patterns which we find around us. Because of this, Szasz ought really to have abandoned one of these arguments. I have already suggested that the argument in the previous section is not all that effective—so Szasz would have been best advised to abandon it.

But this can be put aside. Referring to the way in which scientific theories put forward causal explanations of human behavior, Szasz suggests:

In this way we discover what we should have known all along—that genuine scientific 'causal' theories render the assignment of moral 'blame' to persons unnecessary and, in fact, impossible. If we take physics and its various branches seriously, we conclude, as indeed most people in our society have concluded, that we cannot blame the gods if our crops fail or if our cattle die. Similarly, if we would take psychology and its branches seriously, as very few people seem prepared to do, we might conclude that we cannot blame men for what they do. They, too, have their 'reasons.' But, to 'understand' does *not* necessarily mean that one must 'forgive'. (Szasz, 1958, pp. 191–2, original italics)

How should these words be understood? There seem to be two ways of taking the claim that to understand is not to forgive. First, it could be that when the causes of a person's behavior are revealed, this still leaves the moral grounds of responsibility untouched (and cannot remove them). This is the sort of consideration which motivates the next argument—that science cannot determine what the causes of behavior are—which is considered in the next section. Second, it could be that the sciences do successfully show why a person did something (i.e., give a determinative causal explanation) in such a way that it appears that the person is not morally responsible for his or her acts. But we are left with a challenge—to "re-examine the compulsion under which we labor when we insist that a man must be (morally) responsible for his act before we, society, can punish him" (Szasz, 1958, p. 192).

These two understandings of Szasz's words are inconsistent with one another; but the second one is, I think, less Szaszian (if I may so put it), because it is also inconsistent with other things Szasz says as well—such as that we are all responsible moral agents and the insanity defense flies in the face of this basic fact about us. These are some of the big claims Szasz makes, and while they may not be persuasive in general, we can doubt whether any argument he makes, which is inconsistent with them, reflects his true views.

15.4.3 Scientific explanations of behavior

In the previous section, the idea was mooted that, perhaps even when the causal information about a person's behavior has been unearthed, something is still left unexplained. Here, we explore this underdetermination of behavior by scientifically describable causal factors. We consider two arguments, each of which answers the question of what can sciences such as psychology contribute to the question which seems to be raised by the insanity defense. That is, can sciences such as psychology contribute to telling us if a person was insane at the time of the crime, and so was not responsible for his or her actions, and so is innocent of the crime. Szasz's argument is that science cannot contribute an answer to the question of a person's guilt or innocence, or the person's level of responsibility. Since the insanity defense appears to rely on the idea that science can help to determine level of responsibility, Szasz's objection is quite powerful. A possible rejoinder is that the argument focusing on the science of psychiatry does not help to undermine the existence of versions of the insanity defense that predate the existence of psychiatry. But it seems unreasonable to demand that Szasz's arguments must work against prescientific versions of the insanity defense that even its supporters do not deploy.

Background to Szasz's view: the multifactorial account of human behavior

Before looking at the detail of these arguments, we should emphasize that, while they are consistent with the large metaphysical statements about the nature of the human being that Szasz makes, they are also consistent with a common or garden variety of belief about why people do the things they do. We might call this theory, the multifactorial belief, account, or theory. Szasz expresses it in the following hypothetical case:

> What, then, it may be asked, did cause the killer to shoot these people whom he did not
> even know? This question can be answered, more or less satisfactorily, and psychiatry

can contribute much to providing such answers. But such answers, I hasten to add, are of no use to a jury. In general, the 'causes', as I would conceive of them, of such a 'schizophrenic murder' may be arranged in a temporal hierarchy ranging from the way the patient's parents treated him when he was a child to his experiences five minutes before the shooting. The waitress in the cafeteria where he had breakfast might have been gruff and unfriendly, and this might have been the proverbial 'last straw' that broke his precariously weakened self-concept and self-esteem—thus the paranoid-megalomanic 'crime'. But, provided this sort of theory is psychologically meaningful and correct, this is not the sort of 'cause' that would assist a jury in assigning blame to anyone. Surely, the waitress could not be blamed, nor could the patient. (Szasz, 1958, pp. 191–2)

The explanation here, then, is that the circumstances and events of the person's life up to that point, and his or her own reactions to these, explain why a person did what he or she did. From the point of view of the argument being addressed here, assuming that Szasz's skepticism about the insanity defense follows from this common or garden account of why people do things, it represents a very strong starting point. For unless a person takes an extreme or selective view of the causation of human behavior, it is highly likely that he or she will acknowledge the role of all these factors. It is a starting point that Szasz can rely on, to some degree, to be common ground between him and a good number of those with whom he is engaged in discussion. For example, Read and Bentall (2012) argue that factors including early childhood experiences with abuse and experiences of inequality within society should be taken into account in any explanation of mental health problems.

Notwithstanding, Szasz is prepared to make suggestions, as a psychiatrist or psychologist, about why life may become a challenge for some people, as part of an explanation of what they do. This is from his testimony at the Cromer trial, answering questions put to him by the judge:

Life gets in some way existentially, to use this modern word, life gets a little more difficult after puberty, after fourteen, fifteen, sixteen. Up until that age, it is enough for us to be the son or daughter of whoever we are, to go to school, to be a student. After thirteen, fourteen, fifteen, we have to be somebody. We have to do something. And then if we are not good at basketball, at mathematics, at being a mother, a father, a housekeeper, a something, increasingly our self-esteem deteriorates and increasingly that person's life will turn sour and that person will have difficulty in putting it together. So I do not think one needs any special medical or scientific explanation to account for the difficulties that people run into in their young years, which explains why people after adolescence in their early adulthood, have difficulties with the law, with drugs, with their lives, because that is a crucial period, making something with your life. If you don't do it between the ages of fifteen and thirty you will be in trouble. (Finney, 1982, p. 29)

What Szasz refers to here are the "problems of living" (1963, p. 13) which he believes have to be faced by all, but which people deal with in very different ways.

While many might be prepared to share this starting point with Szasz without demur, he offers reasons to believe that behavior cannot be altogether explained by people's psychology, and that a number of factors lead to it: "Virtually all behavior with which the psychoanalyst and psychiatrist deal is learned behavior. Since such behavior cannot be properly described or analyzed without dealing explicitly with the norms and standards that regulate it, and with the goals it seeks to attain, psychoanalytic theory is foreordained to being unable to offer an adequate account of such conduct" (Szasz, 1974, pp. 153–4).

More narrowly—at least in his focus on crime—Szasz states:

> I prefer a broader, sociopsychological perspective on crime, which accords psychological factors their proper place, but which holds that criminality, as well as society's methods of combating it, reflect the socioethical style of the community. The organized lawlessness connected with bootlegging liquor was an American type of criminality. Likewise, relatively punctilious compliance with income-tax laws is also typically American. In brief, the evidence strongly suggests that criminal behavior is learned, as is noncriminal, lawabiding behavior. Crime is a phenomenon that is ethical, legal, and social-psychological, not instinctual-biological and medical. This view is not novel. It requires emphasis only to counteract the medical-psychoanalytic view that tends to attribute criminal behavior either to genetic and neurological factors, or to early human influences over which the individual has little or no control in later life. (Szasz, 1963, pp. 110-11)

Here, Szasz talks about counteracting the medical-psychoanalytic view, not about replacing it.

Szasz uses two arguments to draw out the implications of the multifactorial account of behavior for the insanity defense: First, he argues that scientific explanations underderdetermine the chosen course of action which a person takes. Second, he argues that, if it were the case that a psychological explanation is determinative, then all other explanations can make the same claim—but this has absurd consequences. Both arguments are fleshed out in the following section.

Underdetermination of behavior by psychological factors

There are two versions of this point to be found in Szasz's writings. The first is that, though the resources of psychology can play a role in the understanding and explanation of behavior that has already happened, just because the theories of psychology are about people in general, they do not provide a full explanation for any particular behavior that has already happened, and do not make one behavior more likely than another. The second is that the sciences of psychiatry deal not with the function of the whole of a person's psyche, but with its part functions. However, part functions do not necessarily determine the course a person takes in life.

The first version of the underdetermination argument is inferred from Sigmund Freud, whom Szasz, in this case, quotes with approval. Freud was asked at one point to offer an opinion on whether the Oedipus complex could incriminate a person in the murder of his father. The case concerned the young Halsmann. Freud wrote:

> If it had been objectively demonstrated that Philipp Halsmann murdered his father, there would at all events be some ground for introducing the Oedipus complex to provide a motive for an otherwise unexplained deed. Since no such proof has been adduced, mention of the Oedipus complex has a misleading effect; it is at least idle. Such disagreements as have been uncovered by the investigation in the Halsmann family between the father and son are altogether inadequate to provide a foundation for assuming in the son a bad relationship towards his father. Even if it were otherwise, we should be obliged to say that it is a far cry from there to the causation of such a deed. Precisely because it is always present,

the Oedipus complex is not suited to provide a decision on the question of guilt. (Freud, 1931; quoted by Szasz, 1963, pp. 104–5)

Freud makes two points here: First, he suggests that it is misleading to appeal to the psychodynamic notion of the Oedipus complex in order to help answer the question whether someone is guilty or not of a crime. The fact that Halsmann had the Oedipus complex contributes nothing—is "idle," as Freud puts it—to answering the question of whether he actually had the motivation to murder his father or did in fact murder him. Second, since the presence of the Oedipus complex is universal among men, it must be linked to all behavior, including all which is linked to a man's relationship with his father. What it does not do is determine what form that behavior will take. The man who reveres his father, the man who is indifferent to him, and the man who murders him, all have the Oedipus complex.

How persuasive are these arguments? Their persuasiveness seems reduced because they rely upon a controversial idea, namely, that the explanations of psychology apply to everyone, whatever their behaviors are. For example, the argument supposes that the Oedipus complex applies to all men, because it is part of a universal theory about male psychology. It is as persuasive only as this claim to universality.

One objection to the claim of universality would be that the sciences of psychology deal with normal psychology differently from the way that they deal with pathologies of the psyche. An argument in support of this claim is that the pathological states with which psychologists and psychiatrists deal are natural kinds. If something is a natural kind, then it would be expected to have an essence distinguishing it from all other kinds. One basis for believing pathologies of the psyche to be natural kinds, with distinct essences, would be if they responded to medications in different ways to similar but nonpathological psychic conditions. For example, it might be thought that depression is a natural kind if depressive symptoms attributable to it were relieved by antidepressant medication, while depressive symptoms not attributable to it, but rather arising in the context of grief or loss, were not relieved by the same medications. About this matter there is considerable and heated debate in the empirical literature, but here it only illustrates an issue.

This seems to raise the question of whether there are indeed pathologies of the psyche taking the form of natural kinds—which seems very like the question of whether there are any mental illnesses or diseases. This route to undermining the insanity defense has already been considered. However, for the purposes of the argument here, the issue can be construed in a slightly different way. Many psychologists affirm that there are unhealthy states of mind, but not that there are categorically discrete mental illnesses, or a discrete general category of mental illness. For example, the British Psychological Society (BPS), responding to the consultation for DSM-V (APA, 2013), argued: "The validity of the basic categories is assumed, rather than evidenced from research into distress across both psychiatric and 'normal' populations which might challenge the appropriateness of the paradigm. . . . by not taking account of the evidence for the dimensional spectrum of psychiatric symptoms such as low mood, hearing voices, unusual beliefs and so on across the general population, retention of a categorical model is a methodological flaw, particularly but not exclusively for 'functional' rather than 'organic' disorders" (BPS, 2012, p. 3).

Views such as these of the BPS raise substantial questions about whether mental illnesses are natural kinds with distinct essences—and this is a skepticism that these psychologists share with Szasz, even if they do not share his skepticism about the whole idea of mental health. These skeptical views further suggest reasons to doubt that there is a special science associated with psychiatry, or (a fortiori) that it contributes to questions about guilt or innocence. Nor is this skepticism restricted to categorical approaches to mental health, but rather reflects the views of at least some philosophers of medicine in general. For example, Lester King questions the distinction between normal and pathological physiology. Physiology as a science, he says, can make no sense of the distinction between the pathological and the nonpathological (King, 1954; Canguilhem, 2007).

But let us suppose that a special science of psychopathology does after all exist, at least in the sense that diseases are thought to be natural kinds. If it does, it runs into two problems: First, it is presumably committed to part-functions of the psyche—but it can be argued that part-functions cannot explain the actions chosen by the person. Second, it presumably holds that psychopathology has some special causal role in explaining human behavior (this being the basis upon which it purports to excuse)—but this claim does not stand up to any scrutiny.

The argument from part-functions emerges in Szasz's commentary on Lady Wootton's views, which he cites approvingly:

> Undoubtedly people who suffer from disturbances of mental part-functions have to carry the burden of those disturbances on top of whatever happens to be their share of the ordinary troubles and difficulties of human life. But so also do those who suffer from migraine or weak digestions. How can we be sure that it is legitimate in the one case, but not in the other, to leap to the conclusion that, for those who suffer from these disabilities, the standards of social expectation ought to be lowered? Why is dishonesty excused as well as explained by depression, but not by indigestion? Why should we accept the plea of diminished responsibility for the unlawful revenges of the deluded against their imaginary persecutors, but not for similar actions perpetrated against real enemies by rational persons, if both parties alike recognize what they do is wrong? (Wootton, 1959, pp. 239–40; Szasz, 1963, p. 102)

This is a particularly interesting argument for Szasz to have advanced, because it accepts a basic tenet of much theorizing about mental disorder, namely, that it involves the dysfunction of some part or parts of the human psyche (Boorse, 1976; Wakefield, 1992). What perhaps should make Wootton's approach less conducive to Szasz is her appeal to the state of knowledge of the perpetrators. But, that aside, Wootton's position is that if mental disorder affects the functioning of a part or parts of the human, then that hardly shows that it must affect a human's ability to reach conclusions about the morality or otherwise of behavior, or to act on those conclusions.

Arguing against the insanity defense on the basis of part-functions does not appear to entail acceptance of any metaphysical position on the nature of the human (except that the human psyche has parts—which may be accepted on all sides of the current dispute). But what it suggests is that the science of psychopathology has to explain how it is the dysfunction of one or more parts can excuse a person from a crime committed, when other part-functions of the mind remain unaffected.

Turning to the argument that psychopathology cannot represent a special case of causality, the argument is that the causal aspect of psychopathology (if there is one) is simply the causal aspect of all psychology. If psychopathology is causal with respect to behavior, then normal (nonpsychopathological) psychology must also be causal with respect to behavior, and so all behavior must be caused by the human being's psychology. This seems to catch apologists for the insanity defense in a dilemma. Either they must hold that all criminal activity is caused by a person's psychology (which seems to undercut the special considerations of the defense) or their approach must hold that psychopathology is causal, whereas nonpsychopathological features are not; but this appears to be simply ad hoc. At the very least, it leaves those supporting the insanity defense having to tell us what justifies the claim that only pathological psychic phenomena cause behavior.

In short, the argument that psychology underdetermines behavior is persuasive. It appeals to ideas which, while not uncontroversial, are shared by very many. Moreover, it has the implication that a psychiatrist cannot answer questions of guilt or innocence by appeal to scientific understandings and explanations of human behavior.

If psychological factors explain and excuse, so do all the others

However, suppose that someone holds onto the claim that psychopathologies of the mind have an explanatory power such that a person can be said to be insane by the psychiatrist in a court of law and excused as a result. It turns out that an absurd conclusion follows if the multifactorial theory of why people do what they do is accepted. Suppose it is (and it seems likely to be widely accepted), then what follows if one factor is said to have caused the crime (in this case, the psychological factor)? An argument would then need to be advanced as to why the psychological factors—and not any of the others—should be granted that causal status. This argument is hard to come by. One reviewer of this chapter notes that the focus on psychological factors follows common sense. Though this seems true to me as a description of our practices, including those we find in the insanity defense, it does not equate to an argument in favor of it. As Szasz notes, part of a narrative why someone killed may involve a very recent and somewhat contingent event, such as a waitress being a bit gruff with him (Szasz, 1958, p. 192). Yet surely we do not hold the waitress accountable for the subsequent killing. M'Naghten is reported as saying that Drummond "gave him a scowling look" (Quen, 1968, p. 47; quoting *The Times*, 1843) prior to his shooting Drummond in the back; but this hardly leads to the conclusion that Drummond provoked his own death. But if it is believed that the psychological part of the story has a determinative force, why should not the waitress's gruffness or Drummond's sneering look be attributed the same force? For Szasz, either we must take all economic, sociological, and other causal theories seriously and accept their necessary implication that people should not be blamed for what they do because they could not have done otherwise, or we must grant that people "always have some choice in how they act—hence they are always responsible for their conduct" (Szasz, 1963, p. 135).

The inclination may be to answer that there is something unusual about psychological explanations; that they are causal in a way that others are not, or that they excuse while others do not. But in the context of this chapter, special pleading for the causal or excusing role of the psychological is circularly linked with the insanity defense. For this seems to be precisely what the insanity defense assumes, and so it is precisely what is at stake.

15.5 Conclusion

Szasz rejects the insanity defense. It is inconsistent both with his claims about human nature, and with his claim that mental illness is a myth. But neither claim is a persuasive basis for Szasz's objection. It asks too much of a disputant—for example, to accept that people's actions are always autonomous or that mental illness does not exist—in order to conclude that the insanity defense is incoherent. However, an argument from the limits of the sciences of psychology and psychiatry is damaging to the insanity defense, and is persuasive. This argument lacks the sweep and metaphysical depths of the other arguments—but that is just where its persuasiveness lies.

Acknowledgments

An early version of this chapter was presented to the postgraduate research forum at the Bioethics Centre at the University of Otago, where there was much interesting discussion. A later draft was read by Dr. Mike King, and I owe him many thanks for his comments and encouragement. The reviewers appointed by the editors made very helpful and challenging comments, which I have both acknowledged and attempted as best I could to respond to. The editors of this volume were extremely helpful in providing support and ideas for the chapter—though I cannot claim to have done them justice.

References

American Psychiatric Association (APA). 2013. *Diagnostic and Statistical Manual of Mental Disorders [DSM-V]*, 5th edn. Arlington, Virginia: American Psychiatric Association.

Boorse, Christopher. 1976. "What a Theory of Mental Health Should Be." *Journal for the Theory of Social Behaviour* **6** (1) (April): 61–84.

British Psychological Society (BPS). 2012. *DSM-5: The Future of Psychiatric Diagnosis (2012—Final Consultation)*. Accessed April 22, 2018. <www1.bps.org.uk/sites/default/files/DSM-5 2012 - BPS response.pdf>

Canguilhem, Georges. 2007. *The Normal and the Pathological*, translated by Carolyn R. Faucett and Robert S. Cohen. New York: Zone Books.

Daniel M'Naghten's Case. 1843. 10 Cl & F 200; 8 ER 718.

Durham v. United States. 1954. 214 F. 2d, 862 (D.C. Circ).

Edwards, Rem B. 1982. "Mental Health as Rational Autonomy." In *Psychiatry and Ethics: Insanity, Rational Autonomy, and Mental Health Care*, edited by Rem B. Edwards, pp. 68–78. Buffalo: Prometheus Books.

Feinberg, Joel. 1970. *Doing and Deserving: Essays in the Theory of Responsibility.* Princeton: Princeton University Press.

Finney, Joseph C. 1982. "The Psychiatrist in Court: People of the State of California v. Darlin June Cromer." *American Journal of Forensic Psychiatry* **3** (1): 5–46.

Freud, Sigmund. 1931. "The Expert Opinion in the Halsmann Case." In *The Standard Edition of the Complete Psychological Works of Sigmund Freud, Volume 21*, pp. 251–3. London: Hogarth, 1961.

Gettier, Edmund L. 1963. "Is Justified True Belief Knowledge?" *Analysis* **23** (6) (June): 121–3.

Hathaway, Mark. 2009. "Comment: The Moral Significance of the Insanity Defence." *Journal of Criminal Law* **73** (4): 310–17.

Hesslow, Germund. 1993. "Do We Need a Concept of Disease?" *Theoretical Medicine* **14** (1) (March): 1–14.

John Hinckley Jr. 2018. Accessed April 8, 2018. <en.wikipedia.org/wiki/John_Hinckley_Jr.>

King, Lester S. 1954. "What is Disease?" *Philosophy of Science* **21** (3) (July): 193–203.

Levine, Robert J. 1988. *Ethics and Regulation of Clinical Research*, 2nd edn. New Haven: Yale University Press.

McGee, Hugh J. 1961. *Hearings on Constitutional Rights of the Mentally Ill Before a Subcommittee of the Senate Committee on the Judiciary*, 87th Cong., 1st Sess., pt. 2. Washington, D.C.: USGPO.

McGee, Hugh J. 1963. *Hearings on S. 935 to Protect the Constitutional Rights of the Mentally Ill Before a Subcommittee of the Senate Committee on the Judiciary*, 88th Cong., 1st Sess. Washington, D.C.: USGPO.

Mill, David van. 1995. "Hobbes's Theories of Freedom." *Journal of Politics* **57** (2) (May): 443–59.

Miller, Bruce L. 1981. "Autonomy and Refusal of Lifesaving Treatment." *Hastings Center Report* **11** (4) (August): 22–8.

Mitchell, Edward W. 1999. "Madness and Meta-Responsibility: The Culpable Causation of Mental Disorder and the Insanity Defence." *The Journal of Forensic Psychiatry* **10** (3): 597–622.

Morse, Stephen J. 1985. "Excusing the Crazy: The Insanity Defense Reconsidered." *Southern California Law Review* **58**: 777–836.

People v. Darlin June Cromer. 1980. No. 70061, Alameda County Super. Ct. (Cal.) (April 18).

Quen, Jacques M. 1968. "An Historical View of the M'Naghten Trial." *Bulletin of the History of Medicine* **42** (1) (January–February): 43–51.

Read, John, and Richard P. Bentall. 2012. "Negative Childhood Experiences and Mental Health: Theoretical, Clinical, and Primary Prevention Implications." *British Journal of Psychiatry* **200** (2) (February): 89–91.

Ryle, Gilbert. 1973. *The Concept of Mind.* Harmondsworth, England: Penguin.

Szasz, Thomas S. 1958. "Psychiatry, Ethics, and the Criminal Law." *Columbia Law Review* **58** (2) (February): 183–98.

Szasz, Thomas S. 1963. *Law, Liberty, and Psychiatry: An Inquiry into the Social Uses of Mental Health Practices.* New York: Macmillan.

Szasz, Thomas S. 1967. "The Insanity Plea and the Insanity Verdict." *Temple Law Quarterly* **40** (3–4) (Spring–Summer): 271–82.

Szasz, Thomas S. 1970. *Ideology and Insanity: Essays on the Psychiatric Dehumanization of Man.* Garden City, New York: Doubleday Anchor.

Szasz, Thomas S. 1974. *The Myth of Mental Illness: Foundations of a Theory of Personal Conduct*, revised edn. New York: Harper & Row.

Szasz, Thomas S. 1991. *Ideology and Insanity: Essays on the Psychiatric Dehumanization of Man*, revised edn. Syracuse: Syracuse University Press.

The Times, 1843. London (March 6).

Wakefield, Jerome C. 1992. "Disorder as Harmful Dysfunction: A Conceptual Critique of DSM-III-R's Definition of Mental Disorder." *Psychological Review* **99** (2) (April): 232–47.

Weinberg, Lee S., and Richard E. Vatz. 1982. "The Insanity Plea: Szaszian Ethics and Epistemology." *Metamedicine* **3** (3) (October): 417–33.

White, Michael. 1997. *Isaac Newton: The Last Sorcerer*. London: Fourth Estate.

Wootton, Barbara. 1959. *Social Science and Social Pathology*. London: George Allen & Unwin.

Chapter 16

Bringing psychopaths into the moral community: Reassessing agency cultivation and social participation

Marisola Xhelili Ciaccio

16.1 Introduction

Recent philosophical literature on moral responsibility makes the case that, among other things, we are moral agents on the basis of our possession of a set of morally spe-cific agential capacities: it is due to the possession of such capacities that we are able to rely on each other to understand moral norms and behave accordingly, and to hold each other morally and legally responsible when we do not adhere to and breach such norms. Interestingly, in both past and contemporary philosophical accounts of moral responsibility, the psychopath features as the paradigmatic exception to any imputed account of "normal" moral agency. Within these accounts, the psychopath has become the symbol of a deranged moral architecture, opening a lacuna within the logic of morality that makes it difficult to know how (or whether) we can hold psychopaths morally responsible.

I would argue that it is irresponsible of any account of moral responsibility to de-velop itself on hasty assumptions about the psychopath as someone who is necessarily morally untrainable and outside the sphere of moral responsibility. This is a matter on which Szasz's work has important insight. The more we push to subsume psychopathy under the mental illness umbrella, the more likely we are to dismiss psychopaths as lost causes—victims of a brain disease—and the less likely we are to seriously consider their agency and the importance of their moral training. The fact that psychopathy is a serious psychological condition and yet does not strictly classify as a mental illness is an interesting illustration of a type of mental disorder that transcends our classifications of disease and, at the same time, challenges us to consider its implications outside psy-chiatry and within the moral-social sphere.

Psychopathy, because it cannot simply dwell within the excuses of mental illness, must of necessity be theorized within the realm of moral agency, if only because it is in this realm that it raises undeniable concerns. If we engage with it as a ques-tion regarding human freedom and morality, instead of regarding the incapacitation of mental illness, we begin to think not through the limitations of the language of psychiatry but through the opportunities of the language of moral responsibility. From this properly Szaszian perspective, we show that we can indeed do something about the moral training and responsibility of psychopaths—and that this requires more complex understandings of psychopathy as a problem in social and ethical living, of the variety of ways in which different people become moral agents, and of the legitimate reasons for holding each other accountable (with and despite our different capacities) in order to become better moral beings.

16.2 Defining characteristics of psychopaths

It is important to clarify from the beginning of this chapter exactly to whom we are referring when we speak of psychopaths, even though clarity in this topic in some ways still eludes us. The definition of psychopathy has differed throughout its history, starting with Hervey M. Cleckley's categorization of traits in the 1940s and 1950s (Hare, 1999, pp. 27–8), but broadly, it refers to individuals with a cluster of personality traits that vary in degree throughout the human population. The Hare Psychopathy Checklist Revised (PCL-R) (Hare, 2011) is most commonly used today to assess psychopathy professionally based on the following traits, which are broken into four facets: interpersonal, affective, lifestyle, and antisocial (see Table 16.1).

According to several recent cross-disciplinary studies, psychopaths are said to lack a number of attributes that are ascribed to ordinary moral agents:

(1) They lack the ability to empathize with the aversive conditions of others.

(2) They do not understand the difference between conventional and moral rules. Conventional transgressions are regarded as rule or authority-dependent; moral transgressions are regarded as rule or authority-independent because they provoke a strong affective response in us (McGeer, 2008, p. 231). Psychopaths fail to distinguish between the two kinds of transgressions.

(3) They do not learn from error in a way that nonpsychopathic persons do.

"These attributes appear to dispose a psychopath toward being able to commit antisocial acts remorselessly, without regard for needs beyond his or her own, in a manner that is otherwise consistent with an ordinary agent, but nonetheless in the presence

Table 16.1 Traits from the Hare Psychopathy Checklist Revised (2011) used to assess psychopathy

Interpersonal	Affective	Lifestyle	Antisocial
Glibness/ superficial charm	Lack of remorse or guilt	Need for stimulation	Poor behavioral controls
Grandiose sense of self-worth	Emotionally shallow	Parasitic lifestyle	Early behavioral problems
Pathological lying	Callous/lack of empathy	Lack of realistic long-term goals	Juvenile delinquency
Cunning/ manipulative	Failure to accept responsibility	Impulsivity Irresponsibility	Revoked conditional release
			Criminal versatility

of a substantially diminished capacity for ordinary moral reasoning" (Fox et al., 2013, pp. 1–2). Studies have also found that psychopaths have trouble with "understanding and processing the affect of others and thus possess an acute lack of empathy, as well as a diminished capacity for aversive conditioning that would ordinarily suppress aggressive behavior" (Fox et al., 2013, p. 7). According to Robert Hare's assessment list, what appears distinct about psychopathy compared to other antisocial psychopathological conditions is the combination of interpersonal and affective traits. "Such traits are not only antisocial, but appear to be great instigators of continued antisocial behavior and blocks to attempts to correct it" (Fox et al., 2013, p. 5). As Adam Fox et al. summarize it: "Psychopaths possess both the personality traits commonly associated with a highly antisocial individual and show an apparent deficit in abilities associated with moral reasoning in non-psychopaths" (2013, p. 14). In addition, psychopaths display deficits in the ability to correct behavior in the face of negative stimuli, such as punishment. Based on these findings, a picture starts to emerge of the psychopath as a person who is impaired in his or her capacity to engage in moral reasoning as well as in his or her capacity to act as a moral agent, leading to the conclusion that they are not capable of moral agency and that we cannot hold them morally responsible (Fox et al., 2013, p. 14).

Most of the aforementioned findings about psychopathy are centered on studies conducted on criminal and incarcerated psychopaths, and it is based on just these findings that accounts of moral responsibility dismiss the psychopath as essentially incapable of it. One of the problems with making the psychopath the exception to moral responsibility based on studies conducted only on criminal psychopaths is that it does not capture the range and the variety of manifestations of psychopathy. Heidi Maibom argues that psychopathy is in fact "a dimensional construct"—meaning that psychopathic traits exist on a spectrum and that the cutoff point for who is classified as a psychopath is rather arbitrary (Maibom, 2017, p. 1110). Many people who fall below the cutoff point still share traits with those who are above—traits that are of high moral relevance (such as lack of empathy, fear, and remorse, and acute displays of callousness, violence, and aggression).

A more complicated understanding of the range of psychopathy therefore comes forth when we look not only at incarcerated psychopaths but at the prevalence of psychopathy in the general population "and its expression in ways that are personally, socially, or economically damaging, but that are not necessarily illegal or that do not result in criminal persecution" (Oliveira-Souza et al., 2008, p. 152). The research of Oliveira-Souza et al., for example, is concerned with people who are at or below the threshold for psychopathy but that are nonviolent, or who are callous but nonetheless successful at participating in the world without being incarcerated for harms they cause. They characterize these individuals as "true community antisocials" or TCAs (otherwise known as successful psychopaths). TCAs are adults who frequently and recurrently violate the rights of others for their own gain (most of these being minor infractions, such as lying or stealing), do not care if they cause harm to their supporters, and fail to acknowledge their role in the suffering they cause others (Oliveira-Souza et al., 2008, p. 156). Oliveira-Souza et al. specifically note the TCAs' bizarre dissociation of *knowing* what is right and wrong from *acting* based on what is right and wrong: "The knowledge of how to behave appropriately [is] expressed only rhetorically and [has] little, if any, impact on their behavioral guidance in real contexts" (2008, p. 157).

Several studies conducted by Blair and others (Blair, 1995, 1997; Maibom, 2017) reveal that psychopathy admits not only of degrees but of subtypes. "People distinguish between the primary, low-anxious, or callous-unemotional psychopath and the secondary, high-anxious psychopath. Many regard secondary psychopathy as a sort of hodgepodge category, which likely contains many distinct types of antisocial and emotionally dysregulated individuals" (Maibom, 2017, p. 1112). Evaluating these studies, Maibom exclaims that secondary psychopaths, "who have relatively spared affective abilities," are typically even more violent than primary psychopaths (Maibom, 2017, p. 1112). At the very least, this evidence should warn us away from making blanket statements about the moral potential of psychopaths based on their diminished affect. More generally, it warns us that swiftly dismissing the "psychopath" as the exception to moral responsibility and trainability is not very helpful, since there is no one paradigmatic example of the psychopath.

Yet this is the way psychopathy has traditionally been theorized: researchers thought—on the basis of the distinct immoral behavior of psychopaths—that psychopathy was a mental illness that one was born with and that was unalterable. This made it a ready candidate for a type of brain disease, and consequently excused the affected agent from moral responsibility considerations. According to Szasz, we typically diagnose brain disease on the basis of symptoms that an individual displays: "We often attribute bad behavior to disease (to excuse the agent); never attribute good behavior to disease (lest we deprive the agent of credit); and typically attribute good behavior to free will and insist bad behavior called mental illness is a 'no fault' act of nature" (Szasz, 1998, p. 108). This is the type of reasoning traditionally applied to psychopathy, leading to the (narrowly mistaken) conclusion that psychopaths are incapable of taking moral actions.

We know now that psychopathy is not strictly genetic but a combination of genetic predispositions and a problematic early environment. More importantly, some of the recent research sampled here has led to the proposal that psychopathy should not even be considered a mental illness at all, and that it is best characterized as an adaptation that captures a subset of human beings who have challenges in exercising their moral agency (Hare, 2011). The second suggestion is more compatible with Szasz's proposal not to reduce problems like psychopathy to brain disease preemptively (and recent research supports this proposal), but to view them instead as agential problems in social and ethical living. In Chapter 6 of this volume, Robert Daly refers to symptoms of mental illness from a Szaszian perspective as "manifestations of *states of ignorance* or misguided practical judgments by a person regarding how to specify and achieve a good life, accompanied by learned habits of disability. They are, in some way . . . a failure of right reason, a problem for which the sufferer, as agent, is ultimately, prospectively at least, responsible." To be in this state, Daly continues, "generates problems in living for the person who suffers such a condition, as well as for others."

What psychopaths demonstrate, then, due to diminished affect and improper reasoning about moral matters, is the wrong type of agency regarding morality. Once we make the paradigmatic shift of seeing psychopathy as an agential problem in ethical living rather than a brain disease, and make use of evolving research on the various ranges and subtypes of psychopathy, I do not believe that we can easily dismiss the psychopath as broadly morally untrainable. Going in this direction has particular implications for how (rather than whether) we ought to entertain the moral training and moral agency of individuals with psychopathic traits. It is to this topic I now turn.

16.3 **Manuel Vargas's "agency cultivation model"**

In *Building Better Beings* (2013), Manuel Vargas presents what he calls the "agency cultivation model" of moral responsibility: an account that justifies praise and blame by their effects of moral training (i.e., we praise and blame individuals as a means to condition them to be more moral). The form of agency required for moral responsibility in the agency cultivation model is specifically an agency responsive to moral considerations (MC). Responding to moral considerations depends on a particular epistemic condition of control, or free will. Free will here is to be understood not as a stable inner capacity in the agent but as a relational property. Also important to note is that we have the capacities required for moral responsibility—detecting moral considerations and regulating our behavior in light of them—whether or not determinism is true; determinism is therefore irrelevant to the kind of free will required for moral responsibility. These capacities are second-order characteristics that respond to specifically moral considerations we find in the world, and are not determined by the physical structures to which our agency in general reduces. At the same time, this account does not postulate anything at odds with a naturalistic conception of the world.

Free will as a relational property means that exercising moral agency by way of responding to moral considerations varies from individual to individual and from context to context, and is variably constituted by each context as different individuals relate to it. Vargas argues against the notion that agents have some stable inner capacity that can cross-situationally pick out and respond to moral considerations. Instead, what he argues for is that there are "multiple agential structures or combinations of powers that constitute the control or freedom required for moral responsibility" (Vargas, 2013, p. 205). We thus have an account of responsible agency (RA) that allows for pluralism about capacities across circumstances as well as pluralism about the mechanisms that constitute these capacities. Agency is therefore not a unified cross-situational capacity everyone possesses, but one that is differently structured to varying degrees by our social and cultural structures. The way we are socialized serves to shape the moral architecture of our communities, which in turn shapes what we are morally sensitive to and how we respond to moral considerations. Agency cultivation is thus dynamic, circumstantialist, and relational—it is something that we do with other people as members of moral communities, not something we possess in isolation. This account of moral responsibility is also pluralistic without being relativistic; Vargas holds that there is a fact of the matter about morality and that moral responsibility is objective. Strangely, this objectivity of moral responsibility is not something we ourselves decide, but something about the world which we know and in terms of which we develop ourselves. So, having the capacity for moral agency is an objective fact about us, but one that is cultivated differently depending on our particular social relationships. The ways in which our moral capacities are trained, therefore, takes different routes for different individuals and is dependent on the moral communities to which individuals belong.

The account, broken into two parts, boils down to this: An agent S is a responsible agent with respect to considerations of type M in circumstances C if S possesses (1) a suite of basic agential capacities implicated in effective self-directed agency (including, for example, beliefs, desires, intentions, instrumental reasoning, and generally reliable beliefs about the world and the consequences of action); and (2) the relevant capacity for both detection of suitable moral considerations M in C and also self-governance with respect to M in C.

As we see, in addition to basic agential capacities, freedom to act responsibly involves the capacities for detection and self-government. Detection is the ability to recognize and respond to moral considerations in a given situation in the world. Vargas writes slightly confusingly on how the relevant similarity between contexts where moral considerations are detected should be nonsubjective, and proposes a "moderate degree of granularity" (Vargas, 2013, p. 219) in detecting contexts of relevant similarity. The point of this is to suggest that a moral consideration to responsible agency (MC–RA) relationship is variable, but not quite so variable as to be entirely subjective. The aim is then (1) to foster an MC–RA that supports a form of agency that we already find in the world and (2) to expand its scope of efficacy, or the range of contexts in which agents have the desired relationship to moral considerations (Vargas, 2013, p. 220), so that our moral practice produces agents who are able to recognize a wide range of moral considerations and to govern themselves accordingly.

A moral agent must have the capacity to self-govern in light of the considerations detected. So Vargas's theory holds that people are moral agents only if they (1) are self-directed agents *and* (2) can both detect and respond appropriately to moral considerations. Blameworthiness, he claims, is in fact restricted to those considerations to which the agent is capable of self-governance. Presumably then, blameworthiness conditions would not apply to a psychopath, who might fit the criteria for (1), but who displays a lack of ability both to detect moral considerations as conventionally understood (though Vargas allows for enough variability here where an argument for the psychopath's ability to detect moral consideration can be made); and to govern her behavior appropriately in light of what she knows to be right and wrong. So the psychopath does not fit part of, if any, of the criteria for (2), and thus cannot be considered a free moral agent.

The agency cultivation account of moral responsibility is, simply put, bound up in the very language of limitation that Szasz found so endemic of psychiatry. This account is also philosophically problematic because, if we consider adults with diminished capacities for detecting moral considerations and guiding behavior as broadly morally untrainable, and if we fail to cultivate moral agency in them due to our belief that they are morally untrainable, then we create a contradiction that deems them part of our moral community insofar as they participate in our normal social practices, while at the same time leaving them outside our moral community by not cultivating moral agency in them. We also eclipse the opportunity of their increased agency with the excuse of their presumed brain disorders.

16.4 **Bringing psychopaths into our moral community: objections and advances**

I consider two reasons why it is reasonable to keep psychopaths inside our moral community. First, I argue that they should be held morally accountable for their harmful deeds because their participation in our social structures makes their activities interdependent with those of other agents who operate with a basic expectation of noninterference or goodwill from others. We have to take more seriously the interdependence of social life when making judgments of blameworthiness and responsibility based on fairness, which requires evaluating fairness from the position(s) of the victim(s) and the community impacted by a psychopath's actions, not just the psychopath's psychic makeup. Second, I suggest that psychopaths might not be entirely morally untrainable—that it is actually our belief that they are so which reinforces our keeping them outside our moral community. To make this case, I look at two types of agents who take nonstandard routes to moral reasoning—highly functioning autistics (HFAs) and mildly mentally retarded individuals (MMRs)—and who we nonetheless consider to be inside our moral community (Shoemaker, 2007). I propose that there is a possibility for the moral engagement of psychopaths despite their deficiencies or inabilities to arrive at moral reasoning in the same way as normally-functioning adults are said to do—that is, by bottom–up affective means rather than top–down cognitive means. I support this proposal by suggesting ways that we can accommodate different modes of moral treatment and training.

Though this whole chapter speaks to the claim that psychopaths ought to be considered part of our moral community, earlier sections concern more the importance of holding psychopaths morally responsible for their deeds in our existing social practices, while the following sections address the possibility of the moral training of psychopaths as participants in our moral community.

16.5 **Is it unfair to hold psychopaths morally responsible?**

One could raise the objection that it is unfair to hold psychopaths morally responsible for harmful deeds because they lack one or several essential capacities for moral reasoning and moral agency. Being a moral agent on R. Jay Wallace's account (1994), for example, means possessing a form of normative competence: the ability to grasp and apply moral reasons, and to govern one's behavior by light of such reasons. Wallace holds that our judgments of moral responsibility depend on our social practices, and that these practices depend on the moral belief of fairness. It is fair, this account has it, to hold people responsible only if they possess the rational power of reflective self-control as indicated. To hold someone morally responsible is "essentially to be subject to a distinctive range of moral sentiments in one's interactions with the person" (Wallace, 1994, p. 8). Taking a narrower view than does Peter Strawson (1962), Wallace limits these moral sentiments or reactive attitudes to resentment, indignation, and guilt, all of which are caused by *beliefs* that an *expectation* to which we hold a person has been breached.

Because it is arguable whether or not psychopaths are moral agents on this account's terms, it is presumably unfair to hold them morally responsible in case they do not possess the rational power of reflective self-control (this being the ability to grasp and apply moral reasons, and to govern one's behavior by light of such reasons). Even if we attitudinally react to the actions of psychopaths, we are supposed to judge that it is unfair to be resentful or indignant toward them, since we cannot expect them to behave morally, and we therefore cannot hold them to moral obligations. Besides relying on an underinformed and static picture of psychopathy, the objection that Wallace's account raises also takes a one-sided view of fairness. Wallace fails to consider from whose point of view, other than that of psychopaths themselves, it is unfair to hold psychopaths morally responsible.

It is unfair to look at only what is fair for one of the involved parties to a wrong when making moral responsibility judgments. This is because the participation of psychopaths in our social world makes their actions interdependent with those of all others. This means that their actions have consequences that affect people other than the agents themselves, such as the direct victims of their deeds and even the community as a whole. We have to keep in mind that moral norms are there for the sake of the better functioning of our social world. As already members of social communities, Margaret Urban Walker claims that we are necessarily linked to others in relations of reciprocity and dependency. As such, "doing justice means not only to give what is due to an individual but to keep benefits and burdens in fair proportion among involved parties" (Walker, 2010, pp. 292–3). As Christopher Kutz (2000) discusses, in any socially realistic account of moral responsibility, there will be multiple stakeholders to a harm. In the same vein, Kutz argues that there is no single, uniquely determined or warranted response to wrongs, since these conditions are always relational and positional. They are relational in the sense that people who stand in different relations to each agent vary in their warranted responses. They are positional in the sense that the warranted accountability responses are functions of the perspectives and positions of those who respond to a harm.

According to Kutz (2000, Chapter 2), any agent who infringes upon the morally protected interests of others, in any way, is to be held morally accountable in some way. Not holding a psychopath morally responsible for a harmful deed may feel unfair from the position of the victim, and a victim's feeling that it is unfair reflects the further feeling that victims' interests are not being adequately considered in general. In this sense, benefits and burdens are not being considered in fair proportion among all the parties involved. The community has a mediating role to play in this respect. As Walker (2006) argues, it is the community's role to reinforce the victim's judgment of wrongfulness. The victim's resentment both expresses a sense of wrong and invites a kind of response, because it "calls out for *assurance of protection, defense, or membership* under norms brought into question by the exciting injury or affront" (Walker, 2006, pp. 133–4, original italics). Living in highly interdependent social structures with psychopaths requires them to be parties to the system, and the moral community needs to communicate that to individuals, even if it does not impose the same responses to accountability on psychopaths as it does on other moral agents. The community may also have its own distinct interests in holding psychopaths accountable, such as an interest in reiterating the normative order. One could even make the claim that we owe it to the agent himself, insofar as we recognize him as a human being, to address him morally. Peter French (2001), for example, argues that punishment (though I am not arguing in favor of any form of punishment here) is beneficial to wrongdoers as a recognition of their personhood and psyche, and as respect for their being better.

A psychopath's moral deficiencies will certainly determine in what way different respondents address him, but responding to and holding someone accountable in some way speaks to the fact that we recognize his agency in our community, and that it matters to us how he exercises it. In sum, we cannot decide whether it is fair to hold a psychopath morally responsible if we do not include, in our perspective, the positions of multiple stakeholders to a harm.

16.6 Is it pointless to hold psychopaths morally responsible?

Another objection to holding psychopaths morally responsible comes from Vargas's account itself, which insinuates that we can leave psychopaths beyond judgments of responsibility if we believe that they lack the necessary capacities to develop into moral agents. But Vargas has too unidimensional an understanding of both moral agency and the function of holding an agent morally responsible. On the surface, his account seems to be broadly encompassing: The cultivation of moral agency is pluralistic and is structured to varying degrees by our social and cultural structures. A problem arises, however, precisely if and because our communities believe that psychopaths lack the capacity to detect moral considerations or the ability to control their behavior in light of these circumstances, or both. As a consequence, we do not proceed to train them in morality. Vargas's account does not tell how we ought to respond to individuals, such as psychopaths, to whom we do not give the opportunity to cultivate moral agency. Therefore his account shows a dead-end method of engaging with someone whom we deem to be mentally disordered.

Szasz was adamantly critical of this type of approach throughout his career: we begin with a narrow internalist category of what it means to be psychopathic, dismiss this person as essentially amoral on this basis, and do not think about what it would mean to expand our existing understandings of moral training and responsibility in light of enhancing the agency of psychopaths along with that of other stakeholders to their harms. Using the language of excuses typical of theorizing mental disorders, Vargas objects that it would be pointless to blame and punish psychopaths if we do not believe them to be morally trainable, because in that case blame and punishment would not serve their functions of moral conditioning. Even if it is true that punishing psychopaths for harmful deeds will not make them better, the problem with this stance remains that the function of blame is limited to the construction of a limited view of individual agency and fails to capture its many other functions as they relate to other agents in the community and to the social order as a whole.

On Marion Smiley's pragmatic model of moral responsibility, in addition to conditioning people to behave differently in the future, blame also expresses disapproval at the breaking of expectations, and serves to regulate our relationships by reinforcing a moral social order (Smiley, 1992, Chapter 2). Perhaps the most important insight to take out of Smiley's work is that causal responsibility judgments and blameworthiness judgments are not distinct from the social and political practices already in place in our communities, which means that they serve whatever functions we put them to. It also means that they are constantly evolving as our social practices change, and that they are not exhausted by the facts to which they are geared at any given moment.

As our knowledge about the psychology of psychopaths increases, our assumptions about what kind of behavior we expect them to exhibit changes, and this in turn shapes how we should hold them accountable for certain harms. A better understanding of who they are and what we can expect from them might also help us to shift focus from blame and punishment for their deeds to specific modes of moral training that cater to their possible abilities to differently recognize moral considerations and govern their behavior accordingly—but not to feel wedded to just one picture of what moral agency looks like.

16.7 **Could psychopaths be moral agents?**

In keeping with Szasz, it is important to reiterate that although psychopaths may have problems in social and ethical living, they do have basic agential capacity: Though their agency departs from that of normally functioning adults in certain respects, they are not altogether devoid of it, nor are they devoid of all moral reasoning (Maibom, 2017, pp. 1114–17). Psychopaths are able to reason about what is right or wrong; the issue stems from the impairment of their ability to *follow through* with what they reason to be right or wrong. As Jana Borg (2008) confirms and Fox et al. describe: "Psychopathy does not impair the ability to understand that a particular act is classified as wrongful; rather, the deficits present in psychopaths impair their ability to understand the concept of moral wrong and *why* a particular act is wrongful" (Fox et al., 2013, p. 3). In other words, like ordinary agents, they appear to understand that some behaviors are not permitted, but do not appear to understand the unique character of a moral wrong (Fox et al., 2013, p. 20). This opens the possibility of the moral engagement and likelihood of moral training of psychopaths based on those capacities they do possess.

As we discover more about brain operations, we also understand more about the varieties of human development and behavior. Based on what we understand about individuals with psychopathic traits, there is a likelihood for them to employ successful moral reasoning without necessarily relying upon emotion. Borg is right to say, of course, that we should be careful not to separate terms like "reason," "emotion," "intellect," and "cognition" arbitrarily, because they are all interrelated to complex neural networks. For example, psychopaths tend to have high IQs, but, because the emotional system affects proper moral reasoning, we cannot say that psychopaths have sound cognition even though we can say they are intelligent (Borg, 2008, p. 162). If it is true that the rest of us rely on our emotive brain systems to make moral judgments (through bottom–up automatic processing), and that psychopaths cannot do this, it does not necessarily mean they cannot make moral judgments at all. Psychopaths may be likely to mediate their judgments through top–down deliberative processing, by relying on their cognitive brain systems to evaluate accessible and commonly articulated rules in their social environment. This means that the moral training of individuals with psychopathic tendencies is possible, but it will need to take a different route than that of normally functioning individuals, a lot of which depends on understanding their altered development and abilities, and importantly, on being willing to enhance rather than diminish or excuse their agency. From early in their lives, we can take advantage of the neuroplasticity of developing psychopaths, and early diagnosis of psychopathy might be important because it can improve the management of TCAs by those with whom they live.

To push that point, I invoke two examples David Shoemaker (2007) considers. He describes two types of individuals that reach moral reasoning by nonstandard routes and who we consider to be moral agents: HFAs and MMRs. HFAs display a nonstandard route to moral reasoning. They are not susceptible to the emotional appeal aspect of moral address but are nonetheless able to reach what Shoemaker calls "identifying empathy" (identifying with the position of another). An HFA is not able to directly pick up the emotional cues of another person but is nonetheless able to reach the relevant emotion through reason, by employing a second-person understanding of the position of the other. Victoria McGeer (2008) clarifies that, unlike psychopaths, who fail to make distinctions between moral and merely conventional rules, autistic individuals *do* make the moral-conventional distinction. However, concern for the well-being of others has very little if anything to do with shaping the moral responses of autistic individuals in relevant situations.

According to Shoemaker (2007), MMRs also display a nonstandard route to moral reasoning. They are able to pick up emotional cues from others and have the capacity for empathy, but they cannot on their own make the transition to "identifying empathy" because they cannot engage in reason-based moral exchange. Unlike HFAs, who are insusceptible to the emotional appeal aspect of moral address, MMRs are insusceptible to the reason-based aspect of moral address. Contrary to HFAs, who reach the moral emotion through second-person reason, MMRs reach moral reasoning through emotion and the mediation of a third party. This latter point accentuates the relational aspect of moral responsibility, where certain kinds of moral agents might need to rely on others to exercise their moral agency. Together, these examples are important in showing us that the conventional route to moral reasoning is not the only route, and point to the possibility that there may be (at least) one route by which psychopaths can reach moral reasoning and hence be recognized as moral agents within our moral communities.

The most challenging question to address regarding the moral training of psychopaths is that of motivation: What—if not affect—could motivate psychopaths to behave morally? In addition to their empathy deficiencies, McGeer reminds us that psychopaths have limited capacities for making affective investments in ends that transcend their immediate interests. But what is commonly known about many psychopaths is that they tend to be concerned with social position and social order. "There is something characteristically human . . . that explains the psychopath's quest for dominance in the social world," McGeer writes (2008, p. 254). Could *this* human characteristic be a motivating factor for their moral training? A psychopathic individual wants to be successful, for example. To reinforce this image or goal of herself, we (caretakers, loved ones, physicians, and importantly, our social systems as a whole) can conventionally tie norms of moral behavior to the achievement of success. This requires the promotion of prosocial traits like cooperation, as opposed to antisocial self-interest, as being intimately related to the achievement of success and social power. So, while empathetic care for others may not itself motivate moral behavior in the psychopath (even though it does in some subtypes of psychopaths), the goal of some type of social standing may. If the achievement of social power based on collaborative traits is socially (conventionally) reinforced, it could result in the instrumental uptake of moral behavior by psychopaths, despite their presumed lack of other-regarding sentiments.

In short, a plausible account of moral cultivation for psychopaths is to link the reinforcement of moral norms to something that moves them. However, keeping in mind the dynamic picture of our social practices, so long as our social structures promote standards of individualistic competition over those of cooperation, it seems implausible that psychopaths could be motivated to be moral in the method I described—but this is a topic for another time.

16.8 **Conclusion**

Szasz's work has brought attention to the importance of critique of the very disciplines through which we theorize. Here, I have taken up a critique of at least one philosophical account of moral responsibility in order to argue that at least one presumably incapable moral agent—the psychopath—can be held morally responsible. Making such an argument requires understanding symptoms of psychopathy as ethical problems pertaining to the right exercise of a person's agential powers. From this perspective, I have argued that it is both fair and worthwhile to hold psychopaths morally responsible. It is fair once we consider not only the diminished agency of psychopaths but also the perspectives of respondents to their harms and how their participation in our social structures makes them part of the moral communities coextensive with them. It is also advantageous to cultivate moral agency in psychopaths, as long as we are not narrow in our conception of moral agency and the shapes that moral training can take. Overall, the potential of the moral training and responsibility of psychopaths urges us to shift away from more internalist accounts of agency to externalist ones, since morality is, after all, something we do with a variety of others.

References

Blair, R.J.R. 1995. "A Cognitive Developmental Approach to Morality: Investigating the Psychopath." *Cognition* **57** (1) (October): 1–29.

Blair, R.J.R. 1997. "Moral Reasoning and the Child with Psychopathic Tendencies." *Personality and Individual Differences* **22** (5) (May): 731–9.

Borg, Jana Schaich. 2008. "Impaired Moral Reasoning in Psychopaths? Response to Kent Kiehl." In *Moral Psychology: Volume 3, The Neuroscience of Morality: Emotion, Brain Disorders, and Development*, edited by Walter Sinnott-Armstrong, pp. 159–64. Cambridge, Mass.: MIT Press.

Fox, Adam R., Trevor H. Kvaran, and Reid Griffith Fontaine. 2013. "Psychopathy and Culpability: How Responsible Is the Psychopath for Criminal Wrongdoing?" *Law and Social Inquiry* **38** (1) (Winter): 1–26.

French, Peter A. 2001. *The Virtues of Vengeance*. Lawrence: University Press of Kansas.

Hare, Robert D. 1999. *Without Conscience: The Disturbing World of Psychopaths Among Us*. New York: Guilford.

Hare, Robert D. 2011. *The Hare Psychopathy Checklist Revised (PCL-R): Technical Manual*, 2nd edn. North Tonowanda, New York: Multi-Health Systems.

Kutz, Christopher. 2000. *Complicity: Ethics and Law for a Collective Age*. Cambridge: Cambridge University Press.

Maibom, Heidi. 2017. "Psychopathy: Morally Incapacitated Persons." In *Handbook of the Philosophy of Medicine*, edited by Thomas Schramme and Steven Edwards, pp. 1109–29. Dordrecht: Springer.

McGeer, Victoria. 2008. "Varieties of Moral Agency: Lessons form Autism (and Psychopathy)." In *Moral Psychology: Volume 3, The Neuroscience of Morality: Emotion, Brain Disorders, and Development*, edited by Walter Sinnott-Armstrong, pp. 227–58. Cambridge, Mass.: MIT Press.

Oliveira-Souza, Ricardo de, Fátima Azavedo Ignácio, and Jorge Moll. 2008. "The Antisocials Amid Us." In *Moral Psychology: Volume 3, The Neuroscience of Morality: Emotion, Brain Disorders, and Development*, edited by Walter Sinnott-Armstrong, pp. 151–8. Cambridge, Mass.: MIT Press.

Shoemaker, David. 2007. "Moral Address, Moral Responsibility, and the Boundaries of the Moral Community." *Ethics* **118** (1) (October): 70–108.

Smiley, Marion. 1992. *Moral Responsibility and the Boundaries of Community*. Chicago: University of Chicago Press.

Strawson, Peter. 1962. "Freedom and Resentment." *Proceedings of the British Academy* **48**: 1–25.

Szasz, Thomas S. 1998. *Cruel Compassion: Psychiatric Control of Society's Unwanted*. Syracuse: Syracuse University Press.

Vargas, Manuel. 2013. *Building Better Beings: A Theory of Moral Responsibility*. Oxford: Oxford University Press.

Walker, Margaret Urban. 2006. *Moral Repair: Reconstructing Moral Relations after Wrongdoing*. Cambridge: Cambridge University Press.

Walker, Margaret Urban. 2010. "The Forum: Autonomy, Beneficence, and Justice in the Wider Context." *Ethics and Behavior* **12** (3): 279–80, 291–3.

Wallace, R. Jay. 1994. *Responsibility and the Moral Sentiments*. Cambridge, Mass.: Harvard University Press.

Chapter 17

Mental illness is not a myth: Epistemic favoritism in research funding

Mona Gupta

17.1 Introduction

I first encountered the work of Thomas Szasz during psychiatry residency training through his best-known and most polarizing book, *The Myth of Mental Illness*. In it, Szasz poses fundamental questions about the nature of psychiatric illness that every psychiatrist must eventually answer for herself, even if only implicitly.

Szasz embraced a biomedical model that affirms that diseases are the result of underlying pathophysiological processes. The physician's job, when confronted with a sick person, is to correctly identify that pathophysiological process (diagnosis) and then prescribe treatment based on the diagnosis. For Szasz, because the term "mental" has no referent in the body, mental illnesses cannot be pathologies of organs or tissues. Therefore, mental illnesses could not be diseases, because a disease has to be grounded in bodily pathophysiological processes. Instead, these forms of suffering must be problems that people experience in living. Offers of help for such problems, therefore, do not require medicines to treat bodily parts; rather, they require voluntary, confidential conversations between consenting adults (therapists and patients) to understand and resolve the problems.

Szasz's critique was conceptual, but as he himself pointed out, it had wider ethical implications. For example, the way in which we define mental illness (as a disease, a problem in living, or something else) determines what counts as an ethical response to those considered to be mentally ill. There may be times when a disease requires exceptional intervention, such as quarantine or even treatment against one's will in the cases of infectious disease. But Szasz maintained that in a democratic society, a person's self-identified problem in living cannot possibly be resolved through involuntary interventions imposed by the very people who are supposed to provide help.

Szasz's analysis has ethical implications for psychiatric research as well as for clinical practice. How we define mental illness affects what counts as legitimate academic inquiry; this, in turn, informs decisions about how to allocate limited research dollars. The psychiatric research enterprise has grown considerably over the last two generations and the quest to link the clinical manifestations of mental illnesses to underlying pathophysiological mechanisms has dominated the research agenda. By convincing funders that this is the central problem in psychiatry, this quest has also dominated the resources available to support research. Implicitly, funders and psychiatric researchers have embraced the challenge that Szasz's analysis poses to the field.

This preoccupation with demonstrating the verity and applicability of the disease model to mental illness has been accompanied by a relative lack of research interest in the nuts and bolts of clinical interactions. Psychiatrists do a great many things in practice for which there exists very little research. On what basis do we insist that residents learn and practice clinical case formulation? Is empathy really necessary for successful treatment? Does it matter that a psychiatrist pays attention to his or her own feelings in reaction to a patient? Although generations of authors and clinicians have asserted that these and other practices are important, even necessary, aspects of the delivery of good psychiatric care, in reality we know little about whether or not they are clinically valid practices. Paradoxically, Szasz's analysis may have pushed psychiatric researchers to prove him wrong at the expense of knowledge that might have enriched the kinds of care he actually valued. The fervent pursuit of a biological basis for mental illness means that relatively less attention has been focused on the quality and utility of those kinds of human interactions designed to help people endure their problems, and even thrive despite them.

In this chapter, I discuss the ethical impact of research funding policies on psychiatric knowledge. I contend that existing policies foster an unwarranted bias in favor of topics and methods appropriate to validating a disease model of mental illness. Because resources for research are limited, privileging certain lines of enquiry necessarily comes at the expense of others (Sadler and Foster, 2011, p. 33). This epistemic favoritism can itself have ethical implications. A given model of mental illness will point toward a certain understanding of people's problems as well as the types of solutions that are logically consistent with that model. Are these the best ways to understand those problems and the right solutions to them? Favoring certain topics or methods may be justifiable, but requires explicit evaluation.

The allocation of resources in research constitutes a problem of research ethics similar to allocation of resources within clinical practice. However, unlike clinical resource allocation, which is a robust subfield of bioethics (and economics and health policy), existing research ethics frameworks such as the influential Tri-Council Policy Statement (CIHR et al., 2014)—that is, of the Canadian Institutes of Health Research (CIHR), the Natural Sciences and Engineering Research Council (NSERC), and the Social Sciences and Humanities Research Council (SSHRC)—focus almost exclusively on downstream ethical issues relating to the conduct of research and do not concern themselves with upstream ethical issues related to the context and funding of research resource allocation. The fact that a researcher's career progress in the nonprivate sector is often dependent on securing research funding means that unchecked, epistemic biases can become self-sustaining. For example, researchers who wish to advance in their careers are unlikely to pursue areas of enquiry where funding is extremely limited. They will research and contribute to knowledge in areas where funding is available. Over time, a growing body of research in more readily funded topic areas can easily be mistaken to indicate that there is more to be discovered or known in that area. Thus, I argue that research funders, particularly when publicly supported, have an ethical obligation to evaluate the outcome of their funding allocations and, where appropriate, support epistemic diversity.

17.2 Psychiatric research in evolution

Over the last hundred years, medical research has led to a vast expansion in our knowledge about the human body, its diseases, and treatments. As a result, we believe firmly that medical research is the route to further knowledge, and further knowledge leads to better health. The twentieth century saw numerous discoveries, such as insulin and antibiotics, that dramatically influenced medicine's ability to intervene effectively for many patients with certain medical conditions. While psychiatry, too, saw certain developments such as the invention of electroconvulsive therapy (ECT) and the discovery of lithium, the therapeutic benefits were more limited and the side effects were considered to be more serious.

The publication of DSM-III in the 1980s heralded a new era in psychiatric research. Using its operationalized criteria sets, researchers had a more explicit basis to define patient populations for research studies. This fostered greater comparability between studies as well as larger sample sizes resulting from collaboration between many sites each using the same diagnostic criteria for recruitment. The contemporaneous arrival of fluoxetine on the market intensified interest amongst commercial funders in new pharmacological strategies for the treatment of many psychiatric conditions. Operationalized diagnostic criteria strengthened the application of the clinical trial method, needed to obtain regulatory approval to bring drugs to market. A key underlying assumption of this type of research concerns the locus of intervention. Pharmacological treatments target individuals; therefore, the responsibility to take them and endure their effects falls to individuals. However, this approach does not pass judgment on the cause of the problem; that is, the cause can be external to the person, even if the treatment falls to the individual.

Meanwhile, evolving imaging technologies over this same period, beginning with computerized tomography (CT), magnetic resonance imaging (MRI), and a host of functional imaging techniques—positron emission tomography (PET), single-photon emission computed tomography (SPECT), and functional MRI (fMRI), permitted more detailed understanding of brain structure and physiology. Such approaches were, and continue to be, applied to psychiatric disorders in hopes that specific pathologic findings may be linked to symptoms or disorders, thereby enabling improved diagnosis and opening avenues for effective treatment. Similar aspirations accompanied the evolution of techniques in molecular biology and genetics. The idea is that identification of faulty genes or genetic mechanisms would suggest proximate causes. In this strand of research, the key underlying assumption relates to pathophysiology: for a mental disorder to express itself, there must be some pathology within the individual that leads to the disorder. There may be upstream insults but these must lead to concrete changes in biological mechanisms (Grob, 1998).

Taken together, these trends over the last two generations demonstrate the growing conviction that mental disorders are best understood as defects within the bodies of individuals. The remainder of this section will present two examples of the power of this conviction to shape research and resultant knowledge about mental disorders. The first concerns the type of research about mental disorder funded by the major public funding agency in Canada, the CIHR. The second is the strategy for funding priorities proposed by the National Institute of Mental Health (NIMH), the major public research funder of psychiatric research in the United States.

17.2.1 Funding by the Canadian Institutes of Health Research

The CIHR was created in 2000, replacing the Medical Research Council of Canada. Its "mandate is to excel, according to internationally accepted standards of scientific excellence, in the creation of new knowledge and its translation into improved health for Canadians, more effective health services and products and a strengthened Canadian health care system" (CIHR, 2013). It allocates one billion Canadian dollars annually toward research at all levels, from students to senior investigators (CIHR, 2016). It is subdivided into thirteen virtual institutes whose role is to initiate and plan strategic priorities in research funding. Some institutes are disease- or system-based (e.g., Institute of Circulatory and Respiratory Health), while others have a transversal focus (e.g., Ageing).

The CIHR (2018) maintains a searchable database of its funded research projects. The current database includes applications that date back eight to ten years, and to funding announcements that go back no further than 2007. This database can be queried along various parameters: by research subject, investigator, location, program, institute/theme, or funding partner. Research concerning mental disorders transcends location, funding partners, and even the relevant virtual institute (Neuroscience, Mental Health, and Addiction); therefore, searching by research subject offers the possibility of identifying the broadest range of projects. One can search using terms from CIHR's list of keywords or one's own keywords, or both. Keywords include both topic areas and broad methodological approaches (e.g., qualitative methods, epidemiology).

There were three terms on the official list which could have identified projects relating to psychiatric disorders: "mental and behavioural disease," "mental disability," and "mental health." However, these turned out to be low-yield terms. "Mental and behavioural disease" yielded no results, while "mental disability" referred to a patient population with developmental delay or other intellectual disabilities. "Mental health" extended well beyond the scope of clinically relevant problems. I generated the search terms "psychiatric disorder," "psychiatric disease," and "mental disease," which also yielded no results. "Mental disorder" and "mental illness" were fruitful terms which generated extensive results relating to psychiatric disorders. I did not restrict my search by type of funding program; therefore, the results included operating grants, salary awards, student awards, etc. I then combined the terms "mental disorder" or "mental illness" with two official keywords that could point to studies involving alternative frameworks of understanding ("societal and cultural dimensions of health") or alternative methods ("qualitative methods").

There are two major mental disorders on the official keyword list: depression and schizophrenia. As psychiatric research is often conducted by disease category,

Table 17.1 The Canadian Institutes of Health Research (CIHR) funding, 2007–2016, of all programs (in Canadian dollars)

Search term combinations	"Societal and cultural dimension of health"	"Qualitative methods"
"Mental illness" OR "Mental disorder"	160,977,222 (578)	0	635,321 (5)
"Depression"	72,778,734 (327)	0	1,039,190 (10)
"Schizophrenia"	123,338,364 (368)	0	1,387,222 (1)

Figure in parentheses = number of successful applications

I searched these two diagnostic categories to see if this would be more likely to identify a broader range of topics or methods. "Depression" is a difficult search term because by itself it yields entities or phenomena that may be nonpsychiatric (e.g., "myocardial depression"); therefore, I combined "depression" with "mental health." Of these 327 results, only three were unrelated to depression as a mental disorder. I then restricted the search to "depression" and "societal and cultural dimensions of health" as well as "depression and qualitative methods." I did not need to combine "depression" with "mental health" in these cases, as there were so few allocations, I could quickly determine whether or not these were related to depression as a mental disorder. I repeated this same strategy with the search term "schizophrenia," which the search showed to be unambiguous. I then repeated the combination search strategies used for "depression."

Table 17.1 presents the results of these searches. Each individual cell provides the total funding allocation in Canadian dollars for the combination of search terms listed in the corresponding row and column. The numbers in parentheses indicate the number of successful applications that were funded by a given allocation. For example, the cell containing "635,321 (5)" means that C$635,321 were allocated to five successful applications concerning "mental illness" or "mental disorder" combined with "qualitative methods." The second column provides the figures for the search terms on the vertical axis alone—that is, not in combination with other terms.

An exercise of this nature is not without its flaws. For example, the official list of keywords is quite limited; thus, the number of projects related to mental illness, depression,[1] or schizophrenia, but that adopt approaches or methods that are nonbiological or quantitative, might be underestimated because these are categorized under investigator-generated keywords instead of those on the list. Furthermore, researchers in nonhealth science disciplines who work in areas of enquiry adopting alternative approaches or topics might be funded through other agencies. Nevertheless, we can make some preliminary observations. First, there is relatively little CIHR-funded research relating to mental illness, depression, or schizophrenia that focuses on societal or cultural aspects of illness or uses nonquantitative methods. It may be that few

---

[1] The results for depression reflect the search term "depression" combined with "mental health" because "depression" by itself yielded numerous results that were unrelated to the psychiatric sense of this word.

researchers approach these topics from alternate perspectives or it may reflect the self-reinforcing phenomenon already discussed: an orientation toward funding certain approaches encourages certain types of research and discourages others. Another way of looking at these results is to note that, as a society, Canadians have invested about C$125,000,000 in schizophrenia research and C$72,000,000 in depression research over the last ten years. Has this investment paid its dividend? Who is entitled to ask and answer this question, and according to what criteria should the answers be formulated?

17.2.2 **The Research Domain Criteria Project**

The National Institutes of Health (NIH) is an entity similar to the CIHR; indeed, the CIHR was modeled on the American structure of government-funded medical research. The NIH is part of the U.S. government's Department of Health and Human Services (DHHS). "NIH's mission is to seek fundamental knowledge about the nature and behavior of living systems and the application of that knowledge to enhance health, lengthen life, and reduce illness and disability" (NIH, 2017).

The NIMH is one of twenty thematic health research institutes, some of which concern disease categories (cancer) and some of which are transversal (child health). In 2009, the NIMH released its Research Domain Criteria (RDoC) Project. The rationale for this project was to foster research that was not constrained by DSM categories. This approach is in line with what some observers have suggested may be necessary—different classification schemes for different purposes. The DSM can be used in clinical practice but a different scheme for researchers, if the area of enquiry does not lend itself to DSM classification (Phillips et al., 2012).

The RDoC is a grid which divides mental life into five domains—negative valence systems, positive valence systems, cognitive systems, social processes, and arousal and regulatory systems—each of which can be further broken down into component constructs (e.g., negative valence systems include the constructs of fear, anxiety, sustained threat, loss, and frustrative nonreward). These five domains are expressed at eight different levels or units of analysis: genes, molecules, cells, circuits, physiology, behaviors, self-reports, and paradigms.

The NIMH has decided to shift a substantial portion of funding toward those projects which conform to the RDoC model. The overview of the September 2016 strategic plan states: "For the Institute to pursue its mission of transforming the understanding and treatment of mental illnesses most effectively, we request that all new and competing applications be targeted to the research priority areas within the four Objectives of the Strategic Plan" (NIMH, 2017a). Under Strategic Objective 1 is the following suggestion regarding applications for research funding: "NIMH encourages research that seeks to define the neural bases of complex behaviors and mental illnesses. . . . The Institute encourages applications that propose to advance scientific discovery through novel methods and approaches, interdisciplinary scientific collaborations, and integration of multi-dimensional data to discover the complex neurobiological architecture of the processes underlying normal brain function" (NIMH, 2017b). Table 17.2 summarizes the research strategies to be used in pursuit of fulfilling these objectives. The NIMH

Table 17.2 The National Institute of Mental Health (NIMH) strategic objectives (updated September 2016)

Strategic objective	Research strategy
1. Define the mechanisms of complex behaviors	1.1. Describe the molecules, cells, and neural circuits associated with complex behaviors
	1.2 Identify the genomic and non-genomic factors associated with mental illnesses
	1.3. Map the connectomes for mental illnesses
2. Chart mental illness trajectories to determine when, where, and how to intervene	2.1. Characterize the developmental trajectories of brain maturation and dimensions of behavior to understand the roots of mental illnesses across diverse populations
	2.2. Identify clinically useful biomarkers and behavioral indicators that predict change across the trajectory of illness
3. Strive for prevention and cures	3.1. Develop new treatments based on discoveries in genomics, neuroscience, and behavioral science
	3.2. Develop ways to tailor existing and new interventions to optimize outcomes
	3.3. Treat interventions for effectiveness in community practice settings
4. Strengthen the public health impact of NIMH-supported research	

(2017a) website shows a detailed list of the research priority areas within each research strategy.

Table 17.2 and the research priority areas outlined by the NIMH in its explanatory section on the RDoC orient research in a certain direction—that is, toward a biological understanding of mental illness.[2] To wit, "NIMH recognizes that manifest mental illnesses are likely the late signs of changes in brain circuits and disruptions in behavior and cognition that began years earlier" (NIMH, 2017c). Furthermore, the RDoC is structured by the assumption that the best way to understand mental illness is through biology and the best way to intervene is by acting upon the bodies of individuals. The NIMH's approach to research funding then serves to reinforce these beliefs.

The problem with this approach is that there are reasons to believe that at least some mental disorders are not merely disorders of individual bodies. At the very least, there is uncertainty about the extent to which external versus internal factors weigh more heavily in fostering the development of major depression in specific cases. This raises the ethical question of whether intervening at the level of individuals is the best or the right thing to do. For example, the development of major depressive disorder is

---

[2] I did not elaborate on the research strategies for Objective 4 as the NIMH strategic plan explains that Objective 4-related research will continue to be carried out under DSM categories.

influenced by a great many external factors, such as financial precariousness or the experience of trauma. Even if financial precariousness leads to major depression by ultimately modifying a bodily mechanism within an individual, it is both an ethical and political choice that the focus of intervention should be the individual rather than circumstances leading to financial precariousness.

But even knowing the pathophysiology of a disease does not commit one to a certain level of intervention, at least not from a macroallocation point of view. Smoking-related pulmonary disease provides a useful example: Though we may understand the causal relationship between cigarette smoking and specific patho-physiologic changes in lung tissue, we could decide that, in the overall health-care budget, relatively more resources ought to be invested in prevention and smoking cessation rather on treatment of pulmonary diseases once they arise. A policymaker would want to know which approach (individual treatment versus prevention) has a greater impact on the decline of smoking-related morbidity and mortality. The question must be asked to be answered; that is, it will be hard to answer this question if research funding targets only projects evaluating individual clinical treatments. A decision to prefer to fund studies of individual interventions sidesteps the question of whether community-level interventions would have a greater impact on specific types of problems.

To its credit, the NIMH explicitly acknowledges the need to evaluate its choice to favor RDoC-related research. In its strategic plan, updated in 2016, the NIMH wrote:

> What are the metrics of success? That is, how will NIMH know whether and when it has met its goals? While the discovery phase of science may not lend itself to timelines and milestones, being more strategic in our planning necessitates accountability. Our success cannot be measured solely by traditional academic 'outputs': the numbers of grants supported or papers published. Our success needs to be assessed by 'outcomes': how well the research we support changes our understanding of brain and behavior, improves our diagnostic system, provides effective treatments, supports prevention of mental disorders, eliminates the disparities in underserved populations, and reduces premature mortality among persons with mental illnesses. (Insel, 2016, original italics)

While this is an important step, these success criteria lack a commitment to a diversity of views. Knowing that a certain medication is more effective than a placebo or another type of biological intervention is useful, but it is also useful to know if it is more effective than a social intervention such as supported housing or an increase in disability support payments. Research that is designed to further the understanding of the brain and behavior will surely influence our understanding of brain and behavior, but this skirts the question of whether this understanding is what is needed to practice psychiatry and to do it well.

17.3 Patterns of funding, islands of ignorance

As previously demonstrated, public funding for research in mental illness heavily favors research of biological, explanatory models and individual-level interventions. Meanwhile, there are many aspects of ordinary psychiatric care and education whose justifications are not well-founded, fostering islands of ignorance. In this section, I discuss two examples that are part of everyday practice: clinical case formulation and psychiatric diagnostic evaluation.

17.3.1 Clinical case formulation

Clinical case formulation is considered to be a core competency in psychiatry (RCPSC, 2015). In Canada, it is not only a requirement that psychiatry training programs must teach this skill, but every candidate appearing for the specialty certification examinations must also be examined in it. In short, a great deal of time and resources are spent teaching, learning, and evaluating a psychiatrist's ability to formulate cases.

A formulation is a hypothesis which attempts to explain why a person, in light of the various factors to which she or he is subject (including biological, psychological, and social factors) experiences the problem for which she or he is seeking care. A formulation attempts to explain something about a person, not only about a diagnosis or a disease. According to Peter Sturmey (2009, p. 8), formulations can be told from individual theoretical perspectives, by attempting to integrate two or more of these, or by borrowing from diverse sources (eclectic approach). However, regardless of theoretical approach, formulations have common elements. They (1) abstract key features of the case; (2) should tie together the onset, development, and maintenance of the problem(s) and should link these ideas to the treatment that should grow out of and relate to the formulation; (3) are tentative and subject to modification in light of new information; and (4) should predict individually designed treatments that will be more effective than treatments that would otherwise have been implemented (Sturmey, 2009, p. 8).

This approach runs counter to that adopted by evidence-based medicine (EBM) and evidence-based psychiatry (EBP), in which clinical trial data, generated through study of populations of patients, are used to make treatment recommendations in individual cases. For example, if one looks at an instantiation of EBP in the form of treatment guidelines, such as the internationally recognized CANMAT (Canadian Network for Mood and Anxiety Treatment) guidelines, one finds decision-making algorithms based on clinical trial data. The guidelines for major depressive disorder match treatment recommendations with diagnostic categories or subcategories. Some consideration is given to demographic facts about patients, such as gender (e.g., women prefer psychological treatment) (Parikh et al., 2016, p. 527) and age (e.g., older age is associated with greater ECT-induced cognitive impairment) (Milev et al., 2016, p. 567). Contrary to Sturmey's claim, however, clinical case formulation is not a determinate of treatment recommendations in CANMAT, nor is it even mentioned as part of the decision-making process in proposing therapeutic interventions. The question thus arises: Why do residents need to learn to formulate cases, and why do we invest in teaching and doing this practice?

Tracey Eells concludes a recent volume (Sturmey, 2009) on clinical case formulation by observing: "In light of the central role attributed to case formulation, it is puzzling that research in the area has not been more extensive. Few authors of the case formulation chapters in the present volume cite research measuring the reliability or validity of their method" (Eells, 2009, p. 294). Given the factors influencing the funding of clinical research already discussed, this is perhaps not so puzzling after all. Who would support this type of research? There is genuine uncertainty about the explanatory or therapeutic value of this practice. Unless the profession undertakes the exercise of researching formulation, it may well be ignored (e.g., CANMAT) and eventually abandoned. The point here is not to defend clinical case formulation, but to illustrate that systemic epistemic biases of the type discussed here may make empirical justification impossible.

17.3.2 Do we need psychiatrists to make psychiatric diagnoses?

If a key aspect of evidence-based practice is to implement high-quality treatment guidelines by matching treatment recommendations to diagnoses, then it is of utmost importance that the diagnoses made in clinical practice be as similar as possible to those made in clinical research studies. Typically, studies make use of standardized diagnostic interview schedules to identify participants who fall into the diagnostic category relevant to a given study. It would seem, then, that patients in clinical practice ought to undergo similar procedures in order to ensure that when psychiatrists (or other clinicians) apply treatment recommendations derived from clinical trials, these patients resemble as closely as possible the trial participants and, thus, stand the greatest chance of benefitting from these recommendations. Average patients in clinical practice may not resemble clinical trial participants in general, but the use of the same diagnostic instruments will at least have the effect of removing clinician variability with respect to diagnosis from the equation.

The Structured Clinical Interview for DSM-V Disorders Clinician Version (SCID-5-CV, hereafter SCID) is a semi-structured interview guide for clinicians' use to make DSM-V diagnoses. This version allows clinicians to assess several disorders either in the present, over the course of the patient's lifetime, or both. These include mood disorders, psychotic disorders, substance use disorders, anxiety disorders, and trauma-related disorders, as well as ADHD. There are also screening questions for a number of other disorders. The SCID offers questions corresponding to each of the DSM criteria of each of the disorders it intends to review. Although the questions are often closed-ended or worded in such a way that the person can respond by saying "yes" or "no," the authors warn that the SCID should not be used in a checklist manner. Indeed, the authors of the SCID *User's Guide* specify that a positive answer to a SCID question about a criterion is not the equivalent of the criterion being met (First et al., 2016, p. 9). Positive (or negative) answers may require the patient to provide examples, or necessitate additional information from others. Furthermore, the *User's Guide* states that the rating of a criterion "ultimately depends on the clinicians making a clinical judgment as to whether or not a diagnostic criterion is met" (First et al., 2016, p. 9). The guide goes on to explain that clinicians may even state that a criterion is absent even if the patient endorses the symptom that lies behind the criterion (and vice versa). After having gone through the entire interview, which is estimated to take from forty-five to ninety minutes, clinicians have a score sheet that allows them to check off which diagnoses have been established during the interview.

The authors suggest that there is a gap between a patient's response to questions about the DSM criteria and knowing that the criteria are met, and that this gap is filled by clinical judgment. But apart from this assertion, no further explanation is provided as to what this entails. This is further complicated by the fact that the SCID can be used by trained nonclinicians to identify patients for research studies in which DSM diagnostic precision is necessary. Therefore, it is unclear what role clinical judgment or even clinical knowledge or skill are playing in the administration of this structured clinical interview. Certain questions arise as a result: What does psychiatric training contribute to the exercise of making a DSM diagnosis? If we compare psychiatrists working as usual and personnel trained in the use of the SCID on their diagnostic evaluations, who would conduct a more accurate evaluation (where accuracy is defined in DSM terms)? Are psychiatrists needed to fulfill this task, and if so, on what grounds?

Resource allocation is a necessary exercise in any health-care system where an insurer, private or public, is responsible to pay the bills for medical care. Ideally, this would be done rationally, where decisions to finance certain services and not others are based on the positive impact of these services on patient care. The SCID seems to suggest that there is genuine uncertainty about whether a psychiatrist is necessary to make a DSM diagnosis. Of course, there are questions about whether a DSM diagnosis is the desired outcome of an initial evaluation in psychiatry and whether there are other tasks that we believe are fulfilled by the psychiatrist. If so, these are not articulated by the authors of the SCID.

My purpose here is not to assert that psychiatrists play no valuable role in diagnostic evaluations or that they play an essential role, but merely to say that this is a researchable question which might provide valuable insights into what additional skill set psychiatrists and psychiatric training bring to these types of evaluations, as well as justify why health-care funding ought to be allocated to psychiatry evaluations. Furthermore, this type of knowledge strengthens training, by making more explicit what is being taught; and it enhances interprofessional collaboration by offering a clearer portrait of each professional's role. Similar to the problem of case formulation, securing funding for such an area of inquiry would be a difficult task in light of the highly limited funds to investigate these types of questions.

17.4 **Conclusions: in search of ethical resource allocation for psychiatric research**

Private research funders will support the types of projects that further their interests. This preference is to be expected (although there are legitimate political questions to be asked about the extent to which private funders have certain obligations to societies that educate their workers, provide financial assistance to facilitate commercial survival, etc.). But what are the interests of a public research funder? I contend that the public funder should serve the public interest. This includes support of legitimate diversity amongst theories, subject matter, and methods. This also includes a balance between what researchers believe to be priority areas and what other stakeholders—patients, families, clinicians—believe to be priority areas.

The process of funding research contributes to the way we understand mental illness: what proportion of the expression of mental illness can be accounted for by a problem in an individual's body versus a problem resulting from his or her social, cultural, or other circumstances? How does this knowledge affect our choices about the right ways to intervene? When we select certain programs of research over others, we are choosing certain ways of understanding and theorizing about these and related issues. While these choices are made on the basis of scientific excellence, through a process of peer review, one cannot ignore the social, cultural, and ethical dimensions that shape funders' ideas about what constitutes important research. To the extent that these dimensions lead to favoritism, and even systematic bias, in research funding, they ought to be considered in an explicit process of assessing fairness in research resource allocation. This process is particularly important for funders allocating public monies in the service of furthering knowledge to benefit, at least in part, the very people providing the financial support. Hitherto, such considerations have not been a dominant part of the landscape of research ethics, but there is no reason why this field must limit itself to the ethics of research conduct rather than the broader context in which research and research funding occur.

The psychiatric research community has spent two generations trying to prove that mental illnesses are underscored by specific pathophysiological processes. This has come at great expense, in monetary terms, and at great cost, in intellectual terms. Has this been worth it? The answer here depends on one's standpoint. Surely one legitimate standpoint is that psychiatry is not, or not merely, brain science, but the science of suffering persons. If this is the case, then public funders ought to adopt a wider epistemic and ethical scope than what underlies current approaches to allocating research funding. In other words, as Szasz himself explained over fifty years ago, the way we define mental illness will affect what we consider to be an ethical response to it.

References

Canadian Institutes of Health Research (CIHR). 2013. "Our Mandate." Accessed April 16, 2018. <www.cihr-irsc.gc.ca/e/7263.html>

Canadian Institutes of Health Research (CIHR), et al. 2014. *Tri-Council Policy Statement: Ethical Conduct for Research Involving Humans.* Accessed April 16, 2018. <www.pre.ethics.gc.ca/pdf/eng/tcps2-2014/TCPS_2_FINAL_Web.pdf>

Canadian Institutes of Health Research (CIHR). 2016. "Health Research for Canadians Infographic." Accessed April 16, 2018. <www.cihr-irsc.gc.ca/e/50217.html>

Canadian Institutes of Health Research (CIHR). 2018. "Funding Decisions Database." Accessed April 23, 2018. <webapps.cihr-irsc.gc.ca/cfdd/db_search?p_language=E>

Eells, Tracey D. 2009. "Contemporary Themes in Case Formulation." In *Clinical Case Formulation: Varieties of Approaches,* edited by Peter Sturmey, pp. 291–315.

First, Michael B., Janet B.W. Williams, et al. 2016. *User's Guide for the Structured Clinical Interview for DSM-5 Disorders: Clinician Version (SCID-5-CV).* Arlington, Virginia: American Psychiatric Association.

Grob, Gerald N. 1998. "Psychiatry's Holy Grail: The Search for the Mechanisms of Mental Diseases." *Bulletin of the History of Medicine* 72 (2) (Summer): 189–219.

Insel, Thomas R. 2016. "National Institute of Mental Health (NIMH) Strategic Plan for Research: Director's Message." Accessed April 16, 2018. <www.nimh.nih.gov/about/strategic-planning-reports/directors-message.shtml>

Milev, Roumen V., Peter Giacobbe, et al. 2016. "Canadian Network for Mood and Anxiety Treatments (CANMAT) 2016 Clinical Guidelines for the Management of Adults with Major Depressive Disorder: Section 4: Neurostimulation Treatments." *Canadian Journal of Psychiatry* **61** (9) (September): 561–75.

National Institute of Mental Health (NIMH). 2017a. "Strategic Research Priorities Overview." Accessed April 16, 2018. <www.nimh.nih.gov/about/strategic-planning-reports/strategic-research-priorities/index.shtml>

National Institute of Mental Health (NIMH). 2017b. "Research Priorities for Strategic Objective 1." Accessed April 16, 2018. <www.nimh.nih.gov/about/strategic-planning-reports/strategic-research-priorities/srp-objective-1/index.shtml>

National Institute of Mental Health (NIMH). 2017c. "Research Priorities for Strategic Objective 2." Accessed April 16, 2018. <www.nimh.nih.gov/about/strategic-planning-reports/strategic-research-priorities/srp-objective-2/index.shtml>

National Institutes of Health (NIH). 2017. "Mission and Goals." Accessed April 23, 2018. <www.nih.gov/about-nih/what-we-do/mission-goals>

Parikh, Sagar V., Lena C. Quilty, et al. 2016. "Canadian Network for Mood and Anxiety Treatments (CANMAT) 2016 Clinical Guidelines for the Management of Adults with Major Depressive Disorder: Section 2: Psychological Treatments." *Canadian Journal of Psychiatry* **61** (9) (September): 524–39.

Phillips, James, et al. 2012. "The Six Most Essential Questions in Psychiatric Diagnosis: A Pluralogue, Part 3: Issues of Utility and Alternative Approaches in Psychiatric Diagnosis." *Philosophy, Ethics, and Humanities in Medicine* **7**: 9. Accessed April 16, 2018. <www.peh-med.com/content/7/1/9>

Royal College of Physicians and Surgeons of Canada (RCPSC). 2015. *Objectives of Training in the Specialty of Psychiatry.* Accessed April 16, 2018. <www.royalcollege.ca/cs/groups/public/documents/document/mdaw/mdg4/%7Eedisp/088003.pdf>

Sadler, John Z., and Daniel W. Foster. 2011. "Psychiatric Molecular Genetics and the Ethics of Social Promises." *Journal of Bioethical Inquiry* **8** (1) (March): 27–34.

Sturmey, Peter (ed). 2009. *Clinical Case Formulation: Varieties of Approaches.* Chichester, U.K.: Wiley-Blackwell.

Chapter 18

Rights, responsibilities, and mental illnesses: A chronology of the Szasz decades

Jennifer Radden

18.1 Introduction

Thomas Szasz was a consistent champion of individual responsibility. A central part of his war with psychiatry, he explained, involves what he calls psychiatrists' "proclivity for coercive paternalism and *aversion to liberty and responsibility*" (Szasz, 2004b, p. 108, italics added). Prompted by that theme in his work, the subject of the present chapter is conceptions of responsibility in relation to mental illness, as reflected in cultural attitudes (i.e., one corner of the constellation of ideas that includes rights and liberties, freedom from coercion, autonomous agency, and human dignity). What follows is not history as such, but an account of a kind of social dialectic involving those attitudes. It is limited to ethical themes in, and growing out of, Szasz's writing rather than his more ontological claims—although some recent developments will be shown to have unmistakably ontological, and very Szaszian, implications. Regardless of any deeper aspects of the slogan, we can say that *if* mental illness is a myth, then ethical consequences ensue—and attention here is on some of the changing conceptions of, and norms governing, individual responsibility during the Szasz decades.

The demands, and meaning, of this individual responsibility expand, and alter, during the second half of the twentieth century. Some of these changes stem from ideas Szasz employs throughout his writing while others have arguably grown out of, and beyond, them. These developments can be loosely identified by decade: first, the stress on mental patients' rights during the 1970s; second, the application of identity politics to mental disability during the 1980s and 1990s; third, the emergence of self-help approaches through recovery, rehabilitation, and other political movements arising in the 1990s and 2000s; and finally, from the 2000s to the present, the trend toward public mental health, and primary prevention, associated with the demands and assumptions of global mental health policies. The claim here is not that Szasz's own developments follow this chronology very closely, but that broader cultural ideas do. Nor is the aim to offer anything approaching a full explanation, cultural or psychological, of this sequence.

Tracing the history of individual responsibility in this manner is also a way of reviewing my own intellectual trajectory during these years. All researchers and theorists within the philosophy of psychiatry and mental health were inescapably affected by these ideas—originally formulated by Szasz, and later challenged, supported, elaborated, and developed by others (see Schaler, 2004; Schramme and Edwards, 2017). This is no less true, as we will see, of those more immediately affected by such ideas, within communities of "survivors," "consumers," and "service users," and patients.

This chapter is organized around the aforementioned variations and developments. The loose chronology of each elaboration on Szasz's theme of personal responsibility is described in Section 18.2, including some of the limitations of these ways of reading such responsibility; while Section 18.3 explores how such changes can be seen to eventually return us to ontology, their models mirroring Szasz's once seemingly incendiary idea that mental disorders are not helpfully distinguished from other problems encountered in everyday life.

18.2 Chronology of changing responsibility conceptions

18.2.1 Mental patients, civil rights, and Millian liberalism

The broadly liberal political philosophy that runs through Szasz's writing requires little introduction. Although associated with philosophical assumptions about free will, it is equally compatible with soft determinist assumptions depicting human agency as a distinct category of determined events. Szasz explicitly identifies his liberalism with that of the U.S. Constitution, as well as the work of John Stuart Mill, emphasizing a range of broadly "civil" rights or liberties.

For example, the right to trial includes being held responsible for wrongdoing, and because the protection provided the mentally ill defendent through the insanity defense foregoes that right, Szasz has consistently and resoundingly rejected the insanity defense. Similarly, in his abhorrence of all involuntary treatment, Szasz appeals to the civil right of any adult to be free from restraint unless guilty (or suspected, with probable cause), of wrongdoing. Honoring the ability to bind oneself through advance planning lies at the heart of liberalism; so Szasz's support for Ulysses contracts or "psychiatric wills" (Szasz, 1965, 1982) involves a kind of autonomy right. The liberties identified here are united by their status as what are sometimes called noninterference rights. (That language can only be employed if we point out that many of Szasz's critics, and much analysis in political philosophy, deny any simple equation between leaving individuals free from interference and affording them autonomy. Relational accounts of autonomy take issue with the conception of individuality underlying such equations; for example, they aim to replace the paucity of traditional liberal or libertarian conceptions with more positive analyses of freedom that point to interventions, relationships, and forms of scaffolding that are compatible with, and might be required for, a true exercise of autonomy (Mackenzie and Stoljar, 2000; Christman, 2015). This is not the place for a full recounting of these and like deficiencies in Szasz's liberalism, however.)

The response to mental patients' rights rhetoric includes some that is negative and vehement: "Rotting with their rights on" (Gutheil, 1980; Gutheil and Appelbaum, 1980) was the egregious consequence of according patients such rights, in Thomas Gutheil's phrase. Liberal principles have also been invoked when treatment is deemed to "liberate the patient from the chains of illness" (Gutheil, 1980, p. 327) or justified because it *restores* autonomy, in the manner of so-called "autonomy-enhancing interventions" that are supposed to bolster, support, or return autonomy, bearing analogies to other forms of scaffolding that help people achieve their goals. *If* enforced treatment is appropriately so construed, then it can be recognized as consistent with the liberal goal of achieving and enhancing autonomy, it is widely held (Griffiths and West, 2015).

Those who seek to restore autonomy in this way point to disorders that render people temporarily incapable of exercising their rights. The liberal model of the responsible, rights-bearing agent includes decision-making capabilities seemingly compromised by disorder. Moreover, some severe symptoms (of depression or catatonia, for example) apparently disable all agency, leaving their subjects temporarily incapable of autonomous response. Attitudes challenging Szasz's stance, such as these, also appeal to the careful qualifications tempering the liberal position expressed by theorists like Mill in *On Liberty*, although Mill's wording there on these points, (restricting the harm principle to those "in the maturity of their faculties" [Mill, 1859, p. 22] and not "in some state of excitement or absorption incompatible with the full use of the reflective faculty" [Mill, 1859, p. 173]), is notoriously ambiguous in its application to the effects of mental disorder (Powers et al., 2012).

Although primarily conducted in philosophical and legal settings, and within nonclinical contexts, these disagreements have continued unabated since the 1970s. But the 1970s also brought changes in public attitudes and law surrounding some of these civil rights, attributable both to the civil rights movement and, in no small part, to the influence of Szasz's and allied writing. Societal recognition of the right to refuse treatment dates to this era, for example—as do the consequent deinstitutionalization policies that so affected the lives of mental patients worldwide. In addition to these rights, a liberal or libertarian position seems to suggest that there is a right to harm oneself, as Szasz insists. For the most part, however, this last right remained unrecognized during the second half of the twentieth century, as Paul Appelbaum (1997) documented in what he construed as a failed libertarian revolution. Supported by the individuals' perceived status as "in need of treatment" and/or a "danger to themselves," most civil commitment legislation justified intervention when there was serious risk of self-harm, using language that parallels that for harm to others (Appelbaum, 1997). Such broadly paternalistic positions continue to govern potential self-harm in civil commitment statutes today throughout the U.S. and Western Europe.

For all adults, including those diagnosed with mental disorder, Szasz consistently endorses each civil right introduced here (trial rights, treatment rights, autonomy rights, and self-harm rights), his support allied with his conception of individual responsibility, when that responsibility involves being fit subjects of praise and blame.

All adults possess and ought to be accorded these rights—we might summarize his position—and should thus be held individually responsible for their decisions and actions, as well as the foreseeable consequences of those decisions and actions. Because all symptoms arise from actions and decisions made by a person, the reasoning goes, their author is fully responsible for them. Even psychotic symptoms, on this analysis, are described in such a way as to suggest voluntary agency. Hallucinations are "disowned self conversations," while delusions are "stubborn errors or lies. Both are *created by* 'patients,' and *could be stopped by them*" (Szasz, 2004a, p. 324, italics added). We will return to this reasoning. Unarguably, his stance is consistent and principled, and Szasz remains the best-known spokesperson for the mental patients' rights ideology of the 1970s. But, as so many of his critics have pointed out, this attitude about responsibility seems implausible, ignoring important moral differences, qualifications, and exceptions.

In some reasoning, individual responsibility is foundational, neither possessing, nor requiring, further theoretical support. Szasz describes the principle of personal responsibility as "*the ground on which* all free political institutions rest" (Szasz, 1974, p. 262, italics added). This order is reversed in his more natural law-based reasoning, however, where individual responsibility is *derived from* natural rights, rather than the reverse. Because we are possessors of rights, we are appropriately held responsible for our actions and decisions.[1]

In subsequent developments, and within the broader culture, Szasz's ideas are expanded and amended. From the 1970s onwards, not only are there additions to the particular rights and the particular kind of rights attributed to those with disorder, but also, individuals' status vis-à-vis those rights seems to alter. To the extent that their humanity, human dignity, or personhood ensure the status of the mentally ill as rights bearers in these early accounts, they are *status-based* rights in the sense of being not earned, but owed. Initially, within the rhetoric and theorizing associated with them, by Szasz and others, there is no reference to any *particular* exercise or exercises of

---

[1] When the category of individual responsibility plays the part of grounding political principle, it is argued that, because we possess the attribute of moral (and legal) responsibility, we are judged fit subjects of praise and blame, appropriately treated as recipients of reactive attitudes, and granted the status of rights bearers. Attributions such as these stem from an *aretaic perspective*, about which, independent of moral accountability, blaming and praising judgments stand as "attributability conditions" serving to ground "certain appraisals of the individual as an agent" (Watson, 2004, p. 266). On the moral theory of reactive attitudes associated with Peter Strawson, responsibility is *constituted* by the attitudes which we think appropriate to adopt toward other agents and ourselves, such as reproach, praise, gratitude, and resentment (Strawson, 2003). Whereas traditional accounts of responsibility have taken these kinds of reactive attitude as a consequence, engendered by seeing others as responsible, Strawson's idea is that to regard oneself or another person as responsible is nothing more than the proneness to react to them in these kinds of ways under certain circumstances; there is no more fundamental matter justifying or grounding these responses. In this sense, the practice does not rest on a theory at all, but rather on "certain needs and aversions that are basic to our conception of being human" (Watson, 2004, p. 220). If we, or others, are not appropriate subjects for those attitudes, then responsibility cannot rightly be attributed.

agency. Such rights are our human due. Later, without losing that sense of rights and liberties as our human due, conceptions of individual responsibility also come to attach to more active features as well.

18.2.2 **Identity politics and recognition rights**

In response to the failure of the community which psychiatry assigned to replace the asylum system, political interest groups have arisen since deinstitutionalization (Anthony, 1993; Sayce, 2000). Sharing concerns and vulnerabilities that in some way distinguish them from the broader population, the members of these groups have formed together not only for social support, but also for the added power of collective action. Modeled on other consumer and liberation groups and political interest communities, mental health political movements emerged through the 1980s, expanding the meaning and scope of individual responsibility for their members.

The identity politics slogan, "Nothing about us without us!" is a revealing example of how individual responsibility becomes implicated in new and different ways. Its focus is on collective action: participating in group efforts to exert or achieve rights, where each individual becomes part of a collective rights-bearing body, and where these rights are attributed to groups of individuals based on some commonality (a trait or identity). The rights sought are also expanded. In addition to the basic civil or noninterference rights of the traditional kind, they involve identity (i.e., they are rights of "recognition") as it has been theorized. Prominent identity and recognition politics theorists include Jürgen Habermas, Axel Honneth, Nancy Fraser, and Mohammed Rashed. Beyond the familiar "redistributive" rights associated with economic justice, recognition rights call for just and equitable cultural patterns of representation, communication, and interpretation, which are required to redress systematic and damaging misrepresentation (Fraser and Honneth, 2003, p. 15). The misrepresentation of people with psychiatric diagnoses also comes to be seen as leaving them, along with other disadvantaged groups, as victims of what has been described as epistemic injustice. That is, they are unfairly deprived of the authority that allows their words to be respected as meaningful and credible (Fricker, 2007). If there is a right to recognition that would expunge these several kinds of injustice (representation, communication, interpretation, semantic authority, and credibility), then those so deprived possess a collective interest in the manner in which their experiences and lives are represented (Radden, 2012; Rashed, 2019).

In one respect, the goal for which recognition rights makes this consumer group collectively responsible had been anticipated by Szasz's call for the dismissal of "mental illness" as a myth. As he saw, beliefs, metaphors, assumptions, and presuppositions affecting patterns of representation, communication, and interpretation about alleged mental illness are bound up with broader cultural norms, values, and power arrangements. The position of epistemic disadvantage from which the central participants here suffer adds to the collective challenge of being heard and accepted as credible knowers.

A new, self-generated effort on the model of other liberation movements now emerges, calling for group member *participation* (Freire, 1997). For the symbolic redefinition of their collective identity, consumers can achieve justice only through active, personal participation. Since the 1980s, such efforts have taken many forms, including powerful first-person accounts and memoirs (Barker et al., 1999; Read and Reynolds, 1996; Hornstein, 2002; Radden and Varga, 2013). Also, there has been renaming, with a range of self-identifications including "survivor," "consumer," "service user," "mentally disabled," "mad," "neuro-atypical," and the like. In light of historically entrenched and pervasive stigma and discrimination associated with mental disorder, however, and the previous voicelessness of its sufferers in public discourse, a mere name change—even if necessary—is insufficient. Also required, it has been recognized, is reconceptualizing aspects of mental ill health, and an extensive re-envisioning of concepts of mental health, illness, sanity, madness, rationality, and competence. Besides surmounting these obstacles, as Szasz recognized, this project involves negotiation over the controversial ideas and contrary perspectives associated with some forms of disorder, such as the freighted category of insight into illness (Radden, 2010).

These more far-reaching political goals involve what I have elsewhere called *reconstructive cultural semantics*: a revision of general ideas, which consumers undertake as central, privileged participants (Radden, 2012). While not an individual obligation, the particular task of cultural reconstruction is a distinctive responsibility, assigned to those positioned as both *uniquely affected and interested*, and *uniquely informed*, from past personal experiences. Szasz always emphasized the extent to which those with power and authority in society control these meanings, dictating what is said and can be understood.

But as well as concepts of individual responsibility, expectations and norms are also enlarging during the last decades of the twentieth century, so that they encompass collective political action of many kinds. The germ of this enlargement of individual responsibility can be found in Szasz's earliest remarks, whatever he may have thought of these developments. As a historical point, however, this enlargement takes on new momentum only after more fundamental civil rights for the mentally ill have come to be protected through legislative action, case law, and custom.

18.2.3 Self-help and self-care

To assert that mental illness is a myth, Szasz takes pains to point out, is not to deny that personal unhappiness and socially deviant behavior exist. Rather: "We have no enemy that we can fight, exorcise, or dispel by 'cure.' What we do have are problems in living—whether these be biologic, economic, political, or sociopsychological" (Szasz, 1970, p. 24). Life is difficult, and problems in living require a response. But rather than employing the spurious remedies and dangerously paternalistic principles offered by psychiatry, on his view, we should address these mistakenly labeled "mental health" problems as we do any other problems we confront—with courage, honesty, ingenuity, and resolve. Individually as well as collectively, we can best each help ourselves.

The decades that follow see increased emphasis on self-help measures: things we can and should do to protect, restore, strengthen, and preserve our mental health in the face of life's inevitable setbacks and disappointments. Thus, added to the collective responsibility for cultural reconstruction, these mental illness-related political interest groups proceed on individual as well as collective fronts, consistently emphasizing autonomy and responsibility *as an individual goal* for their members. Individual responsibility is integrated within the rhetoric and principles of the recovery movement, where the aim of the recovery model is said to be "to have consumers assume more and more responsibility *for themselves*" (Jacobson and Greenley, 2001, p. 483, italics added). Particular responsibilities cited include developing goals, working with providers and others to make plans for reaching these goals, taking on decision-making tasks, and engaging in self-care. In addition, responsibility is stressed as a factor in making choices and taking risks: "full empowerment requires that consumers live with the consequences of their choices" (Jacobson and Greenley 2001, p. 483). More thorough analyses of the notion of recovery are available (Davidson et al., 2005; Pouncey and Lukens, 2010). Recovery from mental illness involves much more than recovery from the illness itself, it has been stressed, bringing additional challenges and the allied responsibilities that they entail. "People with mental illness may have to recover from the stigma they have incorporated into their very being; from the iatrogenic effects of treatment settings; from *lack of recent opportunities for self-determination*; from the negative side effects of unemployment; and from crushed dreams . . . Recovery is what people with disabilities *do*" (Anthony, 1993, p. 15, italics added).

A range of interests and agendas form these movements, and they reflect differing models of disorder. (The individual growth model and the disability inclusion model are distinguishable, for example [Sayce (2000)]. But as notable as the contrasts are, there are overlaps and commonalities; and these include a consistent emphasis on individual responsibility. Reliance on responsibility and agency associated with the recovery movement are similarly infused with stress on rehabilitation over treatment, for example. Emerging during the same era, the purpose of these rehabilitation models was "to overcome disabilities that are barriers toward *realizing one's own wishes and aspirations*," and the "role of all participants" became to "identify goals and work toward them" (Spaulding et al., 2003, p. 17, italics added). The psychiatric rehabilitation model, it has been noted, stresses treating the consequences of the illness rather than just the illness as such, thus bringing further emphasis on individual agency and *self-help*: "*Recovery can occur without professional intervention*. Professionals do not hold the key to recovery; consumers do" (Anthony, 1993, p. 18, original italics). The very shift from the language of "patient" to "consumer" is emblematic here. The consumer (or "service user") is an autonomous partner capable of contracting services, and *responsible for her or his mental health care*.

Many other therapeutic endeavors have also come to emphasize one form or another of self-help. We find it in various twelve-step programs (e.g., Emotions Anonymous, founded in 1971) that proliferated during the era. Thus, although it begins with the admission that one is powerless over alcohol, and that one's life has become unmanageable, the original credo of the Alcoholics Anonymous twelve-step program embodies a call to action: Step 3: Decide to change; Step 4: "Make a searching and fearless moral inventory of ourselves"; Step 9: Make amends to those we have harmed. And also suggesting agency, GROW allows that people become mentally ill through "learned habits of false thinking and disorganised living" (Sayce, 2000, p. 112).

The extent to which these groups' attitudes around individual responsibility trace directly to Szasz's writing may be difficult to ascertain. But at least it seems fair to say that these cultural trends emphasizing individual responsibility as self-help move the culture toward the position which Szasz staked out with his liberal claim that human dignity and freedom demand that we be held responsible for our mental health.

Importantly, self-help also comes to the fore, toward the end of the twentieth century, when forms of cognitive behavioral therapy (CBT) emerge as the primary alternative to psychopharmacological treatments for psychiatric ills. Emphasizing developing strategies by which the individual can deal with dysfunctional thoughts and unwanted feelings, these approaches make the person *responsible for bringing about change*. This turn toward self-help is a return of sorts, although to premodern times. Stoic philosophy exhibits the same combination of cognitive therapy, self-help, and attention to aberrant mood states. But in the modern era, taking responsibility for one's mental health acquires uniquely new vigor and meaning when consumers' groups and cognitive therapeutic techniques are combined.

This trend has not prevailed unchallenged, of course. Self-help imperatives have emerged alongside quite contrary ideas emanating from an increasingly entrenched biological, neo-Kraepelinean diagnostic psychiatry focused on the DSMs. The very existence of responsibility as a moral and metaphysical category has also been challenged during this era (Eagleman, 2011). It can be assumed here, however, since it is by Szasz. These contrary ideas serve to highlight the passivity of the person receiving care. In an effort to reduce self-blame for disorder, biological psychiatry often depicts the sufferer as a blameless victim of brain disease or genetic risk. Due precisely to the totalized passivity that this model implies, it has been resisted as a simplistic and harmful misrepresentation, by theorists, consumers, and patients themselves. The brain disease model of disorder can be credited with bringing "the welcome relief of removing responsibility for the 'illness'", it has been observed, but at the cost of "the terrible drawback of *removing responsibility for everything else*" as well (Sayce, 2000, p. 115, italics added). Even within the setting where biological psychiatry assigns a more passive role to the patient, and prescribes psychopharmacological treatment, the patient is usually, and in varying degrees according to her or his particular circumstances, assigned some responsibility for compliance with the treatment regime. Also, differences between passivity and more assertive responses reflect relative severity as much as ideology—the nature and course of the disorder. While stricken with catatonia, the patient may be entirely passive; but the same patient emerging from successful treatment, or one with different symptoms, will be relatively engaged and active. Nonetheless, biological psychiatry pays less attention to individual responsibility, and accords less of it, than we find in the rhetoric of these political interest groups.

The persistence of such traditional thinking, some hypothesize, lies with the broader economic systems making up today's "Mental Health Medical Industrial Complex (MHMIC)" (Sadler, 2013; Whitaker, 2010). (Contrasting active and engaged mental health treatments with the more passive psychopharmacological interventions associated with traditional psychiatry, John Sadler explains that "active/engaged treatment modalities generally have no lobby, no corporate investment, no potential for profit-generation, no campaign-finance contributions, or other mechanisms to breach the fence of the MHMIC. Moreover, they are generally more expensive than passive, product-based therapies, and therefore have few to no 'friends' among the DSM constituencies with their pharma industry support" (Sadler, 2013, p. 30).)

Emphasis on individual responsibility for self-care finds support from another direction as well. Added to the treatment models of clinical medicine and psychology, the first decades of the twenty-first century have seen an expansion toward a conception of prevention focused not on the treatment of mental illness, but on its *elimination*—and not only on *individual responsibility* for self-care, but also on seeking, promoting and maintaining *mental health* (Muñoz, 2001). Arguably, the political interest groups and unorthodox treatments described here reached these same attitudes and emphases well before the present era, and we today merely witness their increasing recognition within formal medical settings. Nonetheless, that recognition is significant. It seems to mark a profound shift (affecting institutions, rhetoric, and resources) towards an emphasis long absent in Western cultures. Care of the soul (psyche) is familiar from ancient traditions, but has been eclipsed within modern medicine. This new professional focus holds special interest, in addition, since it derives from a less theoretical, and more observational, source.

18.2.4 **Public mental health**

Documents such as the *Comprehensive Mental Health Action Plan 2013–2020* advocate *prevention in addition to treatment*, and the use of public health measures and models (WHO, 2001, 2012, 2013; Saxena et al., 2006). For better or worse, this is a data-driven change. Arguably, to ascertain its message for policy, we must dig beneath the face value of these data to their underlying conceptions of health and ill health (Vilhelmsson et al., 2011). But that is not my goal here.

In recent years, increasing attention has been paid to the extent and costs of mental disability. The dependence of physical on mental health has also been emphasized, and the applicability of universal health-care rights to mental and behavioral disorders recognized (Saxena et al., 2014; WHO, 2008; Prince et al., 2007). Not only do policy imperatives include increasing awareness of such disorders, together with their appropriate diagnosis and care, they also envision the more ambitious goal of eliminating such disorders altogether through early prevention (WHO, 2001, 2012, 2013; Patel and Saxena, 2014; Patel et al., 2013; Saxena et al., 2014; Kohn et al., 2004; O'Connell et al., 2009; Merry et al., 2011; Radden, 2016). In the 1990s, projections drew widespread attention to the magnitude of depression in particular, as a serious and growing public health problem, by measuring and predicting the cost of untreated depression in terms of mortality and morbidity (Murray and Lopez, 1997). (*The Global Burden of Disease* (WHO, 2008) predictions that depressive disorder would rise to second among the causes of disability were confirmed for developed countries by 2002, by which time it ranked first in developing countries.) With recognition that these data reflect global health problems well beyond the scope of Western-style, individually-based treatment and care, comes the application of the population-wide preventive strategies of public health. These policy efforts speak of establishing "herd immunity" through universal inoculation, as they identify and implement preventive pedagogies for mood and be-havioral disorders such as depression and suicide, and early identification, monitoring, and treatment for psychotic disorder.

The prevention applicable here is often the kind known as *primary* prevention (Saxena et al., 2006). It is also, although not exclusively, *universal*, in targeting whole populations, or other groups, not identified on the basis of increased risk. By con-trast, *secondary* prevention seeks to lower the rate of established disorder; *selective* prevention targets individuals or subgroups whose risk of developing a mental dis-order is significantly higher than average; and *indicated* prevention targets high-risk individuals who have been identified as having minimal, but detectable, signs or symptoms foreshadowing mental disorder or biological markers indicating predispo-sition for it, but who do not meet criteria for disorder (Saxena et al., 2006). Each of these approaches to prevention has been the basis for research initiatives and mental health policies (Durlak et al., 2011).

Among the different forms of primary prevention, new pedagogies involving "neuroprotective" cognitive and behavioral skills, and laying emphasis on building re-silience in the young to prevent later mood disorder, best demonstrate the emphasis on self-help and self-care that increases the responsibility accorded to individual sufferers. Primary prevention for psychotic disorder, by contrast, is sought through early screening, monitoring, and treatment with antipsychotic medications—an in-tervention leaving little room for individual responsibility beyond that required for following a psychopharmacological regimen (McGorry, 2015). One example of the application of these sorts of preventive principles to policy is found in Australia's "beyondblue" (Irwin et al., 2010) and Black Dog (2017) programs, launched early in the 2000s and designed to target mood disorders. The Black Dog Institute differs in several respects from beyondblue, but shares its emphasis on preventive meas-ures undertaken within educational settings. As well as promoting early intervention strategies, initiatives are focused around raising awareness and reducing the stigma of depression, supporting consumer and caregiver advocacy, facilitating training for caregivers, and funding strategic and applied research related to mood disorders.

Based on tenets of CBT, these preventive pedagogies associate depression with maladaptive beliefs and cognitive processing styles (i.e., thought patterns that are unwarrantedly global, absolute, and past-oriented, particularly, and beliefs that are inappropriately self-critical). For example, one style of learning emphasizes posi-tive psychosocial adaptation, "depression literacy," self-awareness, and training in self-talk to expunge overly negative cognitive attitudes. Students are taught to recog-nize negative and unhelpful commentary (in others and in themselves as self-talk), identifying cognitive errors such as all-or-nothing thinking, overgeneralization, "mind reading" beyond the evidence, exaggeration in the form of either magnifi-cation or minimization, and "catastrophizing" (Irwin et al., 2010). With frequent reference to aid from digital technologies, emphasis is placed on interventions of "self-management" (Proudfoot, 2013)—a form of self-awareness, monitoring, and critically evaluating one's thoughts—and in that way *taking responsibility* for the feelings that they affect. As another example, several modules of the Black Dog

Institute under the heading, "Getting Help," guide users through educational and therapeutic links to self-talk, self-help, self-tests, resilience, and strategies that can help them become "the gatekeeper of [their] thoughts" (Black Dog Institute 2013b, www.blackdog.org.au).

With increasing focus now on maintaining mental health and *preventing* mental illness in order to avoid having to *treat* it later, a new round of individual responsibilities is thus emerging. We must inform ourselves of the dangers, and adhere to preventive strategies for acquiring resilience through neuroprotective cognitive habits. No longer merely behavioral goals around diet, exercise, and life-style, these strategies address the voluntary control we exercise over cognition—our thoughts and, through those (albeit indirectly), our feelings. Rather than passive patients who have succumbed to disease, we are increasingly seen as self-helpers, proactively and responsibly nurturing and protecting our mental health. In taking responsibility for our health, those of us with disorders are Szaszian autonomous agents, on this analysis, appropriately in charge of regulating our own thoughts, moods, decisions, and actions. Instead of states that assail us, against which we are powerless, our symptoms are aspects of the selves we actively construct, are responsible for, and must tend, in the manner of the classical care of the soul. The techniques and tools are each available. As a treatment modality, CBT has enabled these changes in our era for everyone, its techniques being suitable for achieving the far-reaching goal of primary prevention. Cognitivist theories of emotion and practices that affect regulation employed by CBT are, of course, much older, tracing to Stoic philosophy (Ussher, 2014). Digital technology is increasingly seen as providing ready tools for new forms of self-management (Proudfoot, 2013; Mohr et al., 2013). For example, myCompass, an interactive program designed for users with mood disorder, gives self-monitoring assistance, prompts, reminders, graphic feedback, contextual information, motivational messages, and self-help modules based on CBT, interpersonal therapy, and positive psychological techniques (Proudfoot, 2013).

Casting mental illness as something wrong with a particular person's brain has a stigmatizing effect, suggesting blame and shame over one's condition (Sayce, 2000, pp. 84–99). The universal-type preventive initiatives of public mental health, where the node of intervention is no longer the individual, have the advantage of avoiding this harmful effect. Moreover, like Szaszian ideas, they also presuppose an ecological model, acknowledging the broader context within which disorder occurs, and best captured in a set of typical features, rather than analytic definition, the classic enumeration of which includes: "The promotion of health and prevention of disease and disability; the collection and use of epidemiological data, population surveillance and other forms of empirical quantitative assessment; a *recognition of the multidimensional nature of the determinants of health; and focus on complex interactions of many factors— biological, behavioral, social, and environmental*" (Childress et al., 2002, p. 170, italics added). These characteristic features distinguish public health approaches from the models of ill health associated with much traditional medicine and medical psychiatry (Childress et al., 2002).

With mental disorder, as has been increasingly recognized, such environmental elements act as risk factors and triggers, forming an essential ingredient even when genetic or other idiopathic elements also account for disorder (Saxena et al., 2006; Kirmayer et al., 2015). The surrounding setting, or ecology, that is addressed by public health interventions includes risk and protective factors that may be biological, emotional, cognitive, behavioral, interpersonal, or related to the family or cultural context. Developmental factors will also be part of this enumeration. Nothing short of that broader context, or ecology, is the focus of the "ecosystemic" models of public health. The individual is a biological organism embedded in, and in constant transaction with, the environment. In such "ecosystemic models," individual circumstances combine with broad societal and cultural factors to explain the systems that cause and maintain symptoms, suffering, and disability (Kirmeyer et al., 2015). We will return to ecosystemic models of disorder underlying public health, for they prove to explain and support one of Szasz's key insights.

In a related development, calls for a public health approach to depression are emerging from a perceived failure of individually focused treatments. Limitations and even risk factors associated with antidepressant treatment are taken to "suggest a need for alternative and/or concomitant means of preventing and treating depression" (Ghaemi et al., 2013, p. 92). Preventive efforts ranging from prenatal care to psychosocial interventions lasting into adulthood, working in tandem with pharmacotherapy, are proposed to improve treatment outcomes in those at risk of depression.

Its immense power makes public health potentially coercive, as Szasz would have been the first to recognize. (So too would Michel Foucault.) The role of surveillance in these new resilience-building pedagogies seems to transform self-monitored depressed mood, sleep disturbance, loss of pleasure, impaired concentration, and the like, into further "biomarkers" likely to erode traditional conceptions and expectations of self-mastery and privacy (McLachlan, 2014). Only a public mental health approach honoring the individual rights which are ensured by traditional autonomy-based ethical principles can offer sufficient protection from such abuses (Kass, 2001; Childress et al., 2002; Griffiths and West, 2015; Radden, 2016). The relationship between public health and these rights may involve tension. Often however, the most effective ways to promote public health seems to be to respect general moral considerations rather than violating them: employing voluntary measures rather than coercive ones, protecting privacy and confidentiality, and expressing rather than imposing community (Childress et al., 2002). Although the preventive pedagogies of public mental health have a particular appeal for the Szaszian liberal, for whom noncoercive education remains the only acceptable means for the state to alter how adults behave, *what* is taught, and *how*, remain important ethical questions for such pedagogies (Tenglend, 2012; Griffiths and West, 2015). These preventive pedagogies must avoid the use of scare tactics and dubiously valid empirical studies to endorse conclusions; for example, guarding against groupthink so that genuine differences on matters of opinion can be voiced and discussed.

18.3 Analysis of changes in conceptions of personal responsibility

Liberal principles have been invoked to uphold mental patients' rights; but equally, they are appealed to in support of contrary views, as we have seen. Contested, through the last seventy-odd years of theorizing and attitudes about mental patients' rights, has been the relationship between being bearers of those rights and the extent and nature of their individual responsibilities in relation to their mental and behavioral functioning. But the history of responsibility attributions through these decades apparently suggests a trend, where rights entail the attribution of *increasing* individual responsibility, together with *particular, new* self-care responsibilities. This is a seeming convergence—and one that apparently leads toward the implausible Szaszian position that *we are all, always, fully responsible for disorder and its outcomes.*

How far do we want to go in this direction? First, we do not need to adhere to Szasz's idea that the presence of rights entails full responsibility. Individual responsibility is often attributed, or withheld, by degrees. Its attribution to persons in relation to particular efforts and actions permits a range—from full and complete responsibility, though every stage of diminished responsibility, until none can be attributed at all. By contrast, rights are either attributed or withheld: They are by their nature accorded to persons, or not—there is no middle ground. Similarly, rights fail to be applicable in at least three broad ways: They can fail to be honored, as was true for the rights of the mentally ill before the 1970s; they may be not exercised due to ignorance on the part of their subject, as is likely also true in that era; and finally, they cannot be exercised properly when the rights bearer lacks the appropriate capabilities (e.g., the right to free speech cannot, or cannot easily, be exercised by those who are prevented from speaking by organic dysfunction). None of these impediments contradicts the presence of rights, or their appropriate attribution—they merely explain why those rights are not exercised.

Because responsibility admits of degree, and full responsibility is only accorded to a limited subset of human actions, most people would today accept some version of the collection of rights which Szasz accords to the mentally ill without agreeing that there is full responsibility for all, or even some, psychiatric symptoms—or for their antecedents, or for all the psychic states and behavior subsequently arising from them. Such an uncompromising position in relation to responsibility for all mental disorder seems to be unwarrantedly extreme, whether expressed by Szasz, his followers, or by those at the extreme fringes of the self-help movement. (See, for example, Louise Hay's *You Can Heal Your Life* [1984]). The rhetoric of the alternative medicine and self-help field sometimes steers close to blaming the victim: strength of will and commitment are depicted as alone sufficient to ensure mental health (Coward, 1989; Sayce, 2000). Expecting people to take responsibility for their symptoms during episodes of extreme disorder, or holding them responsible for such episodes and much of their sequelae, seem equally inhumane and unrealistic.

It is tempting to suppose that, at this point, our moral intuitions about individual responsibility simply diverge from the intuitions of others, including Szasz, so that an end has been reached in fruitful exchange, and attributing individual responsibility here is a matter of immovable opinion. But this may not be so. Conceptions of disease have shifted also during the decades when these attitudes about responsibility have become more aligned with Szaszian ones. The new era of public mental health ushers in a way to avoid the individualistic, person-centered conceptions of both disease and responsibility, over which these disagreements occur.

Public health presupposes a conception of disease or disorder contrary to that found in traditional medical psychiatry—and certainly contrary to the exclusively biological interpretation of "disease" maintained by Szasz. (What counts as a disease, for Szasz, is "an objectively demonstrable bodily lesion or process that deviates from an objectively defined biological norm" (Szasz, 2004a, p. 321).) The promise offered by public mental health lies with its emphasis on early, primary prevention, when prevention is understood as interventions (whether universal or targeted) which would serve to avert or avoid later disorder. But this promise rests on a different conception of disorder, or disease. Because of its resources (in monitoring, data collection, and the like), and its attention to whole populations rather than individual cases, the model of disease underlying much preventive public health is broadly *ecological* or *ecosystemic*. On it, a group of elements, environmental as well as biological and social, interacts with aspects of the individual to bring about ill health. Its domain includes the commonalities, the many aspects of the environment that are shared rather than idiosyncratic. (Because its primary focus remains the treatment and care of seriously ill patients, clinical medicine is wedded to the particularities of individual cases. Medicine, in its inescapable individualism, exemplifies the methodological individualism decried by Daniel Goldberg (2012) as problematic for any effort to reduce health inequities.) Inasmuch as the model accords increasing recognition that individual idiopathic risk factors, while present, will require triggers and precipitating causes from among these shared environmental elements, psychiatry is changing also, if slowly (Ghaemi, 2017). Elsewhere though, the node of intervention is no longer the individual (Goldberg, 2012).

The ecosystemic models distinguishing public health approaches and assumptions can be briefly illustrated here in relation to suicide prevention. Suicide is standardly conceptualized in terms of the particular set of problems surrounding its individual victim. Yet visible at the population level, there is clear evidence that membership in certain social groups represents an enhanced risk factor. As a public health issue, such evidence indicates that suicide prevention programs might better be directed toward trying to address these population influences rather than, as they often do now, merely trying to reduce access to the means of suicide by individuals (Dawson and Silva, 2009). On a public health model, suicide ought to be viewed "not merely as a series of clinical events that need to be prevented . . . but also an affront to social justice arising at a population level," which "means that suicide prevention policies must focus on such things as the socio-economic determinants of health, address discrimination, and focus on background causes such as mental illness" (Dawson and Silva, 2009, p. 5). With this shift of approach to one where the node of intervention is no longer the individual, suicidal behavior becomes a different kind of disorder, amenable to a wider, and different, range of responses.

18.3.1 The myth of mental illness?

The public mental health emphasis on early, primary, universal prevention and an ecosystemic model granting multifactorial causation does not directly address Szasz's claim that "mental disorder" is a mythical entity lacking parallels with physical disorders. There is a feature of public mental health that furthers the Szaszian ontological agenda, however. It draws attention to the incommensurability of psychiatric symptoms and the heterogeneity within the broad category of mental disorder. Increasingly, these mental and behavioral problems have come to be regarded as the result of a range of life experiences, even if those experiences act as triggers and affordances for preexisting, individualistic (idiopathic) risk factors. By their nature, many life experiences can be avoided and averted—making them amenable to cognitive and behavioral interventions, and self-help preventive practices.

Heterogeneity is likewise the most marked characteristic of Szaszian "problems in living." The lack of commonality among "mental illnesses" reflects one of the several interpretations of their mythical status. They are not one thing, but many, and as diverse as the problems in living, among which they are best numbered. So, a reading of the multiply ambiguous phrase "myth of mental illness" explodes the idea of a singular and unique entity or type of entity, or a set of such entities. The mythical status of "mental illness" lies with the fact that, like other problems in living, symptoms vary in the extent to which they can be prevented by any efforts of primary intervention, personal or not, such as those aimed to develop neuroimmunity. Problems in living are endlessly heterogeneous, imposing many kinds of relationships around individual responsibility. They are variously, and in various degrees, (i) our personal responsibility, (ii) the responsibility of others, and (iii) the effect of bad luck, which no effort or foresight on our part, or that of those around us, or indeed policy responses, could have averted. The hegemonic thinking that implies mental disorders are one sort of thing is central to the model Szasz so consistently rejected. With the focus on public mental health as prevention, that model seems to be joined, and challenged—if not yet replaced—by one where, like problems in living, "mental illnesses" are so varied, diverse, and multiply caused as to belie their common name.

Where does this leave individual responsibility? The question of how much individual responsibility is appropriately attributed to any response or action, as we have seen, can be a function of the degree of capacity or ability enjoyed by the person in any particular time, be she troubled in mind or the victim of any other troubling circumstance. Some symptoms of disorder, like some problems in living, will be amenable to being changed through personal agency, foresight, self-control, and effort—and *others will not*.

Szasz and his followers may have oversimplified the complex relationship between rights and responsibilities. Yet the focus on public mental health, I suggest, breathes new life into Szasz's slogan. In respect to individual responsibility, at least, mental illness may be mythical.

Acknowledgment

Dr. John Sadler kindly read a draft of this chapter while it was in preparation, and offered helpful suggestions and additions for which I am very grateful.

References

Anthony, William A. 1993. "Recovery from Mental Illness: The Guilding Vision of the Mental Health Service System in the 1990s." *Psychosocial Rehabilitation Journal* **16** (4): 11–23.

Appelbaum, Paul S. 1997. "Almost a Revolution: An International Perspective on the Law of Involuntary Commitment." *Journal of the American Academy of Psychiatry and Law* **25** (2): 135–47.

Barker, Phil, Peter Campbell, and Ben Davidson (eds.). 1999. *From the Ashes of Experience: Reflections on Madness, Survival, Growth*. London: Whurr.

Black Dog Institute. 2017. "Black Dog Institute." Accessed April 24, 2018. <www.blackdoginstitute.org.au>

Childress, James F., Ruth R. Faden, Ruth D. Gaare, et al. 2002. "Public Health Ethics: Mapping the Terrain." *Journal of Law, Medicine, and Ethics* **30** (2) (Summer): 170–8.

Christman, John. 2015. "Autonomy in Moral and Political Philosophy." *Stanford Encyclopedia of Philosophy*. Accessed April 17, 2018. <plato.stanford.edu/entries/autonomy-moral/>

Coward, Rosalind. 1989. *The Whole Truth: The Myth of Alternative Health*. London: Faber and Faber.

Davidson, Larry, Maria J. O'Connell, Janis Tondora, et al. 2005. "Recovery in Serious Mental Illness: A New Wine or Just a New Bottle?" *Professional Psychology: Research and Practice* **36** (5) (October): 480–7.

Dawson, Angus, and Diego Steven Silva. 2009. "Suicide Prevention: A Task for Public Health and a Role for Public Health Ethics." *Journal of Public Mental Health* **8** (3) (November): 4–6.

Durlak, Joseph A., Roger P. Weissberg, Allison B. Dymnicki, et al. 2011. "The Impact of Enhancing Students' Social and Emotional Learning: A Meta-Analysis of School-Based Universal Interventions." *Child Development* **82** (1) (January–February): 405–32.

Eagleman, David. 2011. *Incognito: The Secret Lives of the Brain*. New York: Pantheon.

Fraser, Nancy, and Axel Honneth. 2003. *Redistribution or Recognition? A Political-Philosophical Exchange*, translated by Joel Golb, James Ingram, and Christiane Wilke. London: Verso.

Fricker, Miranda. 2007. *Epistemic Injustice: Power and the Ethics of Knowing*. Oxford: Oxford University Press.

Friere, Paulo, James W. Fraser, Donaldo Macedo, et al. 1997. *Mentoring the Mentor: A Critical Dialogue with Paulo Friere*. New York: Peter Lang.

Ghaemi, S. Nassir. 2017. "Biomedical Reductionist, Humanist, and Biopsychosocial Models in Medicine." In *Handbook of the Philosophy of Medicine*, edited by Thomas Schramme and Steven Edwards, pp. 773–91. The Netherlands: Springer.

Ghaemi, S. Nassir, Paul Alfred Vöhringer, and Elizabeth A. Whitham. 2013. "Antidepressants from a Public Health Perspective: Re-Examining Effectiveness, Suicide, and

Carcinogenicity." *Acta Psychiatrica Scandinavica* **127** (2) (February): 89–93. Accessed April 17, 2018. <onlinelibrary.wiley.com/doi/pdf/10.1111/acps.12059>

Goldberg, Daniel S. 2012. "Social Justice, Health Inequalities, and Methodological Individualism in U.S. Health Promotion." *Public Health Ethics* **5** (2) (July):104–15.

Griffiths, Paul E., and Caroline West. 2015. "A Balanced Intervention Ladder: Promoting Autonomy Through Public Health Action." *Public Health* **129** (8) (August): 1092–8.

Gutheil, Thomas G. 1980. "In Search of True Freedom: Drug Refusal, Involuntary Medication, and 'Rotting With Your Rights On'." *American Journal of Psychiatry* **137** (3) (March): 327–8.

Gutheil, Thomas G., and Paul S. Appelbaum. 1980. "The Patient Always Pays: Reflections on the Boston State Case and the Right to Rot." *Man and Medicine* **5** (1): 3–11.

Hay, Louise L. 1984. *You Can Heal Your Life.* Sydney: Specialist Publications.

Hornstein, Gail A. 2002. "Narratives of Madness, as Told From Within." *Chronicle of Higher Education* **48** (20) (January 25): B7.

Irwin, Stephen, Jeanie Sheffield, and Kristina Holland-Thompson. 2010. *beyondblue SenseAbility Sense of Control Module.* Australia: Beyondblue Ltd.

Jacobson, Nora, and Dianne Greenley. 2001. "What is Recovery? A Conceptual Model and Explication." *Psychiatric Services* **52** (4) (April): 482–5. Accessed April 17, 2018. <ps.psychiatryonline.org/doi/pdf/10.1176/appi.ps.52.4.482>

Kass, Nancy E. 2001. "An Ethics Framework for Public Health." *American Journal of Public Health* **91** (11) (November): 1776–82.

Kirmayer, Laurence J., Robert Lemelson, and Constance A. Cummings (eds.). 2015. *Re-Visioning Psychiatry: Cultural Phenomenology, Critical Neuroscience, and Global Mental Health.* Cambridge: Cambridge University Press.

Kohn, Robert, Shekhar Saxena, et al. 2004. "The Treatment Gap in Mental Health Care." *Bulletin of the World Health Organization* **82** (11) (November): 858–66.

Mackenzie, Catriona, and Natalie Stoljar (eds.). 2000. *Relational Autonomy: Feminist Perspectives on Autonomy, Agency, and the Social Self.* New York: Oxford University Press.

McGorry, Patrick D. 2015. "Early Intervention in Psychosis: Obvious, Effective, Overdue." *Journal of Nervous and Mental Disease* **203** (5) (May): 310–18.

McLachlan, Andrew. 2014. "Preventative [sic] Therapeutics: A Study of Risk and Prevention in Australian Mental Health." *Culture Unbound* **6**: 815–37. Accessed April 17, 2018. <www.cultureunbound.ep.liu.se/v6/a44/cu14v6a44.pdf>

Merry, Sally N., Sarah E. Hetrick, Georgina R. Cox, et al. 2011. "Psychological and Educational Interventions for Preventing Depression in Children and Adolescents." *Cochrane Database of Systematic Reviews* (**12**) (December 7). Accessed April 17, 2018. <minerva-access.unimelb.edu.au/bitstream/handle/11343/59278/Merry%20et%20al%202011.pdf>

Mill, John Stuart. 1859. *On Liberty.* London: John W. Parker.

Mohr, David C. Michelle Nicole Burns, Stephen M. Schueller, et al. 2013. "Behavioral Intervention Technologies: Evidence Review and Recommendations for Future Research in Mental Health." *General Hospital Psychiatry* **35** (4) (July–August): 332–8.

Muñoz, Ricardo F. 2001. "On the Road to a World Without Depression." *Journal of Primary Prevention* **21** (3) (March): 325–38.

Murray, Christopher J.L., and Alan D. Lopez. 1997. "Global Mortality, Disability, and the Contribution of Risk Factors: Global Burden of Disease Study." *Lancet* **349** (9063) (May 17): 1436–42.

O'Connell, Mary Ellen, Thomas Boat, and Kenneth E. Warner (eds.). 2009. *Preventing Mental, Emotional and Behavioral Disorders Among Young People: Progress and Possibilities.* Washington D.C.: National Academies Press.

Patel, Vikram, and Shekhar Saxena. 2014. "Transforming Lives, Enhancing Communities: Innovations in Global Mental Health." *New England Journal of Medicine* **370** (February 6): 498–501. Accessed April 17, 2018. <www.nejm.org/doi/full/10.1056/NEJMp1315214>

Patel, Vikram, Gary S. Belkin, Arun Chockalingam, et al. 2013. "Grand Challenges: Integrating Mental Health Services into Priority Health Care Platforms." *PLoS Medicine* **10** (5) (May). Accessed April 17, 2018. <www.ncbi.nlm.nih.gov/pmc/articles/PMC3666874/>

Pouncey, Claire L., and Jonathan M. Lukens. 2010. "Madness Versus Badness: The Ethical Tension Between the Recovery Movement and Forensic Psychiatry." *Theoretical Medicine and Bioethics* **31** (1) (February): 93–105.

Powers, Cassandra, Valerie A. Hart, et al. 2012. "The Concept of 'The Will to Thrive' in Mental Health." *Issues in Mental Health Nursing* **33** (11): 805–7.

Prince, Martin, Vikram Patel, Shekhar Saxena, et al. 2007. "No Health Without Mental Health." *Lancet* **370** (9590) (September 8): 859–77.

Proudfoot, Judith. 2013. "The Future is in Our Hands: The Role of Mobile Phones in the Prevention and Management of Mental Disorders." *Australian and New Zealand Journal of Psychiatry* **47** (2): 111–13.

Radden, Jennifer H. 2010. "Insightlessness, the Deflationary Turn." *Philosophy, Psychiatry, and Psychology* **17** (1) (March): 81–4.

Radden, Jennifer H. 2012. "Recognition Rights, Mental Health Consumers, and Reconstructive Cultural Semantics." *Philosophy, Ethics, and Humanities in Medicine* **7** (January 13). Accessed April 17, 2018. <www.ncbi.nlm.nih.gov/pmc/articles/PMC3293003/>

Radden, Jennifer H. 2016. "Mental Health, Public Health, and Depression: A Bioethical Perspective." *Ethics, Medicine, and Public Health* **2** (2) (April–June): 197–204.

Radden, Jennifer H., and Somogy Varga. 2013. "The Epistemological Value of Depression Memoirs: A Meta-Analysis." In *Oxford Handbook of the Philosophy of Psychiatry*, edited by K.W.M. Fulford et al., pp. 99–115. Oxford: Oxford University Press.

Rashed, M. 2019. Madness and the Demand for Recognition: A Philosophical Inquiry into Identity and Mental Health Activism. Oxford: Oxford University Press.

Read, Jim, and Jill Reynolds (eds.). 1996. *Speaking Our Minds: An Anthology of Personal Experiences of Mental Distress and its Consequences.* Basingstoke, U.K.: Macmillan.

Sadler, John Z. 2013. "Considering the Economy of DSM Alternatives." In *Making the DSM-5: Concepts and Controversies*, edited by Joel Paris and James Phillips, pp. 21–38. New York: Springer.

Saxena, Shekhar, Eva Jané-Llopis, and Clemens Hosman. 2006. "Prevention of Mental and Behavioural Disorders: Implications for Policy and Practice." *World Psychiatry* **5** (1) (February): 5–14.

Saxena, Shekhar, Michelle Funk, and Dan Chisholm. 2014. "WHO's Mental Health Action Plan, 2013–2020: What Can Psychiatrists Do to Facilitate Its Implementation?" *World Psychiatry* **13** (2) (June): 107–9.

Sayce, Liz. 2000. *From Psychiatric Patient to Citizen: Overcoming Discrimation and Social Exclusion.* New York: St. Martin's Press.

Schaler, Jeffrey (ed.). 2004. *Szasz Under Fire: The Psychiatric Abolitionist Faces His Critics.* Chicago: Open Court.

Schramme, Thomas, and Steven Edwards (eds.). 2017. *Handbook of the Philosophy of Medicine*. Dordrecht: Springer.

Spaulding, William D., Mary E. Sullivan, and Jeffrey Stephen Poland. 2003. *Treatment and Rehabilitation of Severe Mental Illness*. New York: Guilford Press.

Strawson, Peter. 2003. "Freedom and Resentment." In *Free Will*, 2nd edn., edited by Gary Watson, pp. 72–93. Oxford: Oxford University Press.

Szasz, Thomas S. 1965. *Psychiatric Justice*. New York: Macmillan.

Szasz, Thomas S. 1970. *Ideology and Insanity: Essays on the Psychiatric Dehumanization of Man*. Garden City, New York: Doubleday Anchor.

Szasz, Thomas S. 1974. *The Myth of Mental Illness: Foundations of a Theory of Personal Conduct*, revised edn. New York: Harper & Row.

Szasz, Thomas S. 1982. "The Psychiatric Will: A New Mechanism for Protecting Persons Against 'Psychosis' and Psychiatry." *American Psychologist* **37** (7): 762–70.

Szasz, Thomas S. 2004a. "Reply to Bentall." In *Szasz Under Fire: The Psychiatric Abolitionist Faces His Critics*, edited by Jeffrey Schaler, pp. 321–326. Chicago: Open Court.

Szasz, Thomas S. 2004b. "Reply to Fulford." In *Szasz Under Fire: The Psychiatric Abolitionist Faces His Critics*, edited by Jeffrey Schaler, pp. 93–118. Chicago: Open Court.

Tenglend, Per-Anders. 2012. "Behavior Change or Empowerment: On the Ethics of Health-Promotion Strategies." *Public Health Ethics* **5** (2) (July 1): 140–53.

Ussher, Patrick (ed.). 2014. *Stoicism Today: Selected Writings I*. London: Stoicism Today.

Vilhelmsson, Andreas, Tommy Svensson, and Anna Meeuwisse. 2011. "Mental Ill Health, Public Health, and Medicalization." *Public Health Ethics* **4** (3) (November 1): 207–17.

Watson, Gary. 2004. *Agency and Answerability: Selected Essays*. Oxford: Oxford University Press.

Whitaker, Robert. 2010. *Anatomy of an Epidemic: Magic Bullets, Psychiatric Drugs, and the Astonishing Rise of Mental Illness in America*. New York: Broadway Paperbacks.

World Health Organization (WHO). 2008. *The Global Burden of Disease: 2004 Update*. Geneva: WHO. Accessed April 17, 2018. <www.who.int/healthinfo/global_burden_disease/GBD_report_2004update_full.pdf>

World Health Organization (WHO). 2001. *The World Health Report: Mental Health: New Understanding, New Hope*. Geneva: WHO. Accessed April 16, 2018. <www.who.int/whr/2001/en/whr01_en.pdf>

World Health Organization (WHO). 2012. *Risks to Mental Health: An Overview of Vulnerabilities and Risk Factors: Background Paper by WHO Secretariat for the Development of a Comprehensive Mental Health Action Plan*. Geneva: WHO. Accessed April 16, 2018. <citeseerx.ist.psu.edu/viewdoc/download;jsessionid=033C5D034E524676E66D70D8569352F1?doi=10.1.1.691.7072&rep=rep1&type=pdf>

World Health Organization (WHO). 2013. *Comprehensive Mental Health Action Plan, 2013–2020*. Geneva: WHO. Accessed April 16, 2018. <apps.who.int/iris/bitstream/handle/10665/89966/9789241506021_eng.pdf>

Chapter 19

Szasz's legacy and current challenges in psychiatry

Thomas Schramme

19.1 **Introduction**

Szasz's legacy consists in his relentless criticism of careless and overconfident thinking in psychiatric theory and practice. He asks the right questions, even if his answers might not always be the most plausible. To diagnose problems in our common assumptions and to be skeptical about alleged truths is a truly philosophical approach. Hence, Szasz's legacy is one of a philosopher of psychiatry.

Szasz has often been described as a supporter of antipsychiatry. But he was himself strongly opposed to this term and to many of the arguments put forward by so-called antipsychiatrists (Szasz, 2009). What has been called antipsychiatry is itself formed by a multiplicity of perspectives and agendas. What connects the relevant thinkers—such as Franco Basaglia, Michel Foucault, Erving Goffman, Ronald Laing, and Thomas Scheff—with Szasz is their shared skepticism regarding psychiatric theory and practice. I believe that the term "skepticism" is better suited for the purposes of many "antipsychiatrists," at least for Szasz's purposes, as it connotes an inquiring attitude and inquisitive frame of mind. Szasz stands out in this league of theorists and practitioners, in that he developed a level of analytical rigor that no other skeptical psychiatrist reached.

I focus here on a couple of the main concerns that directed Szasz's analyses: (1) his opposition to the concept of mental illness (2) his criticism of coercive care and (3) the problem of psychiatry's identity, the latter being a problem that is less visible but implied in his writings. An overarching theme that emerges from discussing Szasz's work is the need to draw clear theoretical and practical boundaries between psychopathology and nonpsychiatric problems in life; hence to carve out the identity of psychiatry. Many people acknowledge the problem of medicalization and pathologization (Conrad, 2007; Sholl, 2017). Psychiatry seems to take over an ever-increasing area of normal life. To criticize or reject such developments, we need a proper understanding of the concept of mental illness—or of mental disorder, if you prefer that term (which I will use interchangeably).

Szasz paved the way to get a clearer grasp of the most important problems for psychiatry. These are philosophical problems, which have to do with conceptual and theoretical issues. The problems call for a scientific foundation of psychiatry. However, this does not mean, contrary to what is often assumed when the scientific status of a discipline is discussed, that the so-called natural sciences will alone provide an adequate model for psychiatric theorizing. Such reductionist modeling has unfortunately been the dominant way of psychiatry in the last few decades (Cohen, 1993; Andreasen, 1997; Kandel, 1998, 2005). Ironically, the mentioned trajectory can be traced back, at least partially, to the impact of Szasz's criticism of psychiatry. In other words, Szasz's implicit call for a scientific psychiatry has ignited a one-sided and hence wrongheaded account of psychiatric theorizing, which has eventually led to what can be called an identity crisis of psychiatry. The identity of psychiatry has become uncertain because of theoretical challenges to do with the conceptualization of the mind and practical issues that are owed to nonmedical tasks psychiatry needs to fulfill. Revisiting Szasz's writings might therefore help in sorting out this crisis—and perhaps this would be another ironic twist to the story so far.

19.2 **Critique of the concept of mental illness**

Szasz's main contribution to the debate about the concept of mental illness was negative. He criticized and eventually rejected the common interpretation of mental illness as a pathology of the mind. We will return to his specific arguments shortly, but it might be worth pointing out at this point that perhaps it was the very negativity of Szasz's approach that led many to ignore it altogether. How can a society help people in need if we do not use a label that will qualify them for such help in welfare states? In other words, how can we provide the right means of support for people who struggle with their daily lives? It seems that we need some criterion as to why those people should have a claim, as a matter of justice, to gain access to resources provided by efforts of the state. Since Szasz did not really provide an alternative description of the people commonly seen as mentally ill and hence medically needy, which would have qualified them for support by welfare state institutions, his theory was unacceptable to many people for clinical, ethical, economic, and, overall, for political reasons.

It should be straightforward, however, that Szasz's political libertarianism and antipathy toward the welfare state, on the one hand, and critique of the misuse of the concept of mental illness, on the other, are two different and separable aspects of his thinking. There are no principled reasons against accepting claims of justice on other grounds than medical need. Still, it seems to be the simplest route to the provision of support, as pathology is a widely accepted justifying criterion of claims of justice.

It seems that Szasz saw the normative significance of the concept of mental illness mainly from the flip side of such issues of access to welfare state institutions. He was much concerned about the normative implications of using medical terminology for people who did not see themselves as needy or disadvantaged, and hence did not seek support from welfare state institutions. Being ill does not come merely with rights to access resources but also with role responsibilities; for instance, to seek medical help so that one can get back to work (Parsons, 1958; Szasz, 1977, 1994). Being deemed mentally ill also comes with particular assumptions about the afflicted persons' capacities, or lack thereof, to lead their own lives and to decide for themselves. These often disadvantageous consequences of the concept of mental illness need to be taken very seriously, and it is in this respect that Szasz's contribution is so important.

To be sure, it might be argued that the normative implications are not, strictly speaking, part of the concept of mental illness. We do not necessarily need to see any practical implications of calling persons mentally ill, for instance, in terms of their capacities to make their own decisions. Diagnosing someone as a patient and the social norms attached to the role of a patient could be seen as two completely separate aspects. Although I would agree with this defense of the normative neutrality of the concept of mental illness up to a point, I also believe that Szasz was right in pressing the institution of psychiatry to justify its use of the basic notion of mental illness, or mental disorder for that matter. In reality, especially when Szasz started his mission, medicine in general and psychiatry in particular have been deeply entangled with political and societal purposes. "Misfits" and politically unwanted citizens were regularly deemed psychiatric patients because of their deviant behavior.

It seems that the main criterion for justifying the use of medical terminology in psychiatry has always been scientific rigor. Psychiatry, until today, has strived at being a scientific endeavor, thereby at least partially emulating general medicine, which is widely regarded as a scientific enterprise. Although the aim of scientificity is indeed important, it is also liable to confusion.

I have distinguished among different versions of Szasz's argument against the cogency of the concept of mental illness (Schramme, 2004). One influential version is his claim that there can be no *mental* illness, because the criteria that are used for establishing the presence of pathology are not applicable to the mental realm. This argument comes in two steps: First, he defines what illness is, or rather describes what is usually understood as disease or illness; second, he shows that this definition of illness does not apply to the mental realm:

> Psychiatrists and all those steeped in the psychiatric ideology take the decisive initial step of omitting to define illness in general, or bodily illness in particular, and instead *define mental illness* (whatever they mean by it) *as a member of the class called illness.* I reject this approach. Instead of accepting the phenomena called mental illnesses as diseases, the decisive initial step I take is to *define illness as the pathologist defines it—as a structural or functional abnormality of cells, tissues, organs, or bodies.* If the phenomena called mental illnesses manifest themselves as such structural or functional abnormalities, then they are *diseases*; if they do not, they are *not.* (Szasz, 1987, p. 12, original italics)

Maybe it is no surprise that most psychiatrists, until today, have bought into the first part of the argument and accepted the reading of the general notion of disease as somatic dysfunction. Mental illness is then supposed to be brain disease. Obviously, this is an interpretation that has a long history in psychiatry, starting at least with Wilhelm Griesinger (1817–1868). It also seems to guarantee psychiatry's scientific status. But Szasz has an immediate answer that builds the second part of his argument: "Diseases of the brain are brain diseases; it is confusing, misleading, and unnecessary to call them mental illnesses" (Szasz, 1987, p. 49). Ironically, this second step of the argument was also endorsed by several leading psychiatrists, except that they apparently felt that the consequences of the misuse were not as bad as Szasz projected. They did not see the use of the concept of mental illness as confusing, misleading, or unnecessary, though they agreed that mental disorder "could not be a more unfortunate term, preserving as it does an outdated mind-body duality" (Frances et al., 1991, p. 409).

British psychiatrist Robert Kendell is perhaps the best exemplar of the confusion that is built on the attempt to rebut Szasz's claims: "It follows that there is, strictly speaking, no such thing as disease of the mind or mental disorder and that Griesinger was right—mental illnesses are diseases of the brain, or at least involve disordered brain function—because all mental events are accompanied by and dependent on events in the brain. (Thomas Szasz was also right; mental illness is a myth, though not for the reasons he believed.)" (Kendell, 1993, p. 3). But surely, based on Kendell's own statements, Szasz was right—and for the right reasons (Szasz, 1996, p. 96; 2004, p. 321). After all, Szasz allows for brain pathology to exist, but simply denies that this equals mental illness, and hence claims that psychiatry does not have any phenomena to deal with. It is not clear at all where Kendell's point of view differs.

I have elaborated this argument and the surrounding confusion elsewhere (Schramme, 2013). This confusion is based on a widespread misunderstanding of the traditional mind-body problem and related theories within the philosophy of mind. Many contributions to the debate correctly state that a specific form of dualism—so-called Cartesian or substance dualism, where two different kinds of "stuff," mental and bodily, are assumed—has lost its credibility. But this does not mean that we cannot refer to mental phenomena anymore. Surely we have many terms in our language, such as "art" or "courage," that refer to material instantiations of things in the world and still cannot be reduced to a physical description. Szasz himself is unclear about this whole issue, most visibly when he grapples with the mind-body problem in *The Meaning of Mind* (1996). Ronald Leifer (1982) made an important attempt to clarify the problem from the point of view of skeptical psychiatry. Szasz ended up with a view of the general concept of disease as restricted to physiological processes, which is dubious, because we can meaningfully conceptualize and refer to genuine mental phenomena (Reznek, 1991, Chapter 5).

Be that as it may, it was not any misconception of the mind-body problem which eventually led to undermining the very identity of psychiatry. Rather, it was mainly due to the wrongheaded attempt to come to grips with the elusive nature of mental phenomena, put forward by a large and influential branch of psychiatry itself. By desperately avoiding any allegedly dualistic theorizing, and by restricting the task to establish a scientific status for psychiatry to a purely physicalist model, psychiatric thinking lost a whole range of necessary perspectives and, indeed, traditions. If there really is no genuine mental illness, but merely brain disease, then psychiatry is reduced to neurology. No fashionable plea against "mindless" psychiatry (Eisenberg, 1986, 2000) and no popular endorsement of a "biopsychosocial" model will change that (Engel, 1977; Ghaemi, 2017).

It is a mistake to aim at a scientific status for psychiatry by merely emulating somatic medicine. Surely, the very goal of scientificity is valid and, indeed, important. It would be a very important task for the philosophy of psychiatry to discuss what exactly is required for fulfilling this aim when applied to psychiatry. For instance, Szasz (1960, p. 114) asserted, in a variant of his argument against the concept of mental illness, that psychopathology necessarily relies on value judgments, whereas somatic norms of normality and health could be stated by referring to biological facts only. Several philosophers of psychiatry have attacked this argument by doubting the value-neutrality of somatic medicine. In their view, all medical terminology is infused with values (Fulford, 1989; Sadler, 2005; Cooper, 2014; Bolton, 2008). However, this move seems to put the scientific status of all medicine in doubt instead of improving the scientific credibility of psychiatry. It does not ease, but rather intensifies, Szasz's worries about the medicalization of normal conditions.

The boundaries of the concept of mental illness need to be policed very rigidly. It therefore does not seem helpful to claim that the definition of mental illness, and hence which conditions belong to this category, are based on social value judgments. Szasz makes the same initial assumption about the value-ladenness of psychiatric concepts, but it seems only to intensify the worries of medicalization if we expand a value-laden perspective to all medical concepts. We should rather attempt to pursue the notion of a scientific conceptualization of mental disorder. It seems that this alternative way of answering Szasz's challenge has not received the deserved amount of attention (Boorse, 1976; Papineau, 1994; Schramme, 2016; Wakefield, 2017).

We might not be able to avoid reference to social or individual value judgments altogether when establishing what constitutes mental pathology. But we should strive, as much as we can, to avoid medicalization. This aim requires a clear and justifiable model of mental disorder, which is based on findings about the processes and mechanisms of the human organism. We can indeed define mental illness on the basis of a theory of mental dysfunction—and I have defended such a view (Schramme, 2010). Whether or not this is the most plausible route to take cannot be settled here. Still, it is the way that we need to explore if we want to avoid, as far as possible, Szasz's legitimate worry regarding the wrong kind of medicalization and pathologization, which we have seen too often in the actual practice of psychiatry.

One significant challenge for a scientific account of mental illness is how to draw the boundaries among specific categories that we use to refer to different mental disorders. For example, "schizophrenia" is a specific diagnostic entity, operationally defined in DSM-5 (APA, 2013, p. 99) by reference to diagnostic criteria (e.g., the continued presence of delusions, hallucinations, or disorganized speech). It is, however, obvious, and actually acknowledged in DSM-5, that the boundaries of diagnostic entities cannot be determined by "carving nature at its joints", as it is often put in philosophic al parlance. Psychiatry does not deal with, say, chemical elements or biological species. There is a certain level of arbitration required when devising diagnostic entities, especially when setting thresholds of mental functioning or when defining a specific number of sufficient criteria for a diagnostic term to apply. Many categories of disorders that are officially used in psychiatry are "spectrum disorders" (e.g., autism). Hence, certain thresholds regarding the severity of signs and symptoms are usually introduced. But, as with other disorders in medicine, there can always be a reasonable debate where exactly to draw the line between pathology and (sufficient) normality.

Szasz was again right to flag this element of construction in determining diagnostic entities. It has also raised a lot of attention in relation to the recent publication of the DSM-5 (Horvitz and Wakefield, 2007; Frances, 2013). Questionable practices for defining, describing, and including diagnostic entities in the DSM, which Szasz heavily criticized in his writings (Szasz, 1987, pp. 78–81), do not really support the belief in psychiatry's scientific ambitions. A critical stance, such as Szasz developed, is vital to identifying vested interests and hidden agendas (Szasz, 1987, pp. 81–6). The risk of expanding the boundaries of disorder so that normal conditions are deemed pathological is real and should be made explicit. There are well-known historical examples, most notoriously the diagnosis of drapetomania, the alleged mental illness causing slaves to run away from captivity, or the pathologization of masturbation and homosexuality (Szasz, 1970). More recently, the attempt to deem grief over and above a certain expected period of time, pathological, is a case in point. In addition, especially developments in screening for early onsets of specific disorders and relevant dispositions, for instance, regarding depression or personality disorders, have led to a widespread confusion over the boundaries of disorder (Schwartz, 2008).

However, maladapted methodologies in determining disease categories and fuzzy boundaries do not by themselves undermine psychiatry's aspiration to scientific status. After all, the former can be eliminated or at least significantly reduced, and the latter are owed to the nature of medical classification. Nosology needs to combine purposes of theoretical coherence and cohesiveness, compatibility with ongoing empirical research, and pragmatic elements, such as the reliability and comparability of diagnosis in different cultural settings. Obviously, the boundary problem of delineating the concept of mental disorder and distinguishing it from medically normal phenomena raises numerous important issues in relation to the scientific status of psychiatry, which would require a lengthier treatment than can be offered here (Keil et al., 2017).

An important related debate within philosophy of psychiatry concerns the very foundation of psychiatric classification. Traditionally, absolute categories are used; that is, a person either has or does not have a specific disorder. This picture is in line with lay beliefs. It is also relevant in connection with the context of welfare state institutions. After all, whether someone has a claim to the use of medical resources usually depends on a clear-cut statement about the person's health condition, especially given that the status could be challenged in a court case. Here, an absolute (i.e., nongradual) diagnosis appears to be inevitable.

But it also seems correct to stress that disorder is a gradual phenomenon. People show signs and symptoms to different degrees of severity, and the number of diagnostic criteria also varies. It might therefore be better to reflect the gradual nature of disorder by using other types of classification. Partly, this is already reflected in the dimensional approaches to some categories used in DSM-5. But it could also lead to more radical reforms in classifying mental disorders (Sadler et al., 1994; Sadler, 2002; Kendler and Parnas, 2012; Zachar et al., 2015). Again, such disagreements about the best way of classification and the relevant levels of human arbitration when devising diagnostic entities do not prevent a scientific approach altogether. But they should make us wary of the pitfalls when aiming at a scientific conceptualization of mental disorder. Szasz highlighted numerous such pitfalls (e.g., the confusion of value judgments and scientific theories). His writings can hence serve as an important contribution to improving psychiatry's credibility and to reducing its liability to medicalization.

19.3 **Against coercive care**

Now I would like to focus on another major concern of Szasz's work, which is still of present significance: In contrast to the previous discussion of the conceptual underpinnings of psychiatry, the topic of coercive care might be deemed exclusively connected to the practice of psychiatry. Since the practice of psychiatry has changed considerably in the last few decades, Szasz's writings, especially his early publications, might therefore seem outdated to the occasional reader. Such a verdict would be mistaken. Szasz pointed out perennial problems of psychiatry, which do not disappear by a change in practicing psychiatry. In fact, the normative issues underlying coercive care are not merely practice-related, but raise theoretical problems as well.

An important theoretical problem, which is indeed of practical consequence, concerns the very definition of coercion. There are of course straightforward cases of psychiatric coercion, however rare: for instance, where physical force is used to break the will of a patient. It is these extreme cases that have led to vital reforms in psychiatric practice. The level of such extreme coercion has certainly been significantly reduced in many countries, although psychiatric patients in institutionalized settings worldwide apparently still face serious harm. This harm might include even criminal behavior, in cases where individual rights are violated by psychiatric personnel. Also, even general improvements should not ease general ethical concerns about coercive care, which are obviously due to the involved infringement of individual liberty, not simply the aspect of violence or force. There are numerous less extreme practices still very common in psychiatry, which arguably manifest forms of coercive care.

One such example of possible psychiatric coercion is what I have called "interactive coercion" (Schramme, 2012). There is no physical force involved in these cases and the means of coercion might range from clear-cut threats to seductive offers, which exploit the vulnerabilities of patients. The point is that the range of coercion being used in psychiatric practice might be much wider than is commonly perceived. This poses, first and foremost, a conceptual issue about the definition of coercion. It also poses an ethical problem, of course, about the justification of coercive care. Again, Szasz's writings are important here as he presents the perhaps most radical counterposition to defenders of (some) psychiatric coercion.

Szasz's view regarding coercive care is of course at least partly driven by his rejection of the concept of mental illness (Szasz, 2004b, p. 356). After all, the (allegedly) caring aspect of psychiatric coercion aims at improving the health condition of a patient. If there are no psychiatric patients and no pathology to alleviate or cure, then there are no benefactors of psychiatric treatment and hence no justification for coercive care. So much seems straightforward. But even if we do not follow Szasz in his rejection of the reality of mental illness, we should see the significance of his critique. Assuming a pathology might be a necessary element of considering care at all, but this does not as such justify the use of coercion. Medical normality is not the only element of well-being and arguably not even the most important. Individual liberty is obviously of utmost importance to humans; hence, acting against the will of a person needs to be justified not merely by pointing out the medical benefits of psychiatric intervention.

Szasz and others repeatedly show that the thinking and behavior of allegedly mentally ill people does not by itself suffice to justify acting against their will.

Most psychiatrists and lay people would assume that there are nevertheless some mental conditions, whether they are called pathological or not, which undermine the autonomous will formation of people. These conditions might include insufficiently developed intellectual capacities (e.g., in children), or might be due to pathological personal development, or might be caused by circumstantial impact (e.g., unusual stress). In these and similar cases, acting against someone else's will might be justifiable, because there is evidence that the choice of the person is not his or her own in the normatively relevant sense, which under normal circumstances speaks against interference with individual liberty. Still, we cannot simply assume that, due to any mental pathology, the will of a psychiatric patient is impaired and that hence coercive care is justified in every case of mental disorder. Rather, what we need here, when pursuing a justification of coercive care, is a detailed analysis of the conditions that might in general or in specific circumstances undermine the autonomy of patients. Skeptics such as Szasz, therefore, need to be taken seriously.

A similarly worrying, if somewhat unrelated, aspect of psychiatric practice has been its nontherapeutic use of medical and nonmedical means (e.g., sedating or detaining patients who pose threats to other people). Here, the issue is not the infringement of liberty when providing care for a patient, but the employment of psychiatric institutions to serve public interests. Again, Szasz was a hugely important figure in bringing this to light. Psychiatry has a long and sad record of involvement and collaboration with state institutions. This history does not only include criminal deeds of psychiatric personnel in the name of a state or acts in collaboration with despotic regimes (Fulford et al., 1993), but also fully legal and democratically justified interventions into patients' liberty, most importantly, the detention of patients who are deemed dangerous. The latter tasks are usually performed by institutions of law enforcement, especially the police. The fact that psychiatry takes over policing functions comes with its own ethical problems, which deserve a closer look.

There is obviously an important normative difference between psychiatric compulsory detention and forced treatment. Yet, in psychiatric practice there is a close connection between the two, since patients who are either dangerous to other people or under risk of self-harm are often both kept in psychiatric clinics against their will and treated with psychoactive drugs or other medical means. An obvious reason for this practice is that treatment increases the chance of reducing the risk of harm to either third parties or the patients themselves.

The problematic confusion between therapeutic and nontherapeutic tasks in psychiatry has not gone unnoticed and has recently led to some important developments. In Germany, for instance, high court rulings have had a significant impact on the current debate about coercion in psychiatry. The backdrop of these was the problem of the potentially indefinite detention of persons deemed dangerous, but the debate then developed its own trajectory. Indeed, the whole issue of forensic psychiatry causes more normative and theoretical problems than what is covered by these lawsuits. A case in point is the fact that numerous patients in the U.K. are now labeled with the pseudo-medical term "Dangerous and Severe Personality Disorder (DSPD)" (Scott,

2014). Such confusion of criminal behavior and personality disorder—criminality as pathology—would surely not have escaped Szasz.

In Germany, the Federal Constitutional Court ruled in 2011 and the Federal Court of Justice in 2012 that people who are deemed dangerous due to personality or other mental disorders may not be treated against their will, though they may be detained, provided the usual harm-related criteria apply (e.g., regarding proportionality of the intervention). The rulings made explicit the difference between (coercive) detention and (voluntary or involuntary) treatment. This is a distinction that Szasz analyzed long ago (Szasz, 1987, p. 131). Even when psychiatric patients are legitimately detained against their will for the usual reasons of harm to others or self, psychiatric personnel are not automatically allowed to use compulsory means of treatment. At present, the exact criteria and legality of coercive psychiatric treatment is still subject to debate.

This whole issue has caused tension between psychiatric personnel and lawyers, since the new legal rules may prove quite difficult to apply in real psychiatric contexts. According to the courts' view, in busy psychiatric clinics, people who are a nuisance to other patients, who are abusive, possibly aggressive, and so on, may still not be treated against their will, but only restrained. However, these patients might disrupt the stability of a fragile group and may make it impossible for staff to cater sufficiently to the needs of other patients. From a practical point of view, to observe these new legal rules will also very likely increase the duration of restraining measures and thereby extend (amendable) harm to the patient. Such increased need for restraint (e.g., holding techniques) will call for a higher ratio of staff to patients, which is unlikely to be met.

It seems undeniable that patients have the right not to be treated against their will merely for the sake of other patients or the proper functioning of an understaffed institution. This is obviously a sensitive issue, especially in Germany, where psychiatry is still regularly seen under the shadow of the atrocities committed during the Nazi era. Compulsory treatment is a highly problematic intervention and hence is only allowed, according to the new regulations, under very strict conditions, most importantly only if the benefit of this treatment is to the patients themselves and if there are no other means available to prevent serious harm to them. However, there is now a debate as to whether at least imminent danger of severe harm to others might allow compulsory treatment, though this seems not to be in line with the rationale of the court rulings (Zinkler, 2016).

This new situation raises several interesting normative questions that will have to be answered: First, it seems that as far as sectioned—that is, involuntarily committed—patients are concerned, medical staff are reduced to a policing function, since personnel are not allowed to treat these patients if they do not want to be treated. Hence, staff are not allowed, under certain circumstances and possibly when support seems most urgently needed, to do what medical personnel are supposed to do, namely, help people who may be suffering or in distress. This seems unhelpful; in actual practice it may undermine the motivation of psychiatric personnel. Thus there seems to be a potential conflict between a pragmatic point of view in psychiatric practice (i.e., what is doable and desirable in a specific real-life context) and an idealized point of view in legal norms (i.e., what ought to be done under any circumstances).

An interesting suggestion in relation to this problem is to transfer the policing tasks to nonmedical staff. That would have the effect of reducing the problematic, and usually obscure, liaison of medical means and sociopolitical purposes—in other words, of preventing the current situation where psychiatry is serving nonmedical purposes. Such a transfer of tasks might also reduce the financial burden for the medical system. Since detention is, after all, a legal and not a medical task, funds for fulfilling this task should consequently not be taken from medical services. On the other hand, it would probably require psychiatric hospitals to open new wards for detention, in addition to the usual medical divisions.

Second, a difficult decision needs to be made about what counts as psychiatric treatment, as opposed to detention. For instance, if an agitated patient is strapped to the bed, is this a medical intervention that amounts to treatment—which would be illegal when forced on a patient with capacity to make his or her own decisions? Or is it, rather, a form of detention, since the patient does not receive anything that works internally (i.e., on the organism) such as psychoactive drugs? Since both means—straps and drugs—seem to be aimed at dealing with a symptom of a mental disorder, they might not be so different after all. In the end, via the route of reflections on coercion, we arrive back at the problem of the nature and proper aims of psychiatric care.

Third, the legal discussion has introduced a term that was new to the usual ethical debate: The "natural will" of a person. This is a term that has been used in German legal debate for some time. It refers to the intentions, desires, value judgments, and so on, of persons, which are not based on consciously free or autonomous deliberation. The aforementioned court rulings in Germany made explicit that treatment against the will may also be unlawful when directed against the will of a patient who might not be deemed capable of self-determination (under any theory of what that requires). The natural will of patients, according to the legal interpretation, does not require the usual capacities to give informed consent—such as Gillick competence (which is often used in British law)—and yet has normative force. For instance, if patients show signs of evasion and resistance against proposed or initiated treatment, they thereby express their natural will. To be sure, there are still certain strict criteria that may justify treatment even against the natural will of patients, but incompetence is not seen as giving carte blanche for speculation about a patient's supposed wills or as generally transferring the justification of interventions to proxy consent.

This situation raises interesting philosophical queries regarding the very concept of a natural will. In what sense is it natural, and should these volitional expressions actually be called willful? One might wonder why the natural will should have any normative significance and why it ought to be respected. It might be seen as a mere volitional whim, which does not have anything to do with the personal characteristics or the identity of a patient. So, again, the legal perspective seems to be in conflict with the medical point of view.

In summary, in many countries psychiatry currently fulfills a dual function of medically treating and otherwise supporting patients as well as serving the interests of the state and the general public. Such a situation calls for thorough analysis and careful assessment. It involves problems that are not sufficiently covered by the established discussions of medical paternalism. Rather, these are additional normative and theo-retical issues surrounding the notions of treatment and detention, the will of the pa-tient, and the institutional requirements of modern psychiatric practice. As before, when summarizing the quarrel about the concept of mental illness, Szasz's writings can be instrumental as a starting point to an enhanced debate about important theo-retical and normative issues concerning psychiatry. We do not have to agree with him to see the relevance of the questions he raises.

19.4 The identity crisis of psychiatry

So far, I have discussed Szasz's legacy in relation to two topics he explicitly discussed—the concept of mental illness and coercive care. In this final section, I want to stray away from the clearly visible topics in his work and explore a more hidden issue, which however seems to be of utmost importance, not the least because of his lasting influence.

Psychiatry faces a kind of identity crisis. To have an identity, a discipline or pro-fession needs a fairly clear-cut understanding of its remit and boundaries; it also needs to be sufficiently distinct from other specialties, and hence have a genuine mission in its own right. Now, these identity-forming elements seem to be missing from psychiatry. It clearly seems to be a medical profession, but then it also has nonmedical tasks to fulfill. The status of the phenomena with which it deals is un-certain. Are they real medical disorders or, rather, alternative modes of thinking and acting? Attempts to somatize mental illness have not really helped in this re-spect, as they undermine the autonomous character of psychiatric phenomena in relation to somatic medicine.

It should be clear, from the discussion so far, that I do not believe that psychiatry should abandon reference to mental phenomena, the psyche, or other traditional notions that are used when discussing volition, thinking, emotion, etc. Otherwise it will be reduced to a neurological endeavor. I also do not believe that such reference to mental phenomena leads to an outdated mind-body dualism. In fact, a lack of ac-quaintance with philosophical discussions regarding the mind-body problem—which allows for numerous nonreductive physicalist positions—has undermined psychiatry's identity, as the notion of mental illness has been interpreted by many as a kind of em-barrassing aberration.

Theoretical and conceptual discourse hence seems to be a necessary element of building a foundation for psychiatry. Perhaps this is why there is a growing interest in philosophy of psychiatry. After all, it is here that the conceptual conundrums and ethical challenges have been thoroughly discussed for some time. An interesting his-torical example of such an interest is Karl Jaspers's *General Psychopathology* (1913), which still ignites considerable attention (Stanghellini and Fuchs, 2013). Jaspers made explicit that psychiatry is closely connected to philosophical thinking, but that scien-tific method in psychiatry cannot be replaced by philosophical methodology—and that philosophical thinking in psychopathology cannot be reduced to scientific meth-odology. Rather, philosophy here takes a meta-perspective in that it "creates the space for all the operations of our knowledge" (Jaspers, 1913, p. 770).

It seems clear from even a cursory familiarity with the relevant literature that psychiatry will not build its identity by emulating the methodology of general medicine. Exploring and theorizing the human mind calls for specific terminology and a closer connectedness to other disciplines, most importantly psychology and philosophy. In addition, ethical challenges faced by psychiatric practice also require acknowledgment of the specific vulnerabilities and intricacies of the human psyche. Common conceptions of medical ethics, including an idealized model of informed consent, might not be fully adequate in the relevant context of psychiatry. So perhaps, to find its identity, psychiatry even needs its own ethics of the psyche, which would include special conceptual frameworks and theoretical tools to do justice to the specific vulnerabilities and capacities of psychiatric patients (Feuerstein and Schramme, 2015).

Perhaps the most difficult element in forming a stable identity for psychiatry and overcoming its recent crisis is to develop a convincing account of its scientific basis. In this chapter, I have stated my firm belief that psychiatry needs to be founded on science. However, what this means, exactly, has been left very much in question. This is because the problem is too big to be tackled here. There have been some important contributions, but the debate is, of course, still ongoing (Ghaemi, 2003; Murphy, 2006; Walter, 2013; Zachar, 2014). It seems that here psychiatry really has the chance to get past Szasz. In many areas, psychiatry has not made much theoretical progress (Heinz et al., 2017). The models for many relevant diagnostic entities, such as schizophrenia or bipolar disorder, are still very much based on symptoms and not on etiology, and there are fierce debates about the cogency of many alleged mental disorders, such as post-traumatic stress disorder (PTSD). At least partly, this lack of progress has occurred because skeptical voices, such as that of Szasz, have been ignored and the relevant questions have consequentially been left untouched. But Szasz's skepticism regarding psychiatry is itself partly based on an outdated or one-sided account of what it means to do science.

I should stress that scientific methodology does not mean to be restricted to disciplines that are these days called natural or life sciences. The very notion of the mind or *psyche*, to use the traditional Greek term (Wilkes, 1992), requires conceptualization that cannot be adequately dealt with by, say, neuropsychiatry. Indeed, a scientific exploration of the psyche might even, perhaps paradoxically, involve the humanities. Using a scientific methodology and hence achieving scientific status means, among other things, to strive at objectivity, to reduce judgments based merely on contingent, culturally-laden values, and to be open to criticism or conflicting evidence and to be prepared to revise theories accordingly.

Surely, such a scientific foundation does not solve all problems that psychiatry faces. However, it is important to have such a basis for the very reasons that Szasz rejected the actual conceptualizations of psychiatry at the time of his writing. One of the main reasons is that we must not confuse medical disorder with medically normal problems in life, or similarly, moral impairment due to mental disorder with immoral behavior caused by malicious intentions. In other words, we must keep clear boundaries between medical phenomena and social ills of all kinds. To draw such distinctions we need conceptual tools, which again need a theoretical foundation. Therefore, the scientific foundation of psychiatry is necessary when justifying, and at the same time restricting, medicalization. In short, a scientific perspective is needed to draw the proper boundaries of psychiatric concern. Such a foundation is also vital to get a footing for any consideration of coercive care. After all, compulsory treatment necessarily requires an account of what is good for a patient, which involves an understanding of whether the person suffers from a disorder and, if so, what kind.

The aforementioned scientific foundation of psychiatry is only concerned with these very basic problems. Although they are normatively highly relevant, there are nevertheless further questions in psychiatric practice that need to be tackled (e.g., when to use coercive means of treatment). Such additional questions cannot be answered by scientific methods. So I am not defending a reductionist scientific account of psychiatry altogether. There are theoretical and practical questions in psychiatry, and although there is a certain amount of intersection between the two aspects, they differ in scope and hence require different methodologies. It is one thing to ask whether and, if so, what type of disorder a person has, and another thing to ask what this might mean for his or her life, whether it requires psychiatric treatment, and so on. There is also a difference between the problem of what types of actions constitute coercion and the problem of when to use coercive means legitimately.

The way I have introduced the identity crisis in psychiatry should make clear that this crisis is mainly theoretical (i.e., a crisis concerning the theoretical foundation of psychiatry). This calls for a philosophical perspective, which ties in with the currently increased interest in the philosophy of psychiatry to which I have alluded. I end by re-emphasizing that Szasz's work is an invaluable contribution to the philosophy of psychiatry. Obviously, like others before and after him, he did not get it all right. But he raised many important issues in an exemplary way.

19.5 **Conclusion**

In this chapter, I have introduced a few major concerns of psychiatry, which Szasz exposed in a very helpful way. The issues discussed here were the boundaries of the concept of mental illness and the related problem of medicalization, the problem of coercive care, and, finally, the identity crisis of psychiatry. Szasz was mainly pessimistic about psychiatry's resources to get to grips with these concerns. I am more optimistic and have put my main hopes in a scientific methodology, though admittedly the latter has remained rather blurred in my treatment. Whatever your own thinking about these issues looks like, it should be clear that Szasz's legacy certainly consists in asking the right questions. This is, of course, one of the main achievements of philosophical thinking. Studying his writings will eventually help to overcome the identity crisis of psychiatry. Expressed in medical terminology, even if we might not like Szasz's prescriptions and treatment suggestions, he nevertheless provided the right diagnoses.

References

American Psychiatric Association (APA). 2013. *Diagnostic and Statistical Manual of Mental Disorders [DSM-5]*, 5th edn. Arlington, Virginia: American Psychiatric Association.

Andreasen, Nancy C. 1997. "Linking Mind and Brain in the Study of Mental Illnesses: A Project for a Scientific Psychopathology." *Science* 275 (5306) (March 14): 1586–93.

Bolton, Derek. 2008. *What is Mental Disorder? An Essay in Philosophy, Science, and Values.* Oxford: Oxford University Press.

Boorse, Christopher. 1976. "What a Theory of Mental Health Should Be." *Journal for the Theory of Social Behaviour* **6** (1) (April): 61–84.

Cohen, Carl I. 1993. "The Biomedicalization of Psychiatry: A Critical Overview." *Community Mental Health Journal* **29** (6) (December): 509–21.

Conrad, Peter. 2007. *The Medicalization of Society: On the Transformation of Human Conditions into Treatable Disorders.* Baltimore: Johns Hopkins University Press.

Cooper, Rachel. 2014. *Psychiatry and Philosophy of Science.* London: Routledge.

Eisenberg, Leon. 1986. "Mindlessness and Brainlessness in Psychiatry." *British Journal of Psychiatry* **148** (May): 497–508.

Eisenberg, Leon. 2000. "Is Psychiatry More Mindful or Brainier Than It Was a Decade Ago?" *British Journal of Psychiatry* **176** (January): 1–5.

Engel, George L. 1977. "The Need for a New Medical Model: A Challenge for Biomedicine." *Science* **196** (4286) (April 8): 129–36.

Feuerstein, Günter, and Thomas Schramme. 2015. *Ethik der Psyche: Normative Fragen im Umgang mit Psychischer Abweichung.* Frankfurt am Main: Campus Verlag.

Frances, Allen J. 2013. *Saving Normal: An Insider's Revolt Against Out-of-Control Psychiatric Diagnosis, DSM-5, Big Pharma, and the Medicalization of Ordinary Life.* New York: William Morrow.

Frances, Allen J., Michael B. First, et al. 1991. "An A to Z Guide to DSM-IV Conundrums." *Journal of Abnormal Psychology* **100** (3) (August): 407–12.

Fulford, K.W.M. 1989. *Moral Theory and Medical Practice.* Cambridge: Cambridge University Press.

Fulford, K.W.M., A.Y.U. Smirnov, and E. Snow. 1993. "Concepts of Disease and the Abuse of Psychiatry in the USSR." *British Journal of Psychiatry* **162** (6) (June): 801–10.

German Federal Constitutional Court. 2011. "Successful Constitutional Complaint Lodged by a Person Committed to a Psychiatric Hospital Against Compulsory Medical Treatment Legislation in Rhineland-Palatinate Held Unconstitutional." https://www.bundesverfassungsgericht.de/SharedDocs/Pressemitteilungen/EN/2011/bvg11-028.html

German Federal Court of Justice. 2012. "Keine Hinreichende Gesetzliche Grundlage für Eine Betreuungsrechtliche Zwangsbehandlung." http://juris.bundesgerichtshof.de/cgi-bin/rechtsprechung/document.py?Gericht=bgh&Art=en&sid=dc8017b3e31d6709ff01e6eeb6089bb3&anz=1&pos=0&nr=60958&linked=pm&Blank=1

Ghaemi, S. Nassir. 2003. *The Concepts of Psychiatry: A Pluralistic Approach to the Mind and Mental Illness.* Baltimore: Johns Hopkins University Press.

Ghaemi, S. Nassir. 2017. "Biomedical Reductionist, Humanist, and Biopsychosocial Models in Medicine." In *Handbook of the Philosophy of Medicine*, edited by Thomas Schramme and Steven Edwards, pp. 773–91. Dordrecht: Springer.

Heinz, Andreas, Eva Friedel, Hans-Peter Krüger, and Carolin Wackerhagen. 2017. "Philosophical Implications of Changes in the Classification of Mental Disorders in DSM-5." In *Handbook of the Philosophy of Medicine*, edited by Thomas Schramme and Steven Edwards, pp. 1025–39. Dordrecht: Springer.

Horvitz, Allan V., and Jerome C. Wakefield. 2007. *The Loss of Sadness: How Psychiatry Transformed Normal Sorrow Into Depressive Disorder.* New York: Oxford University Press.

Jaspers, Karl. 1913. *General Psychopathology, Volume I*, translated by J. Hoenig and Marian W. Hamilton (1997). Baltimore: Johns Hopkins University Press.

Kandel, Eric R. 1998. "A New Intellectual Framework for Psychiatry." *American Journal of Psychiatry* **155** (4) (April): 457–69.

Kandel, Eric R. 2005. *Psychiatry, Psychoanalysis, and the New Biology of Mind.* Washington, D.C.: American Psychiatric.

Keil, Geert, Lara Keuck, and Rico Hauswald. (eds.). 2017. *Vagueness in Psychiatry.* Oxford: Oxford University Press.

Kendell, Robert Evan. 1993. "The Nature of Psychiatric Disorders." In *Companion to Psychiatric Studies*, 5th edn., edited by Robert Evan Kendell and Andrew K. Zealley, pp. 1–7. Edinburgh: Churchill Livingstone.

Kendler, Kenneth S. and Josef Parnas. (eds.). 2012. *Philosophical Issues in Psychiatry II: Nosology.* Oxford: Oxford University Press.

Leifer, Ronald. 1982. "Psychiatry, Language, and Freedom." *Metamedicine* **3** (3) (October): 397–416.

Murphy, Dominic. 2006. *Psychiatry in the Scientific Image.* Cambridge, Mass.: MIT Press.

Papineau, David. 1994. "Mental Disorder, Illness, and Biological Dysfunction." In *Philosophy, Psychology, and Psychiatry: Royal Institute of Philosophy Supplement 37*, edited by A. Phillips Griffiths, pp. 73–82. Cambridge: Cambridge University Press.

Parsons, Talcott. 1958. "Definitions of Health and Illness in the Light of American Values and Social Structure." In *Patients, Physicians, and Illness*, edited by E. Gartly Jaco, pp. 165–87. New York: Free Press.

Reznek, Lawrie. 1991. *The Philosophical Defence of Psychiatry.* London: Routledge.

Sadler, John Z. (ed.). 2002. *Descriptions and Prescriptions: Values, Mental Disorders, and the DSMs.* Baltimore: Johns Hopkins University Press.

Sadler, John Z. 2005. *Values and Psychiatric Diagnosis.* Oxford: Oxford University Press.

Sadler, John Z., Osborne P. Wiggins, and Michael A. Schwartz. (eds.). 1994. *Philosophical Perspectives on Psychiatric Diagnostic Classification.* Baltimore: Johns Hopkins University Press.

Schramme, Thomas. 2004. "The Legacy of Antipsychiatry." In *Philosophy and Psychiatry*, edited by Thomas Schramme and Johannes Thome, pp. 94–119. Berlin: Walter de Gruyter.

Schramme, Thomas. 2010. "Can We Define Mental Disorder by Using the Criterion of Mental Dysfunction?" *Theoretical Medicine and Bioethics* **31** (1) (February): 35–47.

Schramme, Thomas. 2012. "Paternalism, Coercion, and Manipulation in Psychiatry." In *Menschenwürde in der Medizin: Quo Vadis?*, edited by Jan Joerden, Eric Hilgendorf, Natalia Petrillo, and Felix Thiele, pp. 147–60. Baden-Baden: Nomos.

Schramme, Thomas. 2013. "On the Autonomy of the Concept of Disease in Psychiatry." *Frontiers in Psychology* **4** (July 19). Accessed April 15, 2018. <www.frontiersin.org/articles/10.3389/fpsyg.2013.00457/full>

Schramme, Thomas. 2016. "What a Naturalist Theory of Illness Should Be." In *Naturalism in Philosophy of Health: Issues and Implications*, edited by Élodie Giroux, pp. 63–77. Switzerland: Springer International.

Schwartz, Peter H. 2008. "Risk and Disease." *Perspectives in Biology and Medicine* **51** (3) (Summer): 320–34.

Scott, Susie. 2014. "Contesting Dangerousness, Risk, and Treatability: A Sociological View of Dangerous and Severe Personality Disorder (DSPD)." In *Being Amoral: Psychopathy and Moral Incapacity*, edited by Thomas Schramme, pp. 301–20. Cambridge, Mass.: MIT Press.

Sholl, Jonathan. 2017. "The Muddle of Medicalization: Pathologizing or Medicalizing?" *Theoretical Medicine and Bioethics* **38** (4) (August): 265–78.

Stanghellini, Giovanni, and Thomas Fuchs. (eds.). 2013. *One Century of Karl Jaspers' General Psychopathology*. Oxford: Oxford University Press.

Szasz, Thomas S. 1960. "The Myth of Mental Illness." *American Psychologist* **15** (2): 113–18.

Szasz, Thomas S. 1970. *The Manufacture of Madness: A Comparative Study of the Inquisition and the Mental Health Movement*. New York: Harper & Row.

Szasz, Thomas S. 1977. *The Theology of Medicine: The Political-Philosophical Foundations of Medical Ethics*. New York: Harper & Row.

Szasz, Thomas S. 1987. *Insanity: The Idea and Its Consequences*. New York: John Wiley & Sons.

Szasz, Thomas S. 1994. *Cruel Compassion: Psychiatric Control of Society's Unwanted*. New York: John Wiley & Sons.

Szasz, Thomas S. 1996. *The Meaning of Mind: Language, Morality, and Neuroscience*. Westport, Conn.: Praeger.

Szasz, Thomas S. 2004a. "Reply to Bentall." In *Szasz Under Fire: The Psychiatric Abolitionist Faces His Critics*, edited by Jeffrey Schaler, pp. 321–6. Chicago: Open Court.

Szasz, Thomas S. 2004b. "Reply to Pies." In *Szasz Under Fire: The Psychiatric Abolitionist Faces His Critics*, edited by Jeffrey Schaler, pp. 354–63. Chicago: Open Court.

Szasz, Thomas S. 2009. *Antipsychiatry: Quackery Squared*. Syracuse: Syracuse University Press.

Wakefield, Jerome C. 2017. "Mental Disorders as Genuine Medical Conditions." In *Handbook of the Philosophy of Medicine*, edited by Thomas Schramme and Steven Edwards, pp. 65–82. Dordrecht: Springer.

Wilkes, Kathleen V. 1992. "*Psuchê* versus the Mind." In *Essays on Aristotle's "De Anima,"* edited by Martha C. Nussbaum and Amélie Oksenberg Rorty, pp. 109–28. Oxford: Oxford University Press.

Walter, Henrik. 2013. "The Third Wave of Biological Psychiatry." *Frontiers in Psychology* **4** (September 5). Accessed April 15, 2018. <www.frontiersin.org/articles/10.3389/fpsyg.2013.00582/full>

Zachar, Peter. 2014. *A Metaphysics of Psychopathology*. Cambridge, Mass.: MIT Press.

Zachar, Peter, Drozdstoj St. Stoyanov, Massimiliano Aragona, and Assen Jablensky (eds.). 2015. *Alternative Perspectives on Psychiatric Validation: DSM, ICD, RDoC, and Beyond*. Oxford: Oxford University Press.

Zinkler, Martin. 2016. "Germany without Coercive Treatment in Psychiatry: A 15-Month Real World Experience." *Laws* **5** (1). Accessed April 15, 2018. <www.mdpi.com/2075-471X/5/1/15/pdf>

Epilogue

C.V. Haldipur

Mad call I it, for, to define true madness,
What is 't but to be nothing else but mad?
But let that go.

Shakespeare, Hamlet, II.ii.93–95

Thomas Szasz questioned the nature and definition of insanity, calling it a man-made myth rather than an illness in his magnum opus, *The Myth of Mental Illness* (Szasz, 1961, 1974), a book that propelled him into fame and earned him both obloquy for challenging the very *raison d'être* of psychiatry as a medical specialty and, interestingly for the same reason, encomium, in equal measure. In some ways, his rationale for denying that madness is an illness is appealing in its simplicity: Because no biologic lesion is shown to be the cause of madness, it is not an illness. *Tout court*. Questioning the nature of madness thus became the leitmotif of many of his subsequent works, which spanned over thirty books and many hundreds of articles in scientific and popular periodicals. For him, it became his life's calling: "I could say the same thing over again from roof tops until my message gets through," he once said to me. Isaiah Berlin (2013) suggested that writers and intellectuals are either foxes who know many things or hedgehogs who know one big thing; Szasz clearly would fall into the latter category. Unlike Polonius in Shakespeare's *Hamlet*, he could not "let that go."

He left no doubt that he was passionate about his views and debated with those who disagreed with him, both in person and in print, at every opportunity. He often dismissed his opponents' arguments as legerdemain and, occasionally, he could be brutal to his opponents in debates. He did not suffer fools gladly. His escape from Hungary just before the takeover by Nazis and later by Communists arguably may have contributed to his fierce and, at times, uncompromising libertarian views. He believed that libertarian writers did not go far enough in defending liberty and individual autonomy. Of John Stuart Mill he wrote: "Mill's head was libertarian, but his heart was utilitarian" (Szasz, 2004, p. 93) and that Mill "did not oppose psychiatric imprisonment, as such" but "opposed only the laxity of procedures used to implement the 'lunacy laws'" (Szasz, 2004, p. 84).

It is possible to trace the trajectory of his views from his early psychoanalytic writings to *The Myth of Mental Illness*. His early book, *Pain and Pleasure* (1957b), is a chrysalis of his subsequent writings, especially relating to his assertion that mental illness is a myth. Pols (Chapter 2, this volume) establishes a nexus between Szasz's early psycho-analytic writings and his subsequent view that mental illness is a myth. Pain, to Szasz, is a psychological phenomenon; the underlying physical lesion is secondary. This arguably suggests Cartesian dualistic thinking. Interestingly, when confronted with a person complaining of hearing voices and expressing false ideas—a mad person—he would confer legitimacy to that condition as a disease only if there was an identifiable bodily lesion.

The term, "illness," has broader connotations in general use: It suggests a state largely determined by psychosocial factors giving rise to a subjective feeling of distress—regardless of whether the mental state arises from bodily pathology. Szasz wrote: "*Ill* . . . has a history and a scope that have nothing to do with medicine or disease. It then means, roughly, *bad, unfortunate, tragic*, or something of that sort" (Szasz, 1977, p. 141). We have an intuitive sense when we are ill, often without being able to explain why. A patient walks into a physician's office complaining of loss of sleep, poor appetite, loss of energy, no will to live, and inability to enjoy life. Most physicians will recognize these as symptoms of depression, and using Szasz's afore-mentioned connotation of the term, the patient can be said to be ill. If a physical examination and laboratory tests are normal, should the patient now be told that he is not ill at all?

Disease, in contrast, refers to an unhealthy condition of the body. Consider a situation in a physician's office: A routine blood pressure check reveals high readings. The patient denies any symptoms and protests that she is not ill, but the blood pressure reading points to an underlying disease. It can thus be argued that the title of Szasz's well-known book ought to have been *The Myth of Mental Disease*. This is merely a cavil that overlooks the major impact of his work, for Szasz had a penchant for the *mot juste*; however, this solecism cannot be easily overlooked. Indeed, at least on one occasion, he ruefully admitted that the title could well have been *The Myth of Mental Disease*, but quickly pointed out that, regardless of the term, one ought to look at what society chooses to do with behaviors so deemed—such as exoneration of contumacious actions or deprivation of civil liberties. This is a valid argument. However, *mutatis mutandis*, one could make a case for granting civil liberties and not exonerating illegal acts for individuals suffering from diseases, such as a brain tumor, dementia, or AIDS—all true diseases with demonstrable bodily lesions.

The notion that mental illness, for Szasz, is a myth forms the leitmotif of his philosophy, and it is the focus of Chapter 12 in this volume, by Pies; but every other contributor has also had to address this issue while examining his legacy.

Throughout the history of medicine, we find tendencies to classify signs and symptoms into disease entities. Sadler (Chapter 4, this volume) and Fulford (Chapter 7, this volume) point out that these diagnostic entities are not value-free. Although, at some level, disease process can be explained by biological laws—disease and, for that matter, health are not biological concepts (Brown, 1985, p. 325). In antiquity, two important medical schools, Cos and Cnidos, argued over the importance of classifying diseases: Hippocrates, from the school in Cos, attacked the thesis of the Cnidians that variant signs and symptoms indicated different diseases (Biggart, 1971). Today we have tomes listing mental disorders: DSM and ICD, the vade mecums of mental health professionals, which Szasz derisively referred to as the *malleus maleficarum* of psychiatry.

Defining mental illness

Can we define disease? Should we? F.G. Crookshank chided physicians for refusing "to consider, in express terms, the relations between Things, Thoughts, and Words involved in their communications to others" (Crookshank, 1989, p. 338). Putative disease is what physicians treat. Yet, defining disease is not as easy as one would imagine, partly "due to the nature of our language and concepts in general, and to the nature of medicine in particular" (Brown, 1985, p. 311). Jean Fernel (1554, pp. 1–2) ventured somewhat arcane definitions of disease in a chapter entitled, "Morbi Definitio Quid Affectus, Quid Affectio" ("Definition of Disease, What is Affected, What it Affects"). It is no wonder that few others have had the courage to offer pithy definitions of disease; it is as if, like Hippolytus, physicians were forbidden to ride close to the shores of defining disease lest they incur the fury of Poseidon and eventual death.

Charles Mercier (1917) devotes two essays to the task of defining disease and notes that physicians have formulated no definition of either disease or, for that matter, health in the modern scientific era. How important is it to be able to define disease? Mercier suggests that we consider the following situation: At a cross-examination of an expert on mental diseases, counsel asks the witness (much to the witness's discomfort) to define insanity. If the witness could turn the table and ask counsel for the definition of law, Mercier avers that counsel would be equally confounded. He then asks, rhetorically, "Do we, when we think of a disease, necessarily mean structural damage with its consequences, or may there be diseases in which no structural damage is *known*?" (Mercier, 1917, p. 410, italics added).

Medical students and physicians consider diseases to be entities *ante rem*, ready to be discovered in much the same way astronomers discover planets or Columbus discovered America. We revere the "discoverers" of diseases and are familiar with eponymous diseases (e.g., Tourette's disease, Pott's disease). Mercier defines disease as "a mental construct: the idea of a symptom or group of symptoms, correlated with or by a single intra-corporeal cause, known or postulated" (Mercier, 1917, p. 421). Diseases, like syphilis, are mental constructs or concepts—a necessary figment of imagination. Schizophrenia, depression, and mania are also such constructs and have no referents outside the imagination. One is reminded of the famous philosophical wit Sidney Morgenbesser's remark: "You think there's no such thing as mental illness? You mean it's all in the mind?" (quoted in Crane et al., 2017).

Increasingly, we seem to be saying, like Humpty Dumpty, "When *I* use a word . . . it means just what I choose it to mean—neither more nor less" (Carroll, 1946, p. 94). Never mind that textbooks in medicine, both ancient and modern, starting with no less an authority than Hippocrates (1950), include mental disorders, Szasz avoids all the traps of defining disease and takes recourse to Rudolf Virchow's definition (not surprising for a pathologist) that demonstrable bodily lesions are the desiderata of diseases. Szasz calls it the "Virchowian gold standard of disease" (Szasz, 2009, p. 78). Virchow's definition, however, is not without problems: Is old age a disease, for example? There are clearly ascertainable changes in various body organs, and people in their dotage recognize diminution of various organ systems' function. Furthermore, Virchow dismissed as baseless the claims that diseases of the mind are holy: "When . . . somebody becomes *mentally or bodily ill, which, to our mind, is not essentially different,* we always have before us the same life, with the same laws, only that these become manifest under other conditions" (Virchow, 1985, p. 115, italics added).

Mental illness—or neurological disease?

That we find out the cause of this effect,
Or rather say, the cause of this defect,
For this effect defective comes by cause.
Thus it remains, and the remainder thus.
Perpend.

Shakespeare, Hamlet, II.ii.101–105

Hippocrates wrote that from nothing else but the brain we become mad (1950, p. 190). Plato, through his character Timaeus, similarly stated that "the disorders of the soul, which depend on the body, originate as follows. We must acknowledge disease of the mind to be a want of intelligence; and of this there are of two kinds—to wit, madness and ignorance. . . . that state may be called disease" (Plato, 1973, p. 1206; *Timaeus* 86b). Thus, a case can now be made that Plato was "the first in the Greek medical literature to conceptualize the notion of mental disease as such, i.e., as a disease that, while having organic causes, specifically affects one's . . . relationship to the world" (Sassi, 2013, p. 415).

Gupta (Chapter 17, this volume) notes that the profession is, in some ways, obsessed with proving Szasz wrong by funding research on the biological etiology of mental disorders, which is the perennial will-o'-the-wisp of physicians and scientists—that sooner or later a cause of this malady, and most likely brain pathology, will be discovered. For if someone were to show a specific brain pathology as a cause of madness, would we not then call it an illness? Szasz was confronted with this question on several occasions, and he would aver, with his characteristic panache, with this *aperçu*: In that case, it would no longer be a mental illness but a neurological disease. He would then cite the case of neurosyphilis, once considered to be a mental illness; after the discovery of its true etiology, it was treated not by psychiatrists but by other medical specialists, such as neurologists or infectious disease specialists.

Both Torrey (Chapter 8, this volume) and Frances (Chapter 13, this volume) refer to possible organic (i.e., brain) pathology in the etiology of schizophrenia. Szasz is correct that in most instances the burden of treating schizophrenia, once a brain pathology is established as the cause, may shift to neurologists rather than to psychiatrists. True, this happened with neurosyphilis. But this may not always be true. For example, most of us are likely to turn to over-the-counter analgesics rather than seek psychotherapy for stress-induced headaches.

Let us now consider a situation where we could identify brain pathology, like a tumor, in a patient who hallucinates and expresses false delusional ideas. The patient's brain, on postmortem, could be preserved in a jar of formaldehyde in a laboratory. We could then point to the brain and say with confidence that it is a "diseased brain." But it would be absurd to point to the brain in the jar and call it schizophrenia or a disease called schizophrenia. One would have to turn to the person's psychiatric records and use the sobriquet or diagnosis of schizophrenia, justifying it on the basis of the person's behavior rather than on the brain lesion.

Szasz and psychotherapy

> *Macbeth*: Canst thou not minister to a mind diseased,
> Pluck from the memory a rooted sorrow,
> Rase out the written troubles of the brain,
> And with some sweet oblivious antidote
> Cleanse the stuffed bosom of the perilous stuff
> Which weighs upon the heart?
> *Doctor*: Therein the patient must minister to himself.
> *Macbeth*: Throw physic to the dogs!

Shakespeare, Macbeth, V.iii.42–49

Szasz was fond of quoting this passage from Shakespeare, both in print and in person. Alas, he often omitted Macbeth's dithyrambic response: "Throw physic to the dogs!"

It is generally assumed among mental health practitioners that Szasz was not in favor of biological treatments with drugs or shock therapy, and supported psychotherapy as the only valid modality of treatment. He, on one occasion, described himself as an "equal opportunity" critic. He wrote a trenchant criticism of psychotherapy in *The Myth of Psychotherapy* (1988) and there suggested an alternative term for the enterprise: "iatrologic" (p. 208). But *iatros*, which means "physician" in Greek, once again has medical connotations. Toward the end of his life, he used the lay term "conversation" between two individuals to describe what psychotherapy is all about, thus avoiding any implication of underlying causes of behavior and belying the claim that the enterprise offers "treatment" (a cure) to those suffering from "mental illness" and allows them to cope with (or cure) their "disease." There is no such thing as mental illness, and hence there can be no such thing as psychotherapy.

Chapter 11 in this volume, by Dewan and Kaplan, has, as its main focus, Szasz's thoughts on psychotherapy. Szasz was, after all, a psychoanalyst; his earlier writings have stood the test of time and can be read today as classics in the field. It is worth quoting a portion of the final paragraph of Szasz's essay on transference, which, in one fell swoop, attacks the very foundation of the edifice of psychoanalysis: "Transference is the pivot upon which the entire structure of psychoanalytic treatment rests. It is an inspired and indispensable concept; yet it also harbors the seeds, not only of its own destruction, but of the destruction of psychoanalysis itself. Why? Because it tends to place the person of the analyst beyond the reality testing of patients, colleagues, and self" (Szasz, 1963, p. 443).

In many ways, though, Szasz remained committed to the tenets of psychoanalysis: He considered the contract between the analyst and the analysand as sacrosanct. He saw the contract into which the two individuals entered as akin to a commercial contract with fees for service buttressing the agreement. The two persons were autonomous and with no outside interference—especially from the government or an insurance company. Herein lies his stringent opposition to involuntary psychiatric treatment: Treatment could occur only in circumstances where two individuals entered into such a contract, in the absence of which no treatment was possible. Frances (Chapter 13, this volume) points out that, for most practitioners, there are times when the need for involuntary treatment becomes the only viable option; for example, for patients who cannot enter into a therapeutic contract (e.g., children) or those who cannot afford the fee and are thus unable to access therapy.

One can now see why Szasz remained opposed to state-funded universal health care, which put him squarely in the conservative right-wing section of politics (Sedgwick, 1982). Privately, he never ceased to be amused when told of the many left-wing politicians, and even some communists, who espoused his ideas.

Much has been made of the fact that Szasz did not work with truly disturbed and psychotic patients, because most of them were institutionalized, often involuntarily. Did he really understand, then, what schizophrenics are like and what their personal experiences are? Early in his career, he wrote a paper on schizophrenia that, in my opinion, only a person who had talked to schizophrenic patients might have been able to comprehend—the inner conflict that manifested itself with symptoms familiar to clinicians working with such patients (Szasz, 1957a).

One wonders, though, if a pristine physician–patient relationship, as espoused by Szasz—totally free from any social, cultural, or economic influence—has ever existed.

Szasz on suicide

There is but one truly serious philosophical problem, and that is suicide.

Camus (1955, p. 3)

When one speaks of freedom, it is difficult not to include the right to die, Szasz averred. He argued that free and nontotalitarian societies should offer to individuals what he called "fatal freedom"—the right to suicide, much the same as the right to life, liberty, and the pursuit of happiness. Two chapters in this book are devoted to Szasz's views on suicide: by Annas (Chapter 5) and by Knoll (Chapter 9).

Szasz (2011) railed effectively against "suicide prohibition," which became the title of one of his last books. He also exposed psychiatrists' mendacity: They consider the prevention of suicide as their professional duty and, at the same time, are willing to participate as experts and proffer their opinion when physician-assisted suicide is the law of the land, often in favor of the individual's right to die with a physician's assistance. On one occasion, a student asked Szasz what he would do if a person in his office threatened to jump out of his office window. "I will stop him," he answered, much to the amazement of the students. The person had a right to commit suicide, Szasz averred shortly thereafter, "but not in my office." In the same vein, he questioned whether a person who wanted to commit suicide needed a physician to assist. Szasz advocated free availability of medications that have the potential to kill: The physician's role was to be the educator rather than the controller of access to drugs. "For if suicide is an illness because it terminates in death, and if the prevention of death by any means necessary is the physician's mandate, then the proper remedy for suicide is liberticide" (Szasz 1977, p. 85).

Szasz, the philosopher

> For only "mad doctors" may in these scientific times dabble in philosophy without loss of their reputation as practitioners!
>
> Crookshank (1989, p. 339)

A student about to enter our graduate education program in psychiatry at Upstate Medical University asked Szasz for his recommendation of books he should read while he was in the program. Szasz listed several writers: economists like Ludwig von Mises and Friedrich Hayek, philosophers like Gilbert Ryle and John Stuart Mill, but no psychiatrists—not even Karl Jaspers, who was a psychiatrist as well as a philosopher. Needless to say, the student was perplexed and had to turn to other teachers for their recommendations of textbooks in psychiatry. Indeed, Szasz's own writings are best read as philosophy rather than as psychiatry. After *The Myth of Mental Illness* (1961), all the books in his enormous corpus were devoid of any case histories listing signs or symptoms of patients. His true *métier* was that of a philosopher rather than of a psychiatrist.

Many of the contributors to this volume are philosophers. Luft (Chapter 3) traces some of the philosophers who may have influenced Szasz's views. Church (Chapter 10) suggests that many questions remain about the term "myth" and its application to psychiatry. Radden (Chapter 18) suggests that, if mental illness is a myth, then several ethical consequences follow, regarding rights, freedom, and individual agency. Ciaccio (Chapter 16) brings the discussion of agency and responsibility into sharper focus by looking closely at psychopathy. Individuals diagnosed as psychopaths, though not considered mentally ill, nevertheless are considered not responsible for their actions. She presents forceful arguments suggesting that they should be held accountable. The issue of agency is also a theme for Daly (Chapter 6, this volume).

Szasz and the insanity defense

> Now a man might conceivably commit an act of one of these kinds from insanity, or when so disordered by disease . . . the rest of the sentence shall be remitted.
>
> Plato, 1973, p. 1425; *Laws* 864d–e

Perhaps the earliest recorded insanity defense is in the *Iliad*, XIX.86–88, where King Agamemnon states: "I am not responsible/but Zeus is, and Destiny, and Erinys the mist-walking/who is assembly caught my heart in the savage delusion" (Homer, 1971, p. 394; Robinson, 1996, p. 8).

A casuist in his approach to ethical problems, Szasz began one such discussion with two hypothetical cases: A man has been harassed by his neighbor. After some years of suffering harassment, the man can no longer take the abuse and takes matters into his own hands and assaults the neighbor. Another person falsely believes that a neighbor is plotting against him. In psychiatric argot, he is delusional. He, too, assaults his neighbor. The second person's lawyer is very likely to plead insanity as a defense; the first person is likely to be told that he had no right to take the law into his own hands and assault the neighbor. Both had clear intention—*mens rea*—to harm the neighbor. Persons who believe that they are harassed or truly are harassed still do not have the right to hurt the alleged perpetrator.

Wilson (Chapter 1, this volume) points out that *mens rea* does not always follow *actus reus* (criminal act). He indicates that there is evidence throughout history, certainly from antiquity, that certain individuals were not deemed responsible for their acts if they suffered from madness or, like children, were deemed incapable of acting responsibly. Pickering (Chapter 15, this volume) notes that Szasz denies insanity as well as the *mens rea* defense. Indeed, psychiatric examination cannot prove that a person lacks responsibility or prove *mens rea* when the act was committed. What if a brain lesion were to be demonstrated in an individual who has committed a heinous crime, say murder? The defense now could say that the *force majeure* is the putative brain pathology, and we have an avatar of the insanity defense: "My brain made me do it."

Szasz wrote powerfully against the insanity defense, and it is likely that his writings will have a lasting influence on jurisprudence. He testified in several lawsuits pertaining to the insanity defense and wrote about famous, headline-making cases. All persons, to Szasz, are responsible for their actions. Socrates said that unexamined life is not worth living; for Szasz, irresponsible life is not worth living. His aphorism about psychiatric expert testimony says it best: "mendacity masquerading as medicine" (Szasz, 1973, p. 40).

Szasz's legacy summarized

> Lector, si monumentum requiris, circumspice.
>
> Epitaph of Christopher Wren

It was tempting to offer this volume as a hagiography. Szasz was, after all, to many of this volume's contributors a mentor, friend, and an important intellectual influence. In his lifetime he was perhaps the most controversial psychiatrist. His caustic aphorisms are now in many anthologies. He was also well-known outside the boundaries of English-speaking countries. For example, a visitor from a northern European country visited Upstate New York and met Szasz, a cynosure in Syracuse. As a social scientist, the visitor had observed homeless, mentally ill persons in metropolitan areas and had noted that large mental hospitals in the state had deinstitutionalized and reduced the number of patients to less than one half of the number just forty years prior. Although Szasz's writings were not solely responsible for deinstitutionalization and stricter laws for involuntary treatment of mentally ill, he played a role. There are now more mentally ill persons in prisons than in mental hospitals. After his visit, the social scientist said that the epitaph on Sir Christopher Wren's tomb seemed appropriate to describe Szasz's legacy: "If a monument is necessary, look around."

Szasz railed against involuntary psychiatric treatment and compared involuntary in-patient psychiatric hospitalization to imprisonment. It is in this area of laws governing involuntary treatment that Szasz's writings have had a major impact. Schramme (Chapter 19, this volume) points out how laws in Germany, for instance, were changed

in this regard. In most states in the United States, as well as in many European countries, a person deemed dangerous may be held against his or her will, but treatment
can be administered only with further approval of the courts.

If one were to read critically the over thirty books and several hundred articles that
Szasz wrote, it would not be too difficult to find a few areas to cavil about. Nevertheless,
there are a few, *inter alia*, that deserve mention in examining his legacy. For example,
there is the ongoing controversy about his involvement with Scientology. This group
often heralded his name in its publications. He did not actively support the movement,
but nor did he openly distance himself from the group. I asked him once about this
matter. His response: "My enemy's enemy is my friend."

As previously noted, Szasz considered the contract between the patient and the
physician to be sacrosanct, which *ipso facto* proscribed the psychoanalysis of a dead
person. He often railed against psychobiography or postmortem psychoanalytic examination of persons. Yet, he wrote a book on Virginia Woolf with a catchy title that says it
all: *My Madness Saved Me* (2006). She had been dead for decades; she never consented
to the analysis of her behavior or to her exercise of her right to "fatal freedom."

Soon after their publication, Szasz's books were read by trainees in psychiatry and
its allied disciplines, only to find them of little relevance to their work in clinics, as
Frances (Chapter 13, this volume) eloquently discusses. Szasz was, at times, identified
with the so called "antipsychiatry" movement, from which he distanced himself. Potter
(Chapter 14) points out that he spawned critical psychiatry, which "takes on some of
these realities of human suffering . . . and . . . aims at reforming practices."

It is not hard to adumbrate some of his achievements: limiting the power of
psychiatrists in courts, slowing medicalization of "problems of living," and tightening
laws permitting civil involuntary commitment to mental hospitals in many countries.
In his lifetime he was called a number of things, most benign of which was the *enfant
terrible* of psychiatry. He was truly the conscience or superego of the profession—a
gadfly, as Wilson (Chapter 1, this volume) suggests. Szasz, like Socrates, continued
to sting the steed of state and psychiatry into acknowledging its proper duties and
obligations and, more to the point, its limitations.

References

Berlin, Isaiah. 2013. *The Hedgehog and the Fox: An Essay on Tolstoy's View of History*, 2nd edn.
Princeton: Princeton University Press.
Biggart, J.H. 1971. "Cnidos v. Cos." *Ulster Medical Journal* **41** (1) (Winter): 1–9.
Brown, W. Miller. 1985. "On Defining Disease." *Journal of Medicine and Philosophy* **10** (4)
(November): 311–28.
Camus, Albert. 1955. *The Myth of Sisyphus and Other Essays*, translated by Justin O'Brien.
New York: Vintage.
Carroll, Lewis. 1946. *Through the Looking-Glass and What Alice Found There*.
New York: Random House.
Crane, Tim, David Papineau, and Daniel Dennett. 2017. "Papineau vs Dennett: A
Philosophical Dispute: An Introduction." *Times Literary Supplement* (August 2). Accessed
April 10, 2018. <www.the-tls.co.uk/articles/public/dennett-papineau-debate/>

Crookshank, Francis Graham. 1989. "Supplement II: The Importance of a Theory of Signs and a Critique of Language in the Study of Medicine." In *The Meaning of Meaning*, edited by C.K. Ogden and I.A. Richards, pp. 337–55. New York: Harcourt Brace & World.

Fernel, Jean. 1554. *Joan. Fernelli Ambiani, Pathologiae Lib. vij. De Morbis Eorvmqve Cavsis Lib. I. [Seven Books of Pathology by Jean Fernel of Belgium, Book I: On Diseases and Their Causes]*. Lvtetiae Parisorvm [Paris]: Apvd Andream Wechelvm.

Hippocrates. 1950. *The Medical Works of Hippocrates*, translated by J. Chadwick and W.N. Mann. Oxford: Blackwell.

Homer. 1971. *The Iliad*, translated by Richmond Lattimore. Chicago: University of Chicago Press.

Mercier, Charles. 1917. "What Is a Disease?" *Science Progress* **11** (43) (January): 410–22.

Plato. 1973. *The Collected Dialogues, Including the Letters*, edited by Edith Hamilton and Huntington Cairns. Princeton: Princeton University Press.

Robinson, Daniel N. 1996. *Wild Beasts and Idle Humours: The Insanity Defense from Antiquity to the Present*. Cambridge, Mass.: Harvard University Press.

Sassi, Maria Michela. 2013. "Mental Illness, Moral Error, and Responsibility in Late Plato." In *Mental Disorders in the Classical World*, edited by William V. Harris, pp. 413–26. Leiden: Brill.

Sedgwick, Peter. 1982. *Psychopolitics*. New York: Harper & Row.

Shakespeare, William. 1988. *The Complete Works*, edited by David Bevington. Toronto: Bantam.

Szasz, Thomas S. 1957a. "A Contribution to the Psychology of Schizophrenia." *AMA Archives of Neurology and Psychiatry* **77** (April). 420–36.

Szasz, Thomas S. 1957b. *Pain and Pleasure: A Study of Bodily Feelings*. New York: Basic Books.

Szasz, Thomas S. 1961. *The Myth of Mental Illness: Foundations of a Theory of Personal Conduct*. New York: Hoeber-Harper.

Szasz, Thomas S. 1963. "The Concept of Transference." *International Journal of Psychoanalysis* **44** (October): 432–43.

Szasz, Thomas S. 1973. *The Second Sin*. Garden City, New York: Doubleday Anchor.

Szasz, Thomas S. 1974. *The Myth of Mental Illness: Foundations of a Theory of Personal Conduct*, revised edn. New York: Harper & Row.

Szasz, Thomas S. 1977. *The Theology of Medicine: The Political-Philosophical Foundations of Medical Ethics*. New York: Harper & Row.

Szasz, Thomas S. 1988. *The Myth of Psychotherapy: Mental Healing as Religion, Rhetoric, and Repression*. Syracuse: Syracuse University Press.

Szasz, Thomas S. 2004. *Faith in Freedom: Libertarian Principles and Psychiatric Practices*. New Brunswick, New Jersey: Transaction.

Szasz, Thomas S. 2006. *My Madness Saved Me: The Madness and Marriage of Virginia Woolf*. New Brunswick, New Jersey: Transaction.

Szasz, Thomas S. 2009. *Antipsychiatry: Quackery Squared*. Syracuse: Syracuse University Press.

Szasz, Thomas S. 2011. *Suicide Prohibition: The Shame of Medicine*. Syracuse: Syracuse University Press.

Szasz, Thomas S. 2017. *Faith in Freedom: Libertarian Principles and Psychiatric Practices*. London: Routledge.

Virchow, Rudolf. 1985. "The Epidemics of 1848." In: *Collected Essays on Public Health and Epidemiology, Volume 1*, edited by L.J. Rather, pp. 113–19. Canton, Mass: Science History Publications.

Index

abandonment, 107, 117
abnormality, 6, 76, 100, 126, 149–150, 152, 155, 163–164, 258
aboriginal / indigenous people, 173
abortion, 56, 61–62
Abraham (biblical character), 44–46
absolute / absolutism, 6, 24, 27, 30, 33, 119, 170, 176, 246, 261
abstraction, 7, 28, 100, 104, 174, 176, 200, 232
absurdity, 20, 29, 46, 119–120, 200–201, 204, 207, 276
academia, 84, 104, 134, 174, 177, 179, 181, 224, 231
academic psychiatry, 104, 181
accountability, 61, 68, 207, 212, 217–220, 231, 240, 278
Achilles heel, 98–102
acquirements, 29, 31, 69, 72–73, 77, 244, 247
acquittal, 190–192, 195, 197, 200
action, 28, 32, 36, 41, 45, 58, 65–79, 83, 101, 111, 117, 135, 151, 163, 194, 204, 216, 240–243, 245, 247, 249, 251
activity versus passivity, 132, 139–140, 244–245, 247
actus reus, 6, 279
addiction, 45, 227
Addington v. Texas, 120
Adler, Mortimer, 68
adolescence, 36, 84, 94, 110, 140, 149, 203
aesthetics, 37
affection, 44, 145
affective traits, 144, 212–214, 217, 221
African Americans, 7, 83, 185, 197
Agamben, Giorgio, 67–68
Agamemnon (Homeric character), 278
agency, 32–33, 45, 55, 65–80, 131–132, 135–136, 141, 184, 194, 211–222, 227, 237–241, 243, 251, 278
agency cultivation, 211–222
aggression, 37, 145, 148, 180–182, 213, 264
agnosticism, 41, 43
Alcoholics Anonymous (AA), 243
Alexander, Franz, 12, 99
Alexander, Leo, 55
algorithms, 232
alienation, 67, 75, 163, 193
allegory, 126
alternative medicine, 15, 249
altruism, 29
Alzheimer's disease, 39, 100, 102, 161–162, 171

American Association for the Abolition of Involuntary Mental Hospitalization (AAAIMH), 101
American Law Institute rule, 192
American Medical Association (AMA) Council on Science and Public Health, 158
American Psychiatric Association (APA), 1, 39, 46
analysands, 141–142, 146, 277
analysis (linguistic), 24
analysis (psychiatric), 141–145, 203
analytic philosophy, 83, 94, 135–136
analytic relationships, 66, 144–145
analytic truth, 6, 159
analyticity, 20–21, 41, 59, 71, 86, 107, 110, 117, 124, 127–128, 135, 159, 180–181, 183, 190, 224–225, 229, 238, 240, 243, 247, 249–251, 256, 263–265, 280
anarchy, 20
Anglicanism, 31
Anna O. (patient), 145
Annas, George J., 277
anthropology, 107, 179
anthropomorphism, 33
anti-Semitism, 21–22
antipsychiatry, 17, 124, 136, 152, 175, 177–178, 256, 280
antipsychotic drugs, 100, 116, 246
antiquity, 5, 106, 273, 279
antisocial personality disorder, 37, 39
antisocial traits, 6, 42–44, 47, 212–214, 222
antithesis, 82–94
anxiety, 6, 133, 140, 143, 149–150, 181–182, 214, 229, 232–233
Appelbaum, Paul S., 55, 82, 90, 93–94, 114, 239
Aquinas, Thomas, 23
arbitrariness, 7, 10, 144, 171, 176, 213, 220
Archbishop of Canterbury, 31
aretaic perspective, 240
Arieti, Silvano, 99–100
aristocracy, 30
Aristotle, 26
armed forces, 15, 79
arousal and regulatory systems, 229
art, 25–26, 30, 259
aspirations, 26, 31, 43, 141–142, 226, 243, 261
assent, 115–116
asylums, 6, 241
atheism, 33
Athens, Greece, 5, 10
atrocities, 55, 264